Fatal Flaws

NAVIGATING DESTRUCTIVE RELATIONSHIPS WITH PEOPLE WITH DISORDERS OF PERSONALITY AND CHARACTER

Fatal Flaws

NAVIGATING DESTRUCTIVE RELATIONSHIPS WITH PEOPLE WITH DISORDERS OF PERSONALITY AND CHARACTER

By

Stuart C. Yudofsky, M.D.

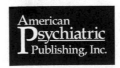

American Psychiatric Publishing, Inc.

Washington, DC
London, England

Copyright © 2005 Stuart C. Yudofsky
ALL RIGHTS RESERVED

Manufactured in the United States of America on acid-free paper
09   08   07   06   05   5   4   3   2
First Edition

Typeset in Adobe's Palatino, The Mix, and Reporter Two

American Psychiatric Publishing, Inc.
1000 Wilson Boulevard
Arlington, VA 22209-3901
www.appi.org

Library of Congress Cataloging-in-Publication Data
Yudofsky, Stuart C.
   Fatal flaws : navigating destructive relationships with people with disorders of personality and character / by Stuart C. Yudofsky.-- 1st ed.
        p. ; cm.
   Includes bibliographical references and index.
   ISBN 1-58562-214-1 (pbk. : alk. paper)
   1. Personality disorders. 2. Personality disorders--Treatment. 3. Psychology, Pathological.
   [DNLM: 1. Personality Disorders. 2. Clinical Medicine--methods. 3. Personality Disorders--Popular Works. 4. Psychotherapy--methods. WM 190 Y94f 2005]
I. Title.

   RC554.Y83 2005
   616.85'81--dc22

                                                                      2004023752

British Library Cataloguing in Publication Data
A CIP record is available from the British Library.

To Beth,
"a summer of wisteria"

—*William Faulkner,*
Absalom, Absalom!

CONTENTS

Part I
FATAL FLAWS

Part II
PERSONALITY DISORDERS

Part III
CONCLUSION

ACKNOWLEDGMENTS

Whatever information and insights are imparted in *Fatal Flaws* derive directly from the kindness, generosity, and patience of my patients, students, colleagues, and teachers—to all of whom I am abundantly and perennially grateful.

I thank, as well, the following people who helped me with the preparation of this book:

- Robert E. Hales, M.D., Editor-in-Chief at American Psychiatric Publishing, Inc. (APPI), my close friend and gracious partner in so many academic projects, who helped me in so many important ways throughout this project. Most of all, Bob helped with the focus and organization of the text.
- Roxanne Rhodes, Senior Editor at APPI and project editor for *Fatal Flaws,* whose careful reading and insightful critique of the manuscript vastly improved the quality, clarity, and impact of the book. Roxanne coordinated all aspects of the preparation of the submitted text and shepherded it to publication.
- Dianna Hobby, editor's editor and grammarian's grammarian, and my dear friend from Houston, who worked tirelessly to vet each word and sentence of the original manuscript for accuracy, precision, and clarity.
- Marianne Szegedy-Maszak, dear friend and inspired and inspiring journalist on behalf of people who suffer from mental illnesses, who gave advice on how to write and structure this book so that it could be useful to clinicians as well as to readers in destructive relationships with people with personality disorders and character flaws.
- Claudia Burns and Lynn Sanders, from my academic office at the Menninger Department of Psychiatry, Baylor College of Medicine, who helped me utilize the marvels of modern information technology to access the

wealth of published data about personality and character disorders that have enriched this volume.

- Joy Yudofsky Behr, my devoted sister, who read carefully the entire manuscript several times and imparted her wise, refined sense of what most readers would find interesting and, more important, what they would not.
- Beth Koster Yudofsky, M.D., my beloved wife, lovely and loving partner, and gifted colleague, whose unswerving support and faith in this book and, *mirabile dictu,* in me, made possible *Fatal Flaws.*

Stuart C. Yudofsky, M.D.
Houston, Texas

The following sources are gratefully acknowledged:

- Faber and Faber Ltd and Harcourt Brace & Company, for permission to reprint excerpts from "The Waste Land" and "The Love Song of J. Alfred Prufrock," from *The Complete Poems and Plays,* by T.S. Eliot (London: Faber and Faber; San Diego, CA: Harcourt).
- Golden Gate National Park Association, for permission to reprint an excerpt from *A Land in Motion: California's San Andreas Fault,* by Michael Collier (Berkeley, CA: University of California Press, 1999).
- Manatt, Phelps & Phillips, LLP, for permission to reprint a lyric excerpt from "You're So Vain," by Carly Simon.
- Hal-Leonard Corporation, for permission to reprint a lyric excerpt from "My Eyes Adored You," by Bob Crewe and Kenny Nolan.
- University of California Press, for permission to reprint two excerpts from *Magnitude 8: Earthquakes and Life Along the San Andreas Fault,* by Philip L. Fradkin (Berkeley, CA: University of California Press, 1999).
- Warner Brothers Publications U.S. Inc., for permission to reprint a lyric excerpt from "Torn Between Two Lovers," by Phillip Jarrell and Peter Yarrow.

INTRODUCTION

No one is perfect. Some among us, however, are far less perfect than others. There are vast numbers of people, impaired by disorders of personality and character, who do not fulfill commitments and who seem incapable of sustaining mature, honest, or constructive relationships. Many people with these conditions are destructive and even dangerous. Because these same individuals also have many assets, I term their personality and character disorders *flaws.* I liken these flaws to imperfections in a building material that can weaken and threaten the stability of an entire structure. When people are unwilling to acknowledge their personality or character problems or are unable to change their damaging behaviors, they are disabled by what I term *fatal* flaws.

Because people with fatal flaws of personality and character also have exceptional abilities and attractive qualities, they engage in all types of relationships and hold a vast variety of positions of responsibility and importance. Ultimately and invariably, their relationships fail and their responsibilities are unmet. These failures are costly to themselves and others and are expensive both emotionally and financially. An example is a husband or wife with narcissistic personality disorder who neglects his or her responsibilities as a spouse and parent while having a long succession of extramarital affairs. The chief financial officer of a large company who has antisocial personality disorder and who lies and cheats to enrich himself or herself at the expense of the viability of the corporation is another all-too-common example. A person with paranoid personality disorder who becomes convinced that you have harmed him in some way and becomes preoccupied with punishing you for your imagined transgressions is a third example. A young woman who makes repeated suicide attempts when she has problems with her boyfriends, a controlling husband who constantly criticizes and finds fault with his wife, and a stranger who stalks and threatens your daughter are three more examples of people who may have serious personality disorders such as borderline, obsessive-compulsive, and schizotypal personality disorders.

In *Fatal Flaws*, I endeavor to present, in a clear and interesting fashion, the rapidly increasing body of clinical and research information about people with disorders of personality and character. By providing, in great detail, representative cases of people whom I have treated during my almost 30 years in the clinical practice of psychiatry, I try to bring their stories to life and to offer a unique view of how biology, life experience, and psychology combine in the development and persistence of personality and character flaws. All of the people presented in this book constitute composites of my many patients and those with whom they have importantly interacted in their lives. *All* identifying facts and relevant details have been changed significantly and sufficiently to protect confidentiality. If you believe that you recognize one of your patients, someone whom you know, or even yourself in these accounts, you are recognizing the psychopathology, not the person.

The clinical course, treatment, genetics, biology, psychology, and destructive consequences of the following conditions are presented in *Fatal Flaws*:

- Hysterical (histrionic) personality disorder
- Narcissistic personality disorder
- Antisocial personality disorder
- Paranoid personality disorder
- Obsessive-compulsive personality disorder
- Addictive personality
- Borderline personality disorder
- Schizotypal personality disorder

Fatal Flaws is an ambitious and unconventional book. It is ambitious in that it is written for an unusually broad audience. It is primarily directed toward mental health students and trainees of all disciplines who aspire to learn more about the clinical features, biology, psychology, assessment, and treatment of people with personality disorders and character flaws. Psychiatry residents, psychology interns, and social work students often begin their training in psychotherapy by treating patients or clients with personality disorders. Even with supervision, they liken this educational experience to trying to learn how to swim by being thrown into the deep end of the pool. There is so much happening at once in the clinical setting and so much to know about the nature of these disorders and their treatments that even highly experienced mental health professionals find the treatment of people with personality disorders to be a major challenge. This book has been especially written to provide the requisite information and sense of the clinical experience to help inform, orient, and support the novice mental health professional treating patients or clients with personality or character disorders.

Fatal Flaws is also crafted so that it may be referred by mental health professionals to their patients and clients who are currently in important and intense relationships with individuals with flaws of personality or character. Used in this fashion, the book is designed to supplement treatment by providing relevant, useful information to patients and clients as they strive to disentangle themselves from flawed, destructive relationships. In this era of the Internet, these patients and clients have access to voluminous information on their conditions. These patients and clients are especially interested in obtaining additional information about the genetics, neurobiology, psychology, and theories of treatment of this category of conditions. However, much of the information they find on Web sites is misleading, inaccurate, exploitive, and even potentially dangerous to them. *Fatal Flaws* was written to complement the professional care of people with personality disorders by providing relevant, respectful, protective, evidence-based information about critical aspects of their conditions and treatment. Finally, the book was written to be useful for people who are uncertain about whether or not they or their loved ones might have a personality disorder and who want to know more about these conditions and their treatments before making a decision about securing professional help.

Fatal Flaws is unconventional for two reasons. First, it is a hybrid: part psychiatric textbook and part self-help manual for patients and clients with personality disorders. Second, I have chosen to write portions of this book in the first person—specifically, as I directly address a patient who either has a personality disorder or is in an important relationship with a person with one of these conditions. I hope that this intimate writing style will bring to life how I and other experienced clinicians think through problems and how we sound as we are treating our patients who have—or are in relationships with people who have—personality disorders and character flaws.

During my medical school education and residency training in psychiatry, it was my privilege to observe and listen while many gifted clinician/educators interviewed and treated patients with psychiatric disorders. I have done my very best to replicate this experience for the reader. The symphony of my mentors' words and the ballet of their movements echo and imprint all of my own interchanges with patients to this very day:

- Hilde Bruch, M.D., smiling knowingly at the sister of a patient with anorexia nervosa and saying, "You seem to be telling me that your sister eats up all the attention in your family."
- Shervert Frazier, M.D., beginning an interview with a serial killer in a high-security prison by declaring, "You needn't be afraid of Dr. Yudofsky and me. We won't hurt you."
- Harold Searles, M.D., bringing laughter to the heart of a withdrawn patient with schizophrenia with his ironic, respectful compliment, "You remind me so much of my own 19-year-old son. Only he doesn't have schizophrenia. He doesn't have it in him."
- Otto Kernberg, M.D., staring intently at the sliced-up forearm of a young woman with borderline personality disorder and asking, "Does that help you figure out where you stop and I begin?"
- Roger MacKinnon, M.D., bringing sobs to a medical resident with obsessive-compulsive disorder by commenting, "Notice that I began our discussion this morning by asking, 'How are you?'; not 'How are you doing?' I believe your father was more interested in how you performed than how you were feeling."
- Robert Michels, M.D., challenging a failing medical student with antisocial personality disorder, "You blame the teacher for being disorganized; you state that the material on the test was never covered in class; you indicate that the teaching assistant is prejudiced against you because of your race. Tell me, now: do you believe that you yourself have any role in your failures?"
- Ethel Person, M.D., while interviewing a depressed young woman who had just made a serious suicide attempt: "You indicate that your only remaining power is over whether or not you live or die. I believe you are confusing 'power' with 'default.' What you're talking about and acting out is misdirected murderous rage toward your disinterested mother and abusive father."

My debt and gratitude to my teachers are far too vast for me to be able to express in words. Applying and passing on their inspired and inspiring lessons through caring for patients, teaching, and writing books like this are the best that I can do.

> And gladly wolde he lerne, and gladly teche.

> —the Clerk of Oxford, in
> Geoffrey Chaucer, *Canterbury Tales*

PROLOGUE

The Dream Home on Shelter Cove: A Parable

Joan and Martin Lawrence found their dream home in the tiny town of Shelter Cove, in Northern California's Humboldt County.

On the days without fog, one can peer through the expanse of windows that form the home's western flank and see miles and miles of roiling purple Pacific. And ample rain ensures that the home's eastern face is perennially framed by thick, green grass with piercings of sturdy pine and oak.

To their happy surprise, the Lawrences found that the sale of their cookie-cutter cottage on its cramped site in a stale Sacramento suburb would more than cover the cost of this gem in its unique setting of purple and green.

But there was one, ever-so-subtle, almost-imperceptible problem: a local fisherman revealed to Martin that picturesque Shelter Cove was in motion. About 14 millimeters, or half an inch each year, toward the purple. This meant that the dream home was also moving—slipping ever so slowly to the edge of the cliff on which it was perched.

"We've worked our entire lives to retire in a place like this. Think of our dream bedroom, newly painted each morning by the amber sunrise," Joan exclaimed.

Martin pointed out to Joan that Shelter Cove slumbers on a northern extreme of the San Andreas fault, before it slices to the west and dives out to sea.

"At half an inch a year, it will take centuries for the home to reach the cliff," Joan reasoned. "And from the kitchen we could watch the surf beating on the rocks while we ate fresh sea trout that you would catch at Black Sand Beach," she persisted.

"But the entire region is unstable. Even a small earthquake could change everything and send our dream home—with us in it—over the cliff and into the sea," Martin lamented.

"Think about the beautiful family room. It would be perfect for our grandchildren. We've always dreamed about a family room," replied Joan.

The reader may choose between two endings of this parable. Each dénouement represents a path a person may take when involved with someone with persistent flaws of personality or character. The two paths lead in very different directions.

Ending #1: "Sand Castle"

Seduced by the beautiful house in its unique setting, Joan and Martin pur-chased their dream home on Shelter Cove. The sunshine warmed their spirits, and the salty breezes preserved their dreams. Everything seemed perfect, at first.

After the tremors came—and they always come—closet doors and kitchen windows wedged and whined in their casings when being opened, while spider-silk fissures threaded through the plaster walls and the cement foundation.

And when the storms came—and they always come—cold wet winds crawled under doors and beneath the Lawrences' blankets to chill their dreams.

A structural engineer was summoned who measured their home's attraction to the beckoning purple—a flirtatious prelude of the wet embrace that was certain to follow.

Only deep-drilled piers and banded pilings might save their dream home. A certain expense for an uncertain remedy. They were advised: "Cut your losses. Don't throw good money after bad decisions."

But they had invested so much, and the house and the setting were almost perfect. So they chose to linger in their dream and hope for best.

Then came the wildfires, followed by the floods and sliding mud. And more tremors. Finally, Joan and Martin watched their home, with softened cliff and abandoned dreams, slip into the sea.

How understandable that anyone might choose to ignore learning about and dealing directly with the personality flaws of someone with whom he or she has invested so much time, effort, and emotion. First of all, one would have to face unpleasant realties regarding that person, who has so many *other* wonderful assets. Second, based on what would be learned, changes would have to be made. How much easier it would be, in the short run, to ignore and live with these problems. However, the destructive problems stemming from personality flaws do not repair themselves. Rather, with the passage of time, the problems only grow worse, undermining the relationship while eroding self-esteem, self-confidence, and self-worth.

Fatal Flaws is not an easy book. It is replete with old wisdom and new, evidence-based concepts that are by no means simplistic or self-evident. Identifying and understanding people with severe flaws of personality and character are not easy tasks. Knowing how to help people with these disorders change themselves, and knowing when and how to help others become disentangled from relationships with these individuals, can be even more difficult. This book harbors the knowledge required to gain this understanding. Although freedom and peace of mind are priceless, changing behavior does not come cheaply. Risks must be taken. Time, effort, and emotions must be committed to make the required changes—a toll of great cost to achieve freedom and equanimity. However, not looking, not learning, not changing, and not acting will exact a far greater toll.

Ending #2: "Paying the Toll"

With Joan's dissent, Martin sought the seasoned wisdom of a structural engineer. He assayed their dream home with steel drills that bored unromantically past the graceful green surfaces to pilfer deep, betraying cores of soil, gravel, and rock. Joyous feelings, sunshine and shadows, were transformed into lengths and levels, weights and numbers, measured scratchings on rolled blue paper.

A tempered verdict for an intemperate fault: "Move the dream home to a new foundation, poured far away from the purple." A golden dream transformed to gray. It could be done, but at what price? Less green and purple, more work and money. While dreams are beyond price, reality has costs.

Martin and Joan chose to preserve their dream at the cost of their leisure. Martin would not retire, and Joan would return to work. Days and weekends in office cells and untold hours gazing at computer screens—a high price for the piers and pilings that would anchor their home of dreams.

But in their early mornings, the amber sunrises glowed and danced for free. And late at night they would lie in their anchored bed and listen to the music of the rock-beating surf. Safe and friendly spray that exacted no further toll upon their house of dreams.

With regard to people with personality disorders, change in self and relationships can only come with great effort, at high cost, and with wrenching trade-offs. By reading *Fatal Flaws* and by understanding and integrating its key principles, information, understanding, and skills can be gained to help willing people make meaningful and liberating changes. There is much work to do, so let's begin.

Part I
Fatal Flaws

WHAT ARE FATAL FLAWS?

The San Andreas is the grinding, growling inter-
face between two great pieces of the earth's crust,
each moving its separate way. This is the fault
that has cleaved volcanoes, opened seaways, and
split mountains. And yet, driving south of Pai-
cines on California Highway 25, I wasn't sure
just where it was.

—Michael Collier, *A Land in Motion:
California's San Andreas Fault*

Defining Fatal Flaws

Fatal flaws are brain-based dysfunctions of thinking and impulse that
lead to persistent patterns of personality and behavior that betray trust
and destroy relationships. Each noun, adjective, and verb in this definition is critical and requires the explanations and amplifications that are
presented in this and subsequent chapters of this book. In these chapters I review the eight personality disorders that most frequently lead to
violated trust, broken commitments, dangerous behaviors, and destructive relationships: hysterical (histrionic), narcissistic, antisocial, obsessive-compulsive, paranoid, borderline, schizotypal, and addictive
personality disorders.

Although their causes and presentations are often hidden and confusing, flawed personalities and character structures create wreckage
that is not at all subtle. The resulting pain and suffering can overwhelm
the lives of those with whom they are importantly associated; and the
related material losses are incalculable. Examples include your fiancée
being unfaithful; your husband gambling away the savings for the chil-

TABLE 1–1.   What makes a flaw "fatal"?

A "fatal" flaw exists if one or more of the following is true:

1. The person with the flaw does not perceive that she or he has a problem.

2. The person with the flaw does not want to change.

3. The nature of the flaw is such that it is not amenable to correction.

4. The nature of the flaw is such that there is the probability of future physical harm occurring to you, to your child, or to others.

5. The nature of the flaw is such that there is the probability of violations of the law by the individual with the flaw.

6. The nature of the flaw is such that there is the probability that the person with the flaw will involve you in the breaking of the law.

dren's college tuition; your employee stealing money from your business; your parent being abused by an attendant in a nursing home; the company for which you work going bankrupt and shutting down because of the greed and dishonesty of the chief executive officer; your child attending school while high on drugs; your wife injuring herself and others while driving while intoxicated from alcohol.

Such consequences may or may not be the results of what I term *fatal* flaws. A goal of this book is to help you to differentiate between people with character and personality flaws that are amenable to change and those whose flaws will never change. My definition of why a particular fault in personality and character is a *fatal* flaw involves 1) its persistence and/or 2) its probability of resulting in serious injury or in violations of the law. *Fatal* flaws have one or more of the qualities listed in Table 1–1.

Defining *Personality, Temperament,* and *Character*

Personality

Personality can be defined in many different ways. The original and oldest definitions found in most dictionaries might surprise you. For example, the popular *Merriam-Webster's Collegiate Dictionary*, 11th Edition (2003), has a rather elusive initial definition of the term: "the quality or state of being a person." I find the corollary definition in this dictionary, "personal existence," to be even more ephemeral and less helpful. *Webster's New Collegiate* also provides two other definitions of *personality* that, I believe, are closer to what most of us understand the term to mean: "the complex of characteristics that distinguishes an individual" and "the totality of an individual's behavioral and emotional characteristics."

C. Robert Cloninger, M.D., a psychiatrist who is a noted authority on personality disorders, makes clear distinctions among the terms *personality, temperament,* and *character* (Cloninger and Svrakic 2000). He believes that the origins of personality are a combination of inheritance (i.e., genetics) and environmental influences (i.e., life experience) (Heath et al. 1999). Central to Dr. Cloninger's definition of personality are the unique ways in which individuals express themselves and adapt to their environments. I believe that his concept of what constitutes personality is best understood by looking at specific *personality traits,* or persistent patterns of how a person perceives and relates to oneself, one's environment, and other people. Examples include such traits as 1) sensitivity, 2) integrity, 3) empathy, 4) conscientiousness, 5) responsibility, 6) reliability, 7) purposefulness, 8) honesty, 9) generosity, 10) kindness, 11) respectfulness, and 12) humility. By placing the word *deficient* before each of these personality traits, you can begin to get a picture of the problems associated with people with fatal flaws of personality and character. *Note that people with fatal flaws of personality and character will have significant problems with several, but not all, of these personality traits.*

Temperament

Dr. Cloninger believes that the term *temperament* should encompass emotional, motivational, and adaptive traits. He includes such traits as harm avoidance, novelty seeking, reward dependence, and persistence. From his perspective, temperament is the "emotional core of personality" (Cloninger and Svrakic 2000). Dysfunctions in these dimensions lead to problems that are conceptualized by Cloninger to occur along a continuum as shown in Figure 1–1.

People with flaws of personality and character have severe problems along the right side of this continuum of temperament. It is interesting to note that people with depression have difficulties along the left side of the continuum. I and other neuropsychiatrists believe that temperament is the component of personality that is most subject to genetic predispositions and to the influence of biological factors in the environment such as alcohol and drugs.

These definitions of personality and temperament point to a constellation of critical behavioral, emotional, and thinking patterns that is unique to a particular individual. If this constellation is impaired in such a fashion that the pattern of the person's inner experience and outward behavior deviates markedly from the person's culture, and if the

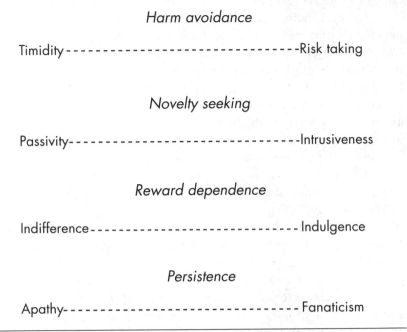

Harm avoidance

Timidity -Risk taking

Novelty seeking

Passivity- -Intrusiveness

Reward dependence

Indifference - Indulgence

Persistence

Apathy- Fanaticism

FIGURE 1–1.   The continuum of temperament.
Source.   Cloninger and Svrakic 2000, pp. 1724–1730.

pattern is persistent and leads to significant distress and relationship problems, this person is said to have a ***personality disorder***. The most disabling and destructive types of personality disorders are comprehensively reviewed in the subsequent chapters of this book. The famed psychoanalyst and authority on personality disorders Glen O. Gabbard, M.D., points out that people with personality disorders usually are not particularly upset by their own flawed patterns of thinking and behavior; however, they can become distressed by the *consequences* of the maladaptive behaviors that get them into so much trouble. Dr. Gabbard contrasts this pattern to that in most other mental illnesses, in which the person with the disorder experiences suffering both from the illness *and* from its consequences (G.O. Gabbard, personal communication, December 2004).

Character

Of the eight major definitions for *character* listed in *Merriam-Webster's Collegiate Dictionary* (2003), most have nothing to do with the considerations of this book. Curiously, the second of these definitions is very

TABLE 1–2.   Cloninger's dimensions of a mature personality

Self-directedness

Disciplined, responsible, purposeful, resourceful, self-accepting

Cooperativeness

Empathic, kind, compassionate, helpful, principled

Self-transcendence

Idealistic, spiritual, intuitive, imaginative, acquiescent

Source.   Cloninger and Svrakic 2000.

similar to a reasonable definition of *personality:* "one of the attributes or features that make up and distinguish the individual." However, it is the final definition that I believe has the greatest relevance for our understanding of fatal flaws of character. This definition is "moral excellence and firmness." Thus people with character flaws would have inconsistencies with and violations of moral behavior.

Behavioral scientists view character as an individual's ability to modulate basic drives and affects such as aggression, hunger and greed, and sexual pleasure. Dr. Cloninger believes that three key dimensions are involved in the concept of character. Dr. Cloninger makes the important point that these dimensions define whether or not a person is a mature adult, as summarized in Table 1–2 (Cloninger and Svrakic 2000).

When the word *not* is placed before each of the descriptions listed in Table 1–2, further traits associated with people with flaws of personality and character are revealed.

As with the components of personality and temperament, *people with character flaws will have problems with some, but not all, of the aforementioned dimensions of character.*

Many people with severe character flaws do whatever they determine is necessary (e.g., lie, cheat, steal, injure) as they exploit others to gratify their own needs. What these people lack is a conscience or an internal sense of values, empathy, and concern regarding the rights of others. In other words, if they seriously harm someone else in the fulfillment of their own needs, they don't worry very much about it. Their concerns are fundamentally self-centered: self-gratification, self-aggrandizement, and self-preservation (e.g., not getting caught or found out). If the last three sentences ring a bell regarding a person with whom you have a current relationship, it is probably worth your while to review and apply the Fatal Flaw Scale as described in Chapter 2, "Does This Person Have a Fatal Flaw?"

Defining Personality Disorders According to DSM-IV-TR

People with personality disorders are considered by American psychiatrists and by many psychologists to have mental illnesses. Mental illnesses are defined in the *Diagnostic and Statistical Manual of Mental Disorders,* Fourth Edition, Text Revision (DSM-IV-TR; American Psychiatric Association 2000). This manual, which is perennially under revision, has revolutionized and standardized the definition and diagnosis of psychiatric disorders. In arriving at the diagnosis of a mental illness by using DSM-IV-TR, no theory of causality is used. Rather, specific criteria—which are clusters of signs and symptoms—are required to be present before a diagnosis of a specific psychiatric disorder can be made. In medicine, *signs* are indications of illness that can be objectively determined, such as fever, pulse irregularity, or aggression; *symptoms* are subjectively experienced indications of illness, as exemplified by pain, anxiety, and anger. Groups of scholars and experts work closely together and utilize research methodologies and epidemiological information to arrive at the DSM criteria for psychiatric disorders. As the knowledge advances, the criteria are refined and improved with successive editions of the manual.

In DSM-IV-TR a distinction is drawn between personality traits and personality disorders. *Personality traits* are defined in DSM-IV-TR as "enduring patterns of perceiving, relating to, and thinking about the environment and oneself that are exhibited in a wide range of social and personal contexts." (American Psychiatric Association 2000, p. 686). In contrast, *personality disorders* are considered persistent patterns of feelings, thinking, and behavior that result in problems with relationships, in controlling impulses, and in functioning in social, school, or occupational settings. People with personality disorders usually, although not always, experience distress with and cause distress for those with whom they are involved. In most cases the abnormal personality patterns appear by the time the individuals are adolescents or young adults. The general criteria for the diagnosis of personality disorders from DSM-IV-TR (American Psychiatric Association 2000) are summarized in Table 1–3.

References and Selected Readings

American Psychiatric Association: Diagnostic and Statistical Manual of Mental Disorders, 4th Edition, Text Revision. Washington, DC, American Psychiatric Association, 2000

TABLE 1–3. General diagnostic criteria for a personality disorder (slightly modified from DSM-IV-TR)

A. An enduring pattern of feeling, thinking, and behaving that deviates markedly from the expectations of the person's culture. This pattern is manifested in at least two of the following areas:

1. *Cognition* (ways of perceiving and interpreting self, other people and events)

2. *Affect* (the range, intensity, volatility, and appropriateness of their emotional responses)

3. *Interpersonal relationships*

4. *Impulse control*

B. This pattern of feeling, thinking, and behaving is inflexible and is exhibited across a broad range of personal and social situations.

C. The pattern of feeling, thinking, and behaving leads to distress in the individual and others and to impairments in interpersonal, social, school, and/or occupation functioning.

D. The pattern of feeling, thinking, and behaving is enduring, and its onset can usually be traced back to childhood, adolescence, or early adulthood.

E. The dysfunctional pattern of feeling, thinking, and behaving is not caused by another type of psychiatric disorder or a consequence of a medical condition such as brain injury.

Source. Adapted from American Psychiatric Association: *Diagnostic and Statistical Manual of Mental Disorders,* 4th Edition, Text Revision. Washington, DC, American Psychiatric Association, 2000, p. 689. Used with permission.

Cloninger CR, Svrakic DM: Personality disorders, in Kaplan & Sadock's Comprehensive Textbook of Psychiatry, 7th Edition. Edited by Sadock BJ, Sadock VA. Philadelphia, PA, Lippincott Williams & Wilkins, 2000, pp 1723–1764

Heath AC, Madden PA, Cloninger CR, et al: Genetic and environmental structure of personality, in Personality and Psychopathology. Edited by Cloninger CR. Washington, DC, American Psychiatric Press, 1999, pp 343–368

Iversen S, Kupfermann I, Kandel ER: Emotional states and feeling, in Principles of Neural Science, 4th Edition. Edited by Kandel ER, Schwartz JH, Jessell TM. New York, McGraw-Hill, 2000, pp 982–996

Merriam-Webster's Collegiate Dictionary, 11th Edition. Springfield, MA, Merriam-Webster, 2003

Phillips KA Yen S, Gunderson JG: Personality disorders, in American Psychiatric Publishing Textbook of Clinical Psychiatry, 4th Edition. Edited by Hales RE, Yudofsky SC. Washington, DC, American Psychiatric Publishing, 2003, pp 803–832

Silk KR: Biology of Personality Disorders. Washington, DC, American Psychiatric Press, 1998

Chapter

2

DOES THIS PERSON HAVE A FATAL FLAW?

Earthquakes are the result of tremendous forces
deep within the earth that are invisible to the na-
ked eye and only dimly understood by the human
intellect.

—Philip L. Fradkin, *Magnitude 8:
Earthquakes and Life Along the San Andreas Fault*

Fatal Flaw Scale

The Fatal Flaw Scale is presented in Appendix A to this chapter. The
scale is in the form of a questionnaire that will help you determine
whether or not a person with whom you have an important relationship
has a fatal flaw of personality or character. If the person is in treatment,
the scale can also be completed periodically by significant others as a
measure of change and progress.

Discussion of the Fatal Flaw Scale and Its Scoring

Structure of the Fatal Flaw Scale

Psychological rating scales can be structured as follows:

- *Subjective rating scales,* in which the individual whose behavior,
  thinking, and/or emotions are being rated fills out the scale himself
  or herself. This type of scale, also called a self-reporting scale, is use-

ful in rating subjective experiences such as anxiety, anger, or sadness of a person who is cooperative, honest, and insightful.
- *Objective rating scales*, in which the behavior and expressed emotions of an individual are rated by another person who has had the opportunity to observe the person being rated.
- *Combination scales*, in which behavior, emotions, and thinking can be rated objectively by a person who has had the opportunity to observe the individual being rated, or subjectively (as a self-reporting instrument) by the person being evaluated.

Clinical Use of the Fatal Flaw Scale

Given the reality that people with flaws of character and personality often do not acknowledge their problems or seek professional help to correct them, I designed the Fatal Flaw Scale to be completed by those who know well and, most commonly, are directly affected by the person being rated. When used in this fashion, the Fatal Flaw Scale is an objective rating scale. Less commonly, when people with character and personality flaws have sought my professional help for diagnosis and treatment, I have suggested that they involve their significant others in completing this scale and that they repeat this process on a regular basis to help monitor their progress in treatment. I recommend having family sessions with the patient with personality and character disorders and his or her significant others, who fill out the Fatal Flaw Scale. On those occasions, the responses to each question are discussed fully.

In the more usual circumstance, the patient is the individual who has a significant relationship with a person with personality and character flaws. As will be discussed throughout this book, many people with severe and persistent disorders of personality or character will not acknowledge their problems or accept professional help. Although it would be my preference—in the clinical setting—to involve the person who was being rated with the Fatal Flaw Scale in the entire rating process, this is usually impractical. Nonetheless, I recommend that the patient consider filling out the scale for a variety of reasons, which I explain. First, just *thinking about* how the questions on the scale may or may not pertain to the significant other is a useful exercise. For example, one patient told me that she had been denying (to herself) how fearful she was of her husband and how concerned she was that he might be abusing her daughter (his stepdaughter) until she thought seriously about answering question 8 in Part A and questions 1 and 3 in Part B of the Fatal Flaw Scale. Second, the Fatal Flaw Scale provides a rough indication of the seriousness or severity of the interpersonal situation in which you are involved. In this circumstance it can serve the function of a "wake-up call" to alert you that you must change the nature of your involvement with the person with serious flaws. Third, as indicated above, the scale can be used to monitor the progress of a significant other who is working elsewhere in therapy to change his or her personality and character flaws. Finally, several of my patients who have successfully disentangled themselves from a destructive relationship with one individual with a personality flaw have used the scale to help them evaluate other suitors. They are correctly concerned that the psychodynamics and blind spots that might have led them into the original dysfunctional relationship might prevail in the newer one. Once burned, twice warned.

How the Fatal Flaw Scale Should <u>Not</u> Be Used

The Fatal Flaw Scale is intended to be a constructive and useful tool for assessment and measurement of change. It is intended to be advocational, not adversarial. As tempting as it might be to do so, you should not use the scale as a weapon to show the person with the putative flaws what a bad or sick person he or she is, or even to give some indication how much the person has harmed you. Because of the nature of the disorder that is measured by the Fatal Flaw Scale, people so afflicted are usually not pleased when others discover this problem in *their* character or personality. Nor, in my experience, have the results of the Fatal Flaw Scale been particularly useful in motivating a person with such flaws to change or to seek professional help.

Should You Attempt to Use the Scale Right Now?

If you believe that a person with whom you have a significant relationship might have serious flaws of personality or character, I see no reason why you should not use the scale as an initial tool to check out this concern. Once you have completed the scale, if the resulting score indicates that it is "possible," "probable," or "highly likely" that the person in question has a flaw, I believe that it is worth your while to read further to learn more about these conditions. The book is designed to provide sufficient information and to present representative examples that will reduce most doubt about whether or not flaws of character and personality are affecting your important relationship. If you have some difficulty in completing the Fatal Flaw Scale on your first attempt, you should review the case studies that are presented in most of the subsequent chapters to see how the scale can be used beneficially.

FATAL FLAW SCALE

Part A

Does this person have a personality and/or character flaw?

Please check the best answer, "Yes" or "No," to the following questions regarding the person with whom you have an important relationship. If you are not sure, mark that answer "No."

1. Do I trust this person? (Yes) (No)
2. Has this person "come through" on important commitments? (Yes) (No)
3. Do I feel better about myself as a consequence of this relationship? (Yes) (No)
4. Does this person consider my needs equally to his or hers? (Yes) (No)
5. Is this person sensitive to and supportive of me? (Yes) (No)
6. Will this person communicate with me honestly on significant issues affecting our relationship? (Yes) (No)
7. Is this person honest with other people and trustworthy in his or her other relationships? (Yes) (No)
8. Do I, and [if applicable] do my children, always feel physically safe with this person? (Yes) (No)
9. Does this person respect rules and obey laws? (Yes) (No)
10. Do *other* people whom I love and trust the most believe this person is good for me? (Yes) (No)

Directions: Total the number of "No" answers that you checked.
Scoring:

A. 0 "No"—<u>Highly Unlikely</u> that this person has flaws of personality and character.
B. 1–3 "No"—<u>Possible</u> that this person has flaws of personality and character.

C. 4–5 "No"—<u>Probable</u> that this person has flaws of personality and character.

D. 5–10 "No"—<u>Highly Likely</u> that this person has flaws of personality and character.

Part B

Does this person's flaw of personality and character qualify as being a <u>fatal</u> flaw?

(Only to be determined if score on Part A is 4 or higher)

Please check "Yes" or "No" for the following questions regarding the person with whom you have an important relationship. For questions 1, 2, and 3, if you are not sure, mark that answer "Yes." If you do not have access to accurate information regarding questions 4, 5, and 6, do not check an answer.

1. Does this person persist in engaging in activities that are impulsive, unnecessarily dangerous, or self-destructive? (Yes) (No)
2. Does this person deny that he or she has a problem? (Yes) (No)
3. Does this person refuse professional help for his or her problem? (Yes) (No)
4. Does the person's problem remain unchanged despite many courses of professional help? (Yes) (No)
5. Is there a good chance that, in the future, this person will physically injure me or my child? (Yes) (No)
6. Does this person persist in engaging in illegal acts? (Yes) (No)

Directions: Total the number of "Yes'" answers that you checked.
Scoring:

A. 0 "Yes"—<u>Highly Unlikely</u> that this person has a <u>fatal</u> flaw.
B. 1–2 "Yes"—<u>Possible</u> that this person has a <u>fatal</u> flaw.
C. 3–4 "Yes"—<u>Probable</u> that this person has a <u>fatal</u> flaw.
D. 5–6 "Yes"—<u>Highly Likely</u> that this person has a <u>fatal</u> flaw.

Chapter

3

NINE PRINCIPLES FOR DEALING WITH PEOPLE WITH FATAL FLAWS

The nine overarching principles presented in this chapter are useful in understanding, relating to, caring for, and helping people with disorders of personality or character. Each of these principles is evidenced in the case examples of the eight personality disorders that are presented in the remainder of the book.

Principle 1

Even though relationships with people with disorders of personality and character are difficult, frustrating, and sometimes destructive and dangerous, people with these conditions should be treated with respect, kindness, and compassion.

Increasing scientific evidence suggests that, as with most other mental illnesses, personality disorders are the result of complex factors, including genetic predispositions, alterations in brain chemistry and structure, and responses to life experiences and stresses. The stigmatization of "borderlines," "hysterics," "narcissists," "sociopaths," "paranoids," and "addicts" mirrors the historic devaluation and persecution of people with schizophrenia, bipolar illness, and learning differences. Note that throughout this book, people are never reduced to the illnesses they suffer. Rather, they are called, for example, "people with border-line personality disorder" to emphasize that there is so much more to the person than his or her illness. Stigmatization, devaluation, and prej-udice intensify levels of misunderstanding and mistrust while obscur-ing opportunities for resolution, remediation, and repair. Diminishing people with personality disorders increases their levels of anger and feelings of alienation and thereby intensifies their focus on retribution and vindication.

Principle 2

Being realistic about the destructive implications of the behaviors of people with disorders of personality and character, establishing and maintaining safe and ethical boundaries with these people, and follow-ing through on fair consequences when your boundaries are violated do not constitute unkind, insensitive, or vindictive behaviors.

You are protecting yourself and helping the person with flaws of per-sonality and character when you do not allow yourself to be exploited or abused. Confusion and resentment inevitably occur when you over-look violations of your trust or accede, at your own expense, to special treatment of people with these conditions.

Principle 3

Disorders of personality and character are frequently the source of se-rious and persistent relationship problems.

Frequently, in my practice of psychiatry, I have been told by my pa-tients, "I wish I had known about the existence of these types of prob-lems before I became so involved with this person." Personality disorders comprise constellations of specific signs and symptoms that lead to grossly impaired relationships. By being aware of the existence of these conditions, their characteristic features, and how these features may be manifested in relationships, a person is empowered to assess the full implications of a troubled relationship. In this book I use a vari-ety of methods—including case histories, official diagnostic criteria, and tables of special problems related to the respective conditions—to help the reader identify specific personality *disorders* in real-life settings and situations. Awareness and acceptance of a problem is the first, es-sential step toward prevention, intervention, and change.

Principle 4

People with disorders of personality and character may also have many attractive qualities, positive attributes, and substantive achievements.

People become involved with individuals with personality disorders and character flaws for good reasons. Many people with these conditions have compelling and engaging qualities that excite and draw others to them. Relationships with such people characteristically get off to a brilliant start but deteriorate over time as the destructive effects of their personality and character flaws are manifested. As illustrated in "The Dream Home on Shelter Cove: A Parable," presented in the prologue of the book, for many people it is difficult to disengage from those with personality disorders or character flaws for several reasons: 1) they focus on the attractive features of the flawed individuals, and they would miss their associations and involvements with these people; 2) they distrust their judgments that their relationships are failing because of the flaws in the other party; they often doubt their own perceptions, because they have endured relentless devaluation and criticism from the person with flaws; 3) they have their own psychological problems and predispositions that make them vulnerable to the exploitations and deprecations of people with personality disorders or character flaws.

Another implication of the coexistence of assets with flaws in people with these disorders is a positive one. Although people with personality or character defects can and do achieve academic, occupational, and financial success, their dysfunctional relationships invariably diminish the level of their achievement and their sense of fulfillment. As indicated in several of the case examples in this book, the good news is that when such people are motivated to engage in treatment, outcomes can be highly favorable in all dimensions of their lives. When the complications, distractions, and chaos resulting from their disorders of personality or character are diminished, the level of their accomplishments and satisfaction is enhanced.

Principle 5

People with disorders of personality and character are excessively self-involved.

Every person has a different personality, and the specific diagnostic criteria for the eight personality disorders presented in this book also are variable. Nonetheless, people with these diverse conditions have certain common features. One feature that people with personality disorders share is intense self-involvement. In particular, they have difficulties understanding and accepting other people's points of view. People with personality disorders often do not even bother to consider how what they say or do might affect the people who are the closest to them or who depend on them. Examples of this self-centeredness are legion across the various personality disorders. People with antisocial personality disorder will inflict severe psychological and physical damage on others to meet their own needs and achieve their own ends. In addition, they do not suffer any pangs of conscience over the damage that they cause to other people. People with borderline personality disorder frequently misrepresent the communications of others, often to serve their own narrow purposes. When differences of opinion arise in relationships, they will not consider the other person's perspective. Rather, in disagreements, they become enraged and launch an attack on the other party. Individuals with paranoid personality disorder and schizotypal personality disorder are so self-absorbed that they distort reality. They are often conflicted about their own angry and sexual feelings, which they unconsciously project onto others. The net result is that, unwarrantedly, they feel threatened and persecuted. If the people with these disorders share their fears and concerns with the others involved, they will not accept the explanations or refutations. People with narcissistic personality disorder take the credit for the accomplishments of others, exaggerate their own achievements, and ignore people whom they believe cannot advance their status. People with this condition generally exploit others to enhance their self-image and self-esteem.

Principle 6

The underlying causes of disorders of personality and character are complex.

When it comes to conceptualizing and describing the likely causes of mental disorders, I believe that theories and explanations should be as simple as possible, *but not simpler than the causes actually are.* Consistent with other psychiatric conditions, personality disorders occur as the result of a complex matrix of biological, psychological, social, and spiritual factors. Prominent among the biological factors are genetic predispositions to these conditions. Although much research work remains to be done relative to the hereditary features of the individual personality disorders, genetic predispositions have been implicated in an individual's vulnerability to alcoholism and certain other addictive disorders, borderline personality disorder, paranoid personality disorder, obsessive-compulsive personality disorder, schizotypal personality disorder, and antisocial personality disorder. Definitive proof of the precise role of genetics in each of these conditions, however, is not yet available. (I believe this avenue of research to be one of the most important frontiers of opportunity in all of medicine and science.) In several of these disorders, abusive treatment by caregivers during childhood interacts with genetic predispositions to give rise to characteristic signs and symptoms in adults with the disorders. For example, people with borderline personality disorder commonly have histories of sexual abuse in childhood, and people with antisocial personality disorder frequently had been physically abused as children. According to many theoreticians, disturbances in interpersonal relationships among mother, father, and child are key factors in leading the child to develop hysterical personality disorder as an adult. People with this condition also, as a rule, are highly suggestible and have characteristic styles of thinking that are impressionistic and deficient in logic—mental states that are likely brain based and genetically determined. Thus, hysterical personality disorder—like other personality disorders—occurs in people with genetic, brain-based predispositions that are *triggered* by life events and particular stresses. The clear implication of the multifactorial causalities of personality disorders is that treatment must, of necessity, incorporate a variety of modalities with evidence-based efficacy.

Principle 7

Many people with personality disorders or character flaws will not accept that they have problems, will refuse treatment, and therefore will not change.

People in dysfunctional relationships often fail to recognize that they are involved with individuals with personality disorders. One reason for this lack of recognition is that their partners in these relationships— people with personality disorders—often refuse to accept that they have any emotional or behavioral problems whatsoever. Many people with personality disorders blame all their relationship problems on the other party. To make the situation even more complex, people with personality disorders often become involved with the most kind, accommodating, and selfless individuals. I do not believe that this is an accident, but rather that such wonderful people are specifically sought out and selected because of their vulnerability to exploitation. Not uncommonly the partners of people with personality disorders will respond to the relentless criticism and devaluation by trying to change and improve themselves—always to no avail. These partners feel that the target (the reason they are being criticized and devalued) is always moving and changing, and therefore their efforts to improve themselves always miss the mark.

If a person with a personality disorder will not accept that he or she has a problem, that individual cannot be helped and most likely will never change. As is clearly indicated throughout this book, many people with personality disorders who are willing to accept that they have problems and to commit to professional treatment can be helped significantly. However, if they will not accept that they have problems and therefore will not commit to treatment, their dysfunctional behaviors will not only persist but usually grow worse. I consider that these people have "fatal flaws." In such a circumstance, any improvement in the relationship or behavioral changes will have to come from the other person in the relationship.

Principle 8

Treatment of motivated people with personality disorders or character flaws can be effective when it is evidence-based and multifaceted.

Much can be learned about the treatment of people with personality disorders from recent scientific investigations of the treatment of those with major depression. Elegant research conducted by neurologist Helen Mayberg, M.D., and co-workers has revealed why people with major depression respond best to treatment with *combinations* of antidepressants and psychotherapy (Goldapple et al. 2004). Her research and that of others has demonstrated the following: 1) major depression has been linked to dysfunctions in different regions of the brain—namely the brainstem and specific areas of the cerebral cortex; 2) treatment of people with depression using antidepressants works by effecting changes in the brainstem, whereas cognitive therapy works by making changes in the cortical areas of the brain; and 3) to achieve and sustain effective treatments of patients with major depression, patients require both modalities. I strongly advocate the use of multiple therapeutic modalities to treat most patients who have personality disorders. Where possible, these treatments should be selected based on scientific evidence of their safety and efficacy. Insight-oriented and cognitive-behavioral psychotherapies are first-line treatments for most people with personality disorders. Because anxiety disorders and mood disorders commonly coexist with personality disorders, psychiatric medications are often another component of the treatment plan. In addition, medications may be helpful in treating serious psychiatric symptoms (such as impulsivity, agitation, and impaired reality testing) that are occasionally associated with some personality disorders. As portrayed in many of the case studies presented in this book, effective treatments are available for people with disorders of personality or character who accept that they have problems and who are committed to changing themselves.

Principle 9

Competent professional care can be very helpful to a person currently in or desiring to relinquish a relationship with a person with a disorder of personality or character.

Psychiatric or psychological care from an experienced, motivated, and competent professional is nearly always useful to a person in a destructive relationship with someone with a personality disorder—whether or not that person must remain in the relationship. That individual can learn how he or she is specifically affected by the stresses of this relationship and can learn interactive skills that will diminish power struggles and the arguments that go nowhere. Treatment will help that person learn how to protect himself or herself from the devaluations, distortions, and exploitations that are endemic in all relationships with people with personality disorders or character flaws. Decisions about how to interact with this individual will be based on solid and specific information about how this person's psychiatric condition affects his or her thinking, emotions, and behavior. If a decision is made to disengage from an individual with a personality disorder, a knowledgeable and practical clinician will help his or her patient or client minimize any danger or damage that might be associated with the breakup. Professional care will also help individuals understand themselves better—particularly why they were especially vulnerable to becoming involved with people with these personality disorders. With this self-awareness will come diminished vulnerability to being attracted to, putting up with, or being preyed on in the future by other individuals with these vexing conditions.

Reference

Goldapple K, Segal Z, Garson C, et al: Modulation of cortical-limbic pathways in major depression: treatment-specific effects of cognitive behavior therapy. Arch Gen Psychiatry 61:34–41, 2004

Part II
Personality Disorders

Chapter

4

HYSTERICAL (HISTRIONIC) PERSONALITY DISORDER

Who is the third who walks always beside you?
When I count, there are only you and I together
But when I look ahead up the white road
There is always another one walking beside you

—T.S. Eliot, "The Waste Land"

And he knows he can't possess me
   and he knows he never will
There's just this empty place
   inside of me that only he can fill
Torn between two lovers, feelin' like a fool
Lovin' both of you is breakin' all the rules

—Phillip Jarrell and Peter Yarrow,
   "Torn Between Two Lovers"
   (recorded by Mary MacGregor)

Essence

Have you ever noticed someone from a distance who seemed so vibrant and inviting that you felt compelled to move in closer? Did she appear to be so brimming with life, suffused with charm, and overflowing in sexuality that you could barely contain your excitement? Did she step to an alluring ballet that drew you nearer while at the same time pushing you away? Were you enticed by her mountainous outpourings over your molehill favors? Were you drawn, mothlike, by her incandescent personality to abandon your customary caution and take leave of your trodden paths? Was your joy unbridled when at last she opened to you and welcomed you in? The burning, blinding exuberance of one who is chosen from the adoring many? Did you inflate with pride to have prevailed over the countless competitors who swarmed and warmed around her, like bees about a swollen rose? Did you then prospect her granite for golden grains of common ground and silver slivers of connecting souls? Did you discover, however, veins of chalk pouring into cold, dark caverns of slate? Probing for depth, did you uncover a vacuum at the center of her volcano? Or was it a lake of ice? Did the fuel of her flame—a consuming interest in how she looked and appeared to others—cast about you a chilling shadow? Would she turn corpse-cold to you in the sudden presence of *certain* others? Did you shiver with rage as she lusted after them in disregard and discard of you? Can you accept that your crimson, full-bloomed, and fragrant flower is barren of pollen and of passion pale? Will you ever swell sufficient strength to abandon your ardor for this paper rose?

The Case of Shelby Fairmont, Part 1: Golden Girl

Discovering Daddy

Bigger Than Life: About Roy Fairmont

When Shelby Fairmont was a luminescent little girl, many who knew her wondered whether she might grow up to be as beautiful as her mother, Colleen, who was widely regarded as one of the most striking women in Houston. Most people who knew Shelby's father, Roy Fairmont, speculated that he had married Colleen, his second wife, mainly because of her great looks. The couple did not seem to have much else in common, other than Roy's ability and willingness to pay for anything Colleen's unrestrained personal shopper at Neiman Marcus ever recommended draping on her statuesque figure. Descended from one of the founding families of Houston, Roy Fairmont had made his own mark as a brilliant jurist and a shrewd businessman. Instead of joining his family's established banking empire, Roy had founded a Houston-based law firm that specialized in the acquisition of oil and gas leases from Texas and Louisiana landholders. Early in his career, Mr. Fairmont invested heavily in natural gas reserves along with many of his wildcatter clients, and, as a result, he became enormously wealthy. Referring to his decision not to make a career in his family's banks, Roy had said, "I would much rather a depositor than a lender be—especially to strangers who would hate my guts when they have to pay me back." And few people in America were capable of making deposits of the size that that Roy Fairmont did each month when the revenue from his oil leases poured in. As Houston became a large city and an international hub of the energy business, Mr. Fairmont's law firm also grew and prospered. Roy Fairmont became a fixture in Texas business and political circles. He helped put together and participated in major business deals and investments at an international level—particularly in off-shore oil well development—and was on the boards of many major corporations and important charitable organizations. Widely acknowledged as one of the leading power brokers in Texas, he was a principal backer of Texas politicians who became governors, senators, and even presidents.

Nobody Is Perfect: Roy Fairmont's Family Life

In contrast to his professional life, Roy Fairmont was not successful in his personal life. When he was in law school he had married Martha, a woman from a prominent Fort Worth family, and it was less than an ideal union. Roy traveled frequently, and when he was in town he worked late hours at his law firm. Roy and Martha had two children, Holcomb and Maureen. The children saw little of their father. Holcomb Fairmont consistently disappointed his father, who proclaimed, "I guess it's not his fault that he is not intelligent, but I cannot excuse him for being so lazy and irresponsible." A poor performer throughout school, Holcomb was constantly in trouble both in and out of the classroom. He was a regular and heavy drinker by the time he was 16 years old, and he was charged with drunken driving on four occasions before his eighteenth birthday. Only his father's powerful political connections kept him out of jail. Although Holcomb was graduated from his private high school at the very bottom of his class, he was admitted to an excellent university—also as a result of his father's influence. However, he did not attend a single class during his first semester of college and was asked to leave. At that point Mr. Fairmont tried to persuade his son to enlist in the army, but both Holcomb and his mother were offended by the suggestion and resisted it. Instead, Holcomb went to work in the construction business of his maternal grandfather, and he continued to drink heavily and get into all types of trouble. Early one morning, driving while intoxicated, he was thrown at a high speed from his overturning car and was killed instantly. Saying "I had written him off many years ago," Mr. Fairmont did not attend his son's funeral. If Roy Fairmont mourned the death of his son, he did so privately. He did not miss a day of work as a result of his son's death, nor did he accept or respond to any expressions of sympathy. His wife believed that Mr.

Fairmont's lifelong disapproval of Holcomb was at the core of her son's problems, and she never forgave her husband. Roy Fairmont blamed his wife for "always being so soft on Holcomb" and for blocking his efforts to have Holcomb enlist in the military. He said, "I think the core of Holcomb's problem was the lack of discipline and motivation, and the army would have straightened him out." On one of the few occasions when Roy and Martha discussed their son's tragic fate, Roy said, "In my mind, you killed our boy with overkindness and good intentions. No different from shooting him in the brain with a bullet from Tiffany's." Several years later, Martha asked Roy for a divorce, to which he acceded in a single utterance: "OK, if that's what you want." Turning the details of his divorce over to trusted attorneys in his firm, Mr. Fairmont never spoke another word to his first wife. Many of their mutual friends in the Houston community likened their parting to the dispassionate dissolution of a large business or the selling of a valuable piece of property. At the time of her parents' divorce, Maureen Fairmont was 21 years old. Although she was never in trouble like her brother, she was also an underperformer who was not close to her father. She chose to move to Fort Worth with her mother and had little further interaction with Mr. Fairmont. She married an accountant in her maternal grandfather's business and lived quietly and comfortably on generous trust funds from both sides of her family. Mr. Fairmont attended his daughter's wedding in Fort Worth but was not present for the christening of her two children. Thereafter he showed no further interest in being part of their lives.

Strike 2: Roy Fairmont Remarries

Like many of his peers who grew up in the mansions along the banks of Buffalo Bayou and abutting the fairways of the River Oaks Country Club, Roy Fairmont attended boarding schools in the East and an Ivy League college. Unlike many of his privileged friends from Texas, Roy eschewed fraternities, secret societies, and sports in favor of an intense immersion in the academic life. He was both intelligent and fiercely competitive. Later in life, a Texas business acquaintance who happened to have been a college classmate was chastising Roy for wanting to include as a partner in a business venture a person who happened to be Jewish:

> **Roy Fairmont's Business Associate:** Now Roy, you know very well that I don't like or trust Jews. We have all the investors we need without inviting those Chicago Jews to come in with us on this deal.

Roy Fairmont: Why not? They've included me in many of their deals, and I have found them to be smart and honest. Their money spends just as well as yours and mine, and they have more of it than both of us.

Business Associate: You've had a thing for Jews since college, Roy. Ever since that hebe from the Bronx beat you out for valedictorian.

Roy Fairmont: Hell, I knew David Sugarman was a lot smarter than I from the first class we took together as freshman. What shocked the hell out of me was that son-of-a-bitch could also outwork me. Bottom line, if you keep the guys from Chicago out of the deal just because they're Jews, you can count me out as well.

Many of Roy Fairmont's closest friends believed that his relationship with Martha had failed because she did not share his deep and diverse intellectual interests or his competitive drive. Therefore, in speculations about what woman might be an appropriate match for the 49-year-old bachelor, intelligence, energy, and worldliness were prominent factors. Some of the most accomplished and interesting women in the country were seen accompanying Mr. Fairmont at charitable balls, social outings, and political events. Houston socialites were shocked when Roy announced that, in a private ceremony attended only by the bride and a justice of the peace, he had married Colleen Killeen, a woman whom none of them had ever heard of. To Roy Fairmont's friends, Colleen did not seem intelligent, ambitious, or worldly. A whispering chorus of Texans inquired, "Who is this woman?" Not daring to ask Roy Fairmont directly about her background, his friends eventually learned that she was an independent publicist who had been doing some work for one of Roy's many businesses. They later found out that she was not from Texas, was 29 years old, had been married twice previously, had no children, and had probably not attended college.

Roy Fairmont Meets His Match

The arrival of baby Shelby 6 months after the marriage was reassuring to Roy Fairmont's friends, who were straining to make some sense of his curious union with Colleen. None, however, had anticipated the remarkable changes in Roy that were to follow. Over the first half-century of his life, many adjectives had been affixed to the persona of Roy Fairmont. Most of these described the traits that led to his financial success and political clout, including *intense, ambitious, assertive, driven, competitive, unyielding, shrewd,* and *dangerous.* However, when it came to his relationship with Shelby, adjectives such as *affectionate, captivated,* and *indulgent* aptly applied. The "armchair psychologists" among his

friends explained his involvement with his daughter as "a search for belonging and to find relevance in his life." They pointed out that with the
death of Roy's parents and his only son, with his alienation from his
first wife and their daughter, and with the little he had in common with
his second wife, Shelby was Roy Fairmont's remaining chance to have
a close relationship with someone in his nuclear family. They added
that Shelby brought purpose to Mr. Fairmont's many business triumphs
and other material successes. They asked, "What else was Roy going to
do with all of that money he made, other than give it away to charity?"
But the most careful observers would have noticed something else: Roy
Fairmont's fondness for his daughter was an acquired emotion. As with
his previous children, he didn't seem that interested in Shelby when she
was an infant, nor did he spend much time with her during the first
3 years of her life. Similarly, Colleen was far more involved in retrieving
and preserving her lithe figure through daily aerobics, weightlifting,
and other types of fitness activities carried out with personal trainers or
at the most luxurious of out-of-town spas (she blamed baby Shelby for
ruining her shape) than in spending time with her little girl. Until she
was 4, Shelby's day-to-day care was relegated to nannies, tutors, and
other paid household workers. During those years, the only time that
Shelby and her parents were seen together was on their Christmas card
picture, from which both mother and daughter—clad in matching red
or gold gowns—radiated blond elegance.

   The careful observer would have noted that the key character in the
first act of this paternal passion play was the golden child herself.
Shelby managed to capture her father's eye and heart, not only with her
sparkling beauty and outgoing personality, but mainly through her unbridled devotion to him. Whenever Roy Fairmont returned from an extended trip—even when he arrived at home late at night—Shelby
would be at the door to greet him. Her long, carefully groomed blond
hair flowed over her newest nightgown as she would stretch open her
arms to be elevated to face level with her father. Embracing him firmly
about his neck and streaming tears of joy, Shelby would exclaim,
"Daddy, I missed you *so* much. I thought about you every single minute
you were away. I almost died of loneliness when you were gone. Promise that you will never, never, never go away without me!" Shelby
would beg to spend the nights that her father was home with him in his
room (adjoining Colleen's), and often he would relent. Shelby would
say, "Daddy, I don't feel safe in this great big old house. I get scared at
night when I can't sleep with you." Certain to be up in the early hours
of the morning when Roy customarily arose, she would follow him to
breakfast and sit adoringly by him as he ate and read the morning

newspapers. Before long, Roy was explaining to his attentive daughter the important articles that he was reading, and Shelby would ask endless questions about his work, travels, political activities, and other interests. She became interested in her father's main interests. If sweatsuited Colleen, en route to some exercise class, would happen by on one of these beatific breakfast occasions, neither father nor daughter would lift an eyelid to cast a glance in her direction. For Shelby, father and his work had significance, whereas, like the well-appointed interiors of their River Oaks mansion, mother was mainly decorative.

Shelby Grows Up

Dancing for Daddy

As a young girl, Shelby experienced a form of power that is associated with the pursuit and hard-won seduction of the "center of her universe"; and, for better and for worse, the ramifications of this "triumph" became the defining conflicts and challenges of the rest of her life. The initial indifference between mother and daughter ripened into a bitter rivalry. Although not the original seed of that battle, its first recognizable bud was the oft-repeated question posed by so many well-intentioned, albeit insensitive, observers of the two blossoms when they occasioned the same bough: "I can't decide which one is more beautiful; they are both so stunning!" Through her formidable exercise, diet, and shopping regimen, Colleen waged an admirable offense, but Shelby countered successfully with an arsenal that included her mother's phenomenal genes for physique and pulchritude, her father's indomitable will to compete, and the inevitability of youth and time.

The daughter was also advantaged by her father's ever-increasing involvement in her intellectual and cultural development. A fixture on the boards of trustees of many of Houston's fine museums and performing arts, Roy would arrange for young Shelby to attend all manner of openings and performances and to be taught and tutored by the leading experts in the areas of her cultural and athletic interest. She was especially captivated by and had talent for ballet, which she practiced daily with ardor and vigor that were unrivaled among her peers. By age 13, Shelby was as long, lithe, firm, and graceful as the professional dancers with whom she trained. None of these professionals, however—not even those in the fabled Houston Ballet—matched the young heiress's transcendent beauty. When performing, Shelby pirated almost every eye in her audience, but it was only her father's approval—in truth, his adulation—that mattered to her. Never missing a recital, Roy

Fairmont was often flanked on each side by dance tutors and ballet experts whom he asked to point out mistakes and opportunities for Shelby to improve. After each of her performances, Mr. Fairmont would wordlessly compliment his daughter with a bouquet of two dozen silent, yellow Texas roses; then he would then communicate to her an array of solicited critiques and recommendations from his invited experts.

And thus the protracted waltz between father and daughter was choreographed and executed: the only approval that mattered to Shelby was that of her father, a man of enormous accomplishment who was not easily impressed and was never satisfied. From Shelby's perspective, Roy frequented the showroom but would never consummate the sale. Nonetheless, his presence in her life and dedication to her development were unhollow victories that were not lost on Roy Fairmont's wife, friends, or daughter.

The "Other Woman"

Tomboy. From childhood, Shelby showed a strong preference for the company of males. If one were to judge by appearance—her delicate facial features and towering beauty; her graceful, gazelle-like movements; and, in the presence of males, her outgoing, appealing, and refined personality—she was the epitome of femininity. However, Shelby did not value or care to commune either with other little girls or with grown women. As a child, she regarded her female peers as being too delicate, frivolous, and uninteresting to warrant her attention. Playing with dolls or playing house, especially if it meant assuming conventional female roles such as cooking or caring for children, held little interest for Shelby. Referring to such play many years later, she would contend, "The other little girls would be horrified when I would much rather arm-wrestle the boys than change diapers on dolls or brew tea for pathetic toy tea sets."

Although many of the girls in her grade school and middle school classes desperately wanted to be her friend (and to be just like her), she was not at all interested in spending time with them. Her best friends were boys, who competed madly for her attention. Boys of her own age had no chance with her. Shelby preferred rough-and-tumble sports such as playing football and baseball with the older boys in her neighborhood, who were always thrilled to include her. She was a superior athlete and was competitive in all sports with the best male athletes of her age group. It was not until high school that any boy in any of her classes could beat her in running or swimming events; and, at that, it was only one or two. Loving horses and priding herself on being fearless, she chose riding rodeo events over showing horses. She characterized the latter as "a stuffy, buttoned-up, and boring pseudosport." Shelby had a fundamental distrust of women; she believed they would be competitive with her and jealous of her and would ultimately try to undermine her. She also believed women to be inherently deceptive, dishonest, and backstabbing. She was convinced that most, if not all, of the women she knew were fawning in her presence while being viciously critical of her behind her back. As an adult, Shelby would say, "I find it revealing and not without great meaning that men shoot their enemies in the chest, while women will put poison in the peach cobblers that they serve with such grace and gentility."

"Daughter, dearest".   By the time Shelby was in the fourth grade she was openly contemptuous of her mother, whom she called by her first name. Power struggles ensued on almost any occasion in which Colleen tried to tell Shelby what to do:

> **Colleen Fairmont:** Shelby, darling, the Club is having a talent show. I think it would be just marvelous if you would do one of your dances. I know you would win.
>
> **Shelby Fairmont (with a sarcastic tone):** Colleen, *dahling,* I think it would be just *mahvelous* if I pass on this *wonderful* invitation.
>
> **Colleen:** Marilynn Oster tells me that all the girls in your group will take part. Her daughter Kirby will be singing. I know that it would be fun to be in the show with her.
>
> **Shelby:** I would hate to be in anything with Kirby. She is a complete moron, and I despise her. She always sings that disgusting song "Feelings" and looks like she has fallen in love with herself. She sings like a sick frog. It makes me want to vomit.
>
> **Colleen:** Just this one time, Shelby. Please do just one little thing that your mother asks you to.
>
> **Shelby:** I wouldn't dance in that stupid show if my life depended on it. And why do you even care? It's not like you have ever once gone to my ballet recitals. You won't even drive me to the rehearsals.
>
> **Colleen:** We have a full-time driver at your disposal. There is no need for me to be your chauffeur. All of your friends from school are going to take part. Just one time, can't you be like everyone else?
>
> **Shelby:** I don't want to be like everyone else. If I did, I'd be just like you. I want to be just like me.
>
> **Colleen:** I know that if your father had asked you, you would dance in the show.
>
> **Shelby:** Daddy would never ask me to do something that dumb. You're wasting my time. Now run along and do something really important to you, Colleen, like getting your nails done.

Shelby and her pride.   About 6 feet tall by age 12, with a lion-thick, long blond mane and a fully developed figure, Shelby had an imposing presence. Standing amidst the girls in her age group, Shelby appeared to be a woman among children. She was a leader without being either popular or well-liked. Although most of her peers wanted to be just like Shelby and yearned to be liked by Shelby, neither wish was very often fulfilled. Like vulnerable cubs, they attended to the moods and movements of this beautiful, worldly, and supremely confident lioness, whom they emulated, followed, and feared. Every so often an overconfident classmate or an uninitiated new student would challenge Shelby for her position at the pinnacle of the school's social hierarchy, and that person would pay dearly for her miscalculation and hubris. In the ninth grade, Lauren Bearing, who had the highest grade-point average in the class, ran against Shelby for class president, an office that Shelby had held since kindergarten. In most of the previous elections, Shelby had run unopposed. Two weeks before the election, Shelby's birthday was celebrated. Roy Fairmont leased the Houston Center for the Performing Arts for the occasion. With cost being absolutely no object, all manner of entertainment and favors were provided for the teenage guests. The leading rock group of that era was flown in from Los Angeles, and the band performed a full-fledged concert that ordinarily would have been presented before a sold-out audience at the largest venue in any major city. Shelby's entire class was invited, attended, and was enthralled, with the exception of Lauren Bearing and her campaign manager, neither of whom received an invitation. Shelby won the election by a landslide. There was great speculation that the next year Mr. Fairmont would fly the class to London on his private jet to celebrate Shelby's sixteenth birthday. Her classmates were careful not to be too friendly with Lauren Bearing or to invite her to their parties, or, most assuredly, Shelby would remove them from the invitation list for her "sweet sixteen" birthday bash.

Men, sex, and secrets.   *Celibate goddess.*   Throughout middle school and high school, Shelby's relationships with boys in her age group were exclusively platonic. Although she dressed and danced seductively, the boys who were sufficiently fortunate to be permitted by Shelby to escort her to a dance or to some other type of event instinctively knew not to try anything with her. Consistent with her assertive personality, if Shelby wanted them to touch her, she would let them know. And she flashed no green lights for them. In high school, Shelby was asked out by the most eligible and confident of Houston's college-age bachelors. No serum alcohol level or degree of sexual experience with other women was ever high enough to impart the courage for the young men to make a sexual advance toward Shelby. Somehow they understood that her heady brew of attraction and intimidation could lead only to flaccidity. Shelby's sexual proclivities remained a mystery and a source of endless speculation among her peers. All agreed that her open enmity toward women most likely precluded a homosexual orientation. Many theorized that she was asexual by choice: a type of goddess who transcended the sexual needs and interests of mere mortals. After all, wouldn't her choosing to cavort with some male inherently involve compromise, a lowering of herself to consort with unequals? And wouldn't such a descent also stifle the omnipresent attention of the masses of other adoring men?

The secret.   From the time that she was a baby, Shelby would spend every summer and most holidays at her father's 100,000-acre ancestral ranch in Wyoming. Irreverently named the Flying-F Ranch by Roy Fairmont's wildcatter father, the pristine property was where Shelby's love of horses, mountain climbing, skiing, hunting, and fly fishing was spawned. The adjoining ranch had been owned for more than a century by the Merritts, a wealthy and politically prominent Northeastern family. The neighboring families had been best friends for two generations. In fact, Wallace Merritt, who became the president and chief executive officer of his family's vast financial, mining, and real estate empire, had been Roy's closest friend since childhood. As children, Roy and Wallace hunted the wild elk and fished native brown trout that shared their ranches. The two friends attended the same college, where they arranged to be roommates, were co-captains of the lacrosse team, and became members of the same eating club and secret society. As adults they collaborated on many important business deals and were "joined at the hip" in supporting candidates for national political offices. In at least one realm, however, Wallace and Roy were different: they did not share the same work ethic. Whereas Roy worked diligently to excel in every course that he took in college, Wallace appreciatively accepted the "gentleman's C" that was granted for just showing up for classes by this Ivy League college before it descended to a meritocracy. This difference did not diminish over their lifetimes. Wallace had a passion for outdoor sports, and he would spend almost the entirety of the summer recreating on his ranch, whereas Roy would continue to work tirelessly through the summer and fly in only for an occasional weekend as business permitted.

Wallace Merritt served in loco parentis for Shelby during the many winter and spring holidays and summer vacations that she spent on the ranch. Not long after she learned to walk, "Uncle Wally" taught her how to ski the steep mountain trails that snaked down to their ranches and melted into the iodine-purple lakes. By her tenth birthday he had taught her to be an expert marksman with rifle and shotgun. She learned how to identify that day's insect hatch and to tie fishing flies, which she expertly flicked above murky pockets in frothing streams to entice wary native trout. With her first sexual stirrings at age 12, Shelby thought it to be most fitting, consistent, and even natural that her faithful mentor introduce her to this fundamental aspect of nature. With the very keenness of observation that Uncle Wally had helped her to sharpen when they tracked together the winter elk or searched the deep holes for shadowy silhouettes of trout, Shelby had caught Uncle Wally's quick, uneasy gaze upon her newly swelling breasts and sinewy, hollowing thighs. With the very stealth and cunning that the teacher and pupil had baited and stalked the rapacious bears that preyed on their glistening, first-day foals, Shelby chose the moments and fashioned the opportunities to expose her mentor to her new-woman nakedness and hidden willingness. Almost instinctively, Shelby understood the power of having her very prey believe himself to be the predator. Both understood that the betrayed father would either kill this traitorous lifelong friend or ensure his lifetime imprisonment for statutory rape. Nonetheless, Wallace Merritt had no more chance of detecting or resisting the ploys of wily Shelby than did her private-school classmates, who lusted helplessly and hopelessly for her from behind the insecurities of their ordinariness and indolent complacencies that neither their family wealth, bravado, nor booze could disguise. From her thirteenth to her twentieth year, Shelby engaged in full, frequent, exclusive, and (from her account) fulfilling sex with her father's closest friend.

College Days

Real Competition

Having worked so hard to win her father, Shelby preferred to be pursued by all others. With no exception, colleges sought out Shelby, rather than vice versa. A high achiever without exerting noticeable effort, Shelby was graduated salutatorian of her class, was a National Merit Scholarship finalist, and had justifiably earned a national reputation as a promising young ballet dancer. Although she briefly considered attending the Juilliard School, Shelby ultimately acceded to the intense recruitment efforts of the selective Ivy League university that had been attended by her father and Uncle Wally. Both alumni were generous contributors to this university and also served on its board of governors. Determining that devoting several hours a day to ballet practice was "mindless and a complete waste of my time," Shelby, to the surprise of many, abandoned dance in her freshman year of college. Always a swift and technically gifted swimmer, she walked onto the women's water polo team and soon became one of the team's strongest and most feared players. Commenting to her father about this change of interest, Shelby said, "I much prefer competing openly with other women—as we do in water polo—than having some empty-headed, anemic dancer furtively check me out in hopes that I gained some weight over the weekend. Another benefit is that we get to work out regularly with the men's team. Trust me, Daddy, the men on the water polo team are quite different from the men in my ballet classes." Shelby became great buddies with many of the men on the water polo team and with other male classmates; however, no individual male student succeeded in drawing close to her.

Thinking that she might become an attorney like her father, Shelby majored in government and political science. Her proximate goal was to be chosen, by virtue of high grades and faculty recommendations, for the highly competitive and renowned undergraduate honors program in political science. Although scores of her fellow classmates sought admission to this 2-year program, only five from the class would be selected. Professor Malcolm Bluestein was the faculty coordinator of the program, and rumor had it that he personally selected those who would eventually be admitted. All concerned agreed that one essential step in this process was to take and excel in Professor Bluestein's introductory survey course in "Poly Sci," which Shelby took in her sophomore year. To her surprise, she received a grade of 87 on her midterm examination and a B+ on her the first paper. Alarmed and outraged, she made an appointment to speak with Professor Bluestein.

Shelby Fairmont: I am enjoying your course immensely, but I am upset and bewildered that I am getting the worst grades of my life. I carefully went over all of the so-called corrections of your teaching assistant, and I don't agree with any of them. I came to ask you to consider changing my grade.

Professor Bluestein: First of all, it makes no difference to me whether or not you are enjoying the course, Ms. Fairmont. My classes are for enlightenment, not entertainment. Secondly, in preparation for this meeting, I reviewed both your test and your paper. I believe that you did an excellent job on both, and that is accurately reflected in the grades that you received.

Shelby: My grades in your course are simply disastrous and absolutely unacceptable to me. I want you to tell me what is wrong with my work and what I do to have my grade changed.

Professor Bluestein: There is a possibility that you can bring your grade up by doing better on the next paper and final, but I agree completely with how the T.A. scored your work so far. You got most of the facts correct, but your independent thinking and how you defend your premises are problematic.

Shelby: If I understand what you are saying, I got everything right that wasn't a matter of opinion.

Professor Bluestein: Perhaps, but in this course it is my opinion that counts. The two main problems of your paper and in your test are hyperbole and lack of specificity. You have a penchant for making sweeping, emotionally laden proclamations without careful substantiation. I don't believe that Moses delivered the Ten Commandments with a greater sense of importance and authority.

Shelby: What do you suggest I do?

Professor Bluestein: I don't believe that you have the background to earn an A in this course. I suggest that you take Professor Berry's introductory writing course. He will teach you how to organize your thinking and how to advance and substantiate a thesis. You have to understand, Ms. Fairmont, that some of your classmates are more advanced than you are, at this point, in these skills.

For the first time in her memory, Shelby desperately wanted something that she was uncertain that she could attain for herself. Seized by a panicky feeling that she had not experienced since she was a little girl, she called her father and explained her problems in the Poly Sci course and with Professor Bluestein. Not by nature a reassuring person, Roy Fairmont told his daughter that he would look into her problem and get back to her.

Roy Fairmont: I called several people, including the university president, about Professor Bluestein. Everybody I spoke with assures me that he is tough but fair. They also say that he is a great teacher, which is the most important thing.

Shelby: That's all well and good, Daddy, but can't you do anything about my grade? I'm surprised that you didn't call Professor Bluestein yourself. I don't think he has a clue who you are.

Roy: I don't believe that a call from me to Professor Bluestein is either wise or indicated. You can be certain that he knows that I am on the Board of Overseers and have given several chairs and a lot of money for other projects to the university. However, professors vigorously guard their academic freedom, and appropriately so. Any pressure from me would likely backfire. Just listen to his advice, work hard, and try to do your best.

Shelby: I can't believe you are taking a stranger's side against your own daughter. You're the one who always tells me how important it is to be the very best at whatever you choose to do. All I have ever wanted is for you to be proud of me. Now, when I need your help, you won't do anything!

Fiercely competitive, Roy Fairmont also believed in fairness and competing on level playing fields. Although he could have easily relied on his inherited wealth and family connections, he had excelled through intelligence and hard work in college, law school, and business. He supported the university out of gratitude for his education there and because he believed deeply in their missions of education, research, and service to others. The very last thing he would do would be to use his influence to advance the interests of his daughter. Shelby, however, viewed her father's refusal to help her in the precise way that she wanted as betrayal and weakness. Furious, she dropped out of Professor Bluestein's course, changed her major to art history, and abandoned her ambition to become an attorney.

Expanding Horizons

Although Wallace Merritt tried vainly to dissuade her, Shelby decided to participate in her college's junior year abroad program in London. She was assigned to the Victoria and Albert Museum, where she worked as an apprentice to Professor Jaime Pardes, a scholar of twentieth-century European decorative arts. Shelby became immersed in the research and gained expertise in the European arts and crafts movement of the turn of the century, particularly the works of John Knox and William Morris of England, Charles Rennie Mackintosh of Scotland, and Joseph Hoffman of Austria. A resurgence of interest in this period was taking place at that time, and Professor Pardes was also serving as a paid consultant to wealthy collectors, many of whom were in the American and British film and entertainment industries. The professor's striking student did not go unnoticed by his clients, including Nelson, a famous British rock musician. Shelby accepted Nelson's invitation to accompany him to a chic London nightclub. Much to the rock star's amazement, the tall, elegantly dressed American was an incredible dancer and attracted as much attention from the omnipresent paparazzi as did he. Over the next several weeks, Shelby accompanied Nelson to several of his concerts and, as his date, to many high-profile events. When it became known that Shelby was herself a wealthy heiress, she became increasingly admired, sought after, and included by the international set of young partygoers and thrill seekers who, like the pigeons of Trafalgar Square, flocked and swirled about these revelries. For the first time in her life Shelby began to drink alcohol regularly and heavily, but unlike most of the others, she limited her taking of so-called recreational drugs to cocaine and prescription stimulants. As Shelby's picture began to appear regularly and prominently in glossy periodicals in the company of celebrities, she herself became famous—for being famous.

Shelby stayed in London for the entirety of her junior year of college. When she returned to the United States, she broke off her 7-year sexual relationship with Wallace Merritt. Shelby silenced his unrelenting protests by threatening to inform her father of his best friend's violations. During that summer, she stayed in her father's New York City apartment while taking an internship at an international art and antiques auction house. On returning to college in the fall, Shelby continued to frequent nightclubs and parties in New York City with many of the same people whom she had met in London. In addition, she traveled with them in their private planes to elite events at high-profile destinations like Aspen, Cancún, and Paris. Consequently, for the first time in her life, she was sometimes unprepared for tests and late in handing in many of her assigned papers. Somehow she managed to complete her senior thesis on the Roycrofters, a utopian society that created arts and crafts–style furniture in the early 1900s. Shelby was graduated cum laude and was the best-known member of her senior class.

Real Life

Career

No stranger to being pursued, Shelby had many job opportunities and offers upon graduation. Elite modeling agencies offered her millions of dollars just to sign contracts with them. Cosmetic companies and fashion designers approached her individually to be an exclusive representative of their products. She was tempted by offers from television broadcasting companies, most of which wanted her to be a reporter or anchorperson for their entertainment news programs. Ultimately Shelby accepted a far less remunerative position as an assistant director for twentieth-century decorative arts with the arts and antique auction firm where she had worked the previous summer. She made this decision largely because it afforded her more freedom and open time to spend traveling and partying with her friends. One other factor influencing Shelby's decision was that she was involved in an intense relationship with a professional athlete who was commonly classified by the media as being in the superstar category. The fact that he was married and had two young children did not deter the glamorous pair from appearing together publicly after his athletic events or traveling as a couple on highly publicized skiing and beach holidays.

Going Home Again

Eight months after her graduation, Shelby received a call from her father requesting that she return to Houston to speak with him in person about an important matter. With reservations and trepidation, she complied.

> **Shelby Fairmont:** What did you have to tell me in person that you couldn't communicate over the phone? I have a lot going on, Daddy.
>
> **Roy Fairmont:** I have been reading the papers, Shelby. You certainly seem to have "a lot going on," but I am quite concerned about where you are going.
>
> **Shelby:** I'm not sure what you are talking about. You really must be upset. This is the first time I can recall your being less than direct with me.
>
> **Mr. Fairmont:** I don't understand what you are doing with your life, Shelby. I always held out the hope that you would be my one child who was serious—who would do something relevant with her life.
>
> **Shelby:** What are you talking about, Daddy? I have a serious career in art. Some people believe that art is at least as important as the practice of law and a lot more important than making a bunch of money in business.
>
> **Mr. Fairmont:** You are running around with losers and poseurs, most of whom are living off the wealth and notoriety of their families. I fear that you are wasting your enormous gifts and potential.
>
> **Shelby:** Many of my friends are self-made people. I think you're jealous of them because they are more famous than you are.
>
> **Mr. Fairmont:** I never wanted to be famous, Shelby. On balance, I have always felt it to be a disadvantage to be well known.
>
> **Shelby:** Anyway, Daddy, being around rich and influential people is a big part of my job. I've gotten many of them interested in collecting fine arts and have got a lot of business for the auction house.
>
> **Mr. Fairmont:** If that's your job, you should think about doing something else. I don't want to quibble. There is another matter that I want to discuss with you. I'm dying. I just learned that I have prostate cancer. It's a particularly virulent cell type. It's gone to my lungs and brain. My doctors told me that radiation and chemotherapy will be palliative but not curative.
>
> **Shelby (sobbing):** Oh, Daddy. I'm so sorry. I love you so much. You are the only person I have ever really loved. Isn't there something that the doctors can do?
>
> **Mr. Fairmont:** They can prolong my life for a year or so, but they can't save it. I've had a better run than most people, Baby. I would like to prevail on you spend a bit more time in Houston. I must get my affairs together over the next several months. The family finances are quite complicated, and I want you to understand exactly

what's going on. You will be responsible for a huge estate once
I am gone. We have great advisors, Shelby, but I want you to be in
a position to call the shots. It will take some time for me to teach
you. I know you are capable in that regard, but I must confess that
my greatest fear is about your state of mind. I fear you are losing
your way, losing yourself.

Flooded with feelings, Shelby did exactly what her father asked. She
took a leave of absence from her job in New York City and moved back
into the River Oaks home of her childhood to be close to and to care for
her father. It was the first time in her life that she had taken care of another person. The most difficult part for Shelby was watching her beloved giant's power waning incrementally. Shelby began to feel very
anxious and sad. She had problems sleeping and had little energy. Fear-
ing that she might have the flu or some other contagious disease that
could compromise the well-being of her father (whose immune system
was being suppressed by the chemotherapy for his prostate cancer),
Shelby consulted the family internist, who examined her carefully and
ordered many laboratory tests. Shelby's physical examination and laboratory test results both being normal, the internist concluded that she
must be depressed and prescribed an antidepressant for her. Three days
later, while caring for her father, Shelby experienced what was later determined to be a grand mal seizure. During the seizure, she fell and sustained a deep laceration to her scalp. Shelby was transported by
ambulance to the neurology service of the Methodist Hospital, and
I was later called by Dr. Curtis, her neurologist, to consult on her case
when no abnormalities in brain structure or physiology could be found.

I found Shelby to be alert and cooperative, although weak and anxious and distracted by a severe headache. It did not take long to determine the probable source of her seizure. Three weeks before the seizure,
her internist had given her a prescription for the antidepressant bupropion (Wellbutrin) and had correctly advised her not to drink alcohol
while the dosage of this medication was being increased. Shelby complied with his instructions. However, this physician failed to ask her
several key questions and thereby did not gain vital information that
was essential to guide diagnosis and treatment. He did not ask about
Shelby's drinking patterns and therefore did not know that she had
been drinking about a bottle of champagne and several strong mixed
drinks each day for the past year. He was also unaware that ever since
middle school Shelby had had disordered eating patterns consisting of
cycles of bingeing on chocolates and other sweets, purging, and going
on starvation diets. The abrupt withdrawal of alcohol can lower the
brain's threshold for seizures, as can bupropion. In addition, this med-

ication has been reported to be associated with an increased incidence of seizures in women with a history of bulimia, a form of eating disorder involving bingeing and purging. The internist was correct in his diagnosis of depression and anxiety, so I discontinued the bupropion and prescribed a different antidepressant that was not associated with the elicitation of seizures. Given the strong likelihood of her seizures being the result of alcohol withdrawal and the antidepressant side effect, both of which had been satisfactorily addressed, I also recommended that her anticonvulsants be discontinued and that she be discharged from the hospital in my care. Shelby agreed to see me as an outpatient the next day in my office.

Treatment Begins

Initial Appointment

The day after her discharge from the hospital, Shelby Fairmont arrived at my outpatient office at the appointed hour. Although she was readily recognized by my office staff from her pictures in magazines and from television coverage, she gave no indication to them of her celebrity status. I had scheduled a 2-hour intake interview with Shelby. During the interview I was taken by her combination of intelligence, cooperativeness, and honesty but noted the paradoxical absence of psychological mindedness. For example, she readily acknowledged having symptoms of depression, alcohol abuse, anxiety, and bulimia, but she could not relate any of these problems either to current stress or to past experiences. This dichotomy led to poor insight—an unrealistic understanding of the nature and degree of her psychiatric problems and of the level of treatment required for her to make significant improvement.

> **Shelby Fairmont:** I admit that I have a problem with bingeing, anxiety, and depression. You told me that the medication should help me with all of these. I also know for certain that I can stop drinking any time I want to. Anyway, booze is fattening. So my question is, why do you think I need therapy?
>
> **Dr. Y.:** You seem to perceive your symptoms as external problems that are just happening to you or are being imposed on you. Don't you have interest in understanding your role in these conditions?
>
> **Shelby:** Not really. As long as I get better. Are you saying I won't get better unless I get psychotherapy?
>
> **Dr. Y.:** I am not saying that you cannot get better without psychotherapy. However, I strongly recommend that you invest, at minimum, the next several months in psychotherapy to determine whether or not this form of treatment has benefit for you.

Discussion of My Treatment Strategy for Shelby Fairmont

Each human being has a unique biology, temperament, and life experience. When psychological problems develop, these also are unique and distinctive. Therefore, there should be no formulaic psychiatric treatment approach for all patients, no matter the diagnosis. One size definitely does *not* fit all. From my initial evaluation of Ms. Fairmont, it was clear to me that she had difficulty making direct connections between her emotional responses to important life experiences and her key life choices. Consequently, her own role in and responsibility for her psychological symptoms and other life problems were almost entirely unrecognized by her. Aware that certain defensive structures and personality profiles (and personality disorders) are associated with deficient insight and lack of psychological mindedness, I crafted and communicated my treatment recommendations to Ms. Fairmont accordingly. Even though she was undeniably intelligent and could be assertive and energetic in many other realms of her life, Ms. Fairmont was not ready to assume responsibility for understanding herself or for changing her psychological problems. She chose to defer such choices and decisions to an authority figure. The "Catch-22" of this clinical situation is that the very unconscious conflicts and processes that led to her passivity would require effective treatment *before* Ms. Fairmont would be able to assume requisite initiative and "ownership" of her problems and her treatment. For this reason, even though I understood that there would be deleterious therapeutic trade-offs later (such as her trying to transpose the responsibility for the work of psychotherapy to me), it was necessary for me to make an unequivocal recommendation that she engage in twice-weekly psychotherapy over the next 6 months. She agreed. This directive approach would have been unwise for a person with obsessive-compulsive personality disorder, as it would have led to endless power struggles and distrust. In this latter circumstance, I would encourage the patient to ask as many questions as occurred to him or her about psychotherapy, which I would try to answer factually and fully. It is critical for people with this condition to assume control by making an independent decision about engaging in psychotherapy.

I began Ms. Fairmont's treatment by taking a detailed history of her life experiences, of which many of the most important elements are recounted above. Given her stress and insecurities related to the serious illness of her father, I also continued to provide guidance and support in the early months of treatment. I reasoned that as Ms. Fairmont became more familiar and comfortable with the process of treatment and more trusting of me, she would gradually become more assertive in her psychotherapy. However, I anticipated that transference issues would revolve around her conflicts over feeling dependent on me. The untoward intensity of these feelings would provide useful opportunities for her to gain insight in the role of her early life experiences with her father and mother in her personality makeup and psychological disorders. In addition to her mood, eating, and substance use disorders, I was concerned that Shelby also had a personality disorder. From my initial evaluation, it was clear to me that although she met DSM-IV-TR diagnostic criteria for histrionic personality disorder (American Psychiatric Association 2000, pp. 711–714), her psychiatric history, many of her symptoms, and her unconscious conflicts were more consistent with hysterical personality disorder as classically and currently conceptualized by many leading psychoanalytic theoreticians and clinicians. Hysterical personality disorder has been replaced in the DSM by the diagnosis of histrionic personality disorder.

About Hysterical (and Histrionic) Personality Disorder

Hysterical Personality Disorder Versus Histrionic Personality Disorder

As discussed in Chapter 1 ("What Are Fatal Flaws?"), the DSM editions have enabled standardized psychiatric diagnoses worldwide through a *nontheoretical* approach to categorizing mental illnesses. Clusters of signs and symptoms are grouped together to constitute specific diagnoses without regard to what may or may not have led to the disorders. This approach has certain advantages and certain disadvantages. One advantage is that the approach provides a common, universal language so that clinicians and scientists can communicate with one another and conduct research at multiple sites. A second advantage is that inaccurate theories—such as that bad mothering can cause schizophrenia—will not unfairly ascribe blame as to causality or unduly influence treatment. There are significant disadvantages to this system as well. In most of medicine, to the extent possible, diagnosis is based on underlying biological pathology. For example, heart pain (angina pectoris) stemming from occluded arteries that feed the heart is called coronary artery disease, and brain cancers such as astrocytoma are classified by the abnormalities of the specific cell types. Because this level of specificity is not yet possible for psychiatric conditions, theoretical considerations are *occasionally* the next-best approach for determining a particular diagnosis. I and other psychiatrists believe this to be the case with several psychiatric conditions, including hysterical personality disorder, a diagnosis that no longer has official status in DSM or with the American Psychiatric Association.

DSM-I, the first diagnostic manual of the American Psychiatric Association, published in 1952, had no diagnostic categories related to hysteria. DSM-II (American Psychiatric Association 1968) featured two categories of hysteria. One diagnosis, *hysterical neurosis,* referred to involuntary psychologically based loss of sensation or motor function. Also included under this category was *dissociation,* which was defined as alterations in the patient's state of consciousness or identity that give rise to symptoms including amnesia, fugue, and multiple personalities. The second DSM-II diagnosis was *hysterical personality,* a condition that predominantly affected women and was characterized by self-dramatization, immaturity, vanity, dependence on others, excitability, emotionality, overreactivity, and attention-seeking behaviors. When DSM-III was first published about 25 years ago (American Psychiatric Association 1980), the DSM-II diagnosis of hysterical personality was replaced with *histrionic personality disorder,* in part to reduce the almost exclusive association of this condition with women. The terms *hysteria* and *hysterical* come from the Greek word meaning "womb," and there is a long and unfortunate history of belittling and devaluing women by use of this terminology, and of using these terms to dismiss their pain and suffering. DSM-III not only changed the name of this personality disorder but also, by excluding psychodynamic considerations, altered the basic criteria for making the diagnosis. The net result is a cluster of signs and symptoms connoting much more severe psychopathology, and a departure from what many experts believe to be the essence of the disorder. Psychoanalyst Glen O. Gabbard expressed significant reservations about these changes:

> The staunchly atheoretical nature of the personality disorder criteria in DSM-IV [American Psychiatric Association 1994] is particularly problematic when considering patients with hysterical or histrionic tendencies. To determine the appropriate treatment for this diverse group of patients, a careful psychodynamic assessment is far more crucial than a descriptive cataloging of overt behaviors. One primary source of confusion in the related literature has been a tendency to rely on behavioral characteristics instead of dynamic understanding. (Gabbard 2000, p. 518)

I agree with Dr. Gabbard that the previous diagnosis of hysterical personality disorder that was derived from a psychoanalytic theoretical framework (reviewed later in this chapter under "Psychology of Hysterical Personality Disorder") has conceptual and practical advantages

---

TABLE 4–1. Diagnostic criteria for histrionic personality disorder (slightly modified from DSM-IV-TR)

The person exhibits a pervasive pattern of excessive emotionality and attention seeking, which begins by early adulthood and presents in a variety of contexts, as indicated by five (or more) of the following:

1.   The person is uncomfortable in situations in which he or she is not the center of attention.

2.   The individual's interaction with others is often characterized by inappropriate sexually seductive or provocative behavior.

3.   The person displays rapidly shifting and shallow expression of emotions.

4.   He or she consistently uses physical appearance to draw attention to self.

5.   The person exhibits a style of speech that is excessively impressionistic and lacking in detail and specifics.

6.   The individual is excessively dramatic, theatrical, and emotional.

7.   The person is suggestible and easily influenced by others or circumstances.

8.   He or she often considers relationships to be more intimate than they are in actuality.

Source.   Adapted from American Psychiatric Association: *Diagnostic and Statistical Manual of Mental Disorders,* 4th Edition, Text Revision. Washington, DC, American Psychiatric Association, 2000, p. 714. Used with permission.

in the clinical setting, and, at the very least, is complementary to the current DSM-IV-TR categorization of histrionic personality disorder, as outlined in Table 4–1 (American Psychiatric Association 2000, p. 714). On the basis of biopsychosocial theories of causality of hysterical personality disorder, I have taken the liberty of devising and suggesting diagnostic criteria for this condition, as outlined in Table 4–2. Both approaches to these diagnoses have advantages and limitations.

Dr. Gabbard's differentiations between hysterical personality disorder and histrionic personality disorder (Gabbard 2000, p. 521) are outlined in Table 4–3.

Histrionic Personality Disorder

Diagnostic Features
(Slightly Modified From DSM-IV-TR, pp. 711–712)

The essential feature of histrionic personality disorder is pervasive and excessive emotionality and attention-seeking behavior. This pattern

---

TABLE 4–2.   *Unofficial* diagnostic criteria for hysterical personality disorder, based on psychodynamic and other theoretical models of causality

---

The person with this disorder has a childhood history of a non-nurturing, nonsupportive, and antagonistic relationship with the parent or caregiver of the same gender and an intense, overinvolved relationship with the parent or caregiver of the opposite gender. The stress and unconscious representations of these symptoms, along with predispositions of cognition and temperament, are hypothesized to lead to the following interpersonal, behavioral, and emotional problems. Five or more of these criteria are required for a person to qualify for this diagnosis.

1. Hostile and competitive relationships with peers and others of the same gender.

2. Intense, idealized, inappropriate, and maladaptive relationships with parental figures of the opposite gender.

3. Childlike, overly dependent relationships with idealized parental figures.

4. Attention-seeking, exhibitionistic, sexually suggestive, flirtatious, and seductive behaviors directed toward people of the opposite gender; or, if homosexual orientation, toward people of the same gender.

5. Immature, nongratifying sexual relationships with mature, age-appropriate, available partners.

6. Emotional immaturity, volatility, and excessive enthusiasm.

7. Impressionistic cognitive style that is diffuse, nonspecific, devoid of detail, and expansive.

8. High suggestibility that results in the person's being overly influenced by perceived authority figures and by current fashions and trends.

---

begins by early adulthood and is present in a variety of contexts. Individuals with histrionic personality disorder are uncomfortable or feel unappreciated when they are not the center of attention. Frequently lively and dramatic, they tend to draw attention to themselves and may initially charm new acquaintances by their enthusiasm, apparent openness, or flirtatiousness. Over time these qualities wear thin, as the individuals continually demand to be the center of attention and commandeer the role of the life of the party. If they are not the center of attention, they may do something dramatic (e.g., make up stories, create a scene) to draw the focus of attention to themselves. This need is often apparent in their behavior with a clinician (e.g., flattery, bringing gifts, providing dramatic descriptions of physical and psychological

TABLE 4–3. Dr. Gabbard's differentiation between hysterical personality disorder and histrionic personality disorder (slightly modified)

Hysterical personality disorder	Histrionic personality disorder
1. Heightened emotionality, but with elements of restraint	1. Florid, unrestrained emotionality
2. Excessive need to be noticed and loved	2. Need for attention and prioritization is a "bottomless pit"
3. Sexually exhibitionistic	3. Sexually provocative, demanding, and inappropriate
4. Good impulse control	4. Poor impulse control
5. Seductive in an engaging, socially appropriate fashion	5. Crude, repelling seductiveness
6. Competitive and ambitious	6. Unfocused and not self-sufficient
7. Although often complicated by third parties, relationships can be mature and fulfilling	7. Primitive, clinging, dependent, sadistic, and masochistic relationships
8. Can tolerate separation from loved ones	8. Feels abandoned, anxious, and overwhelmed when separated from loved ones
9. Actions, decisions, and choices usually guided by mature sense of conscience	9. Actions, decisions, and choices guided by primitive, self-centered drives and fears
10 Sexual feelings toward psychotherapist usually develop gradually and are perceived as unrealistic and inappropriate	10 Rapid, intense development of sexual feelings for psychotherapist, which are viewed by patient as realistic and appropriate expectations

Source. Adapted from Gabbard GO: "Cluster B Personality Disorders: Hysterical and Histrionic," in *Psychodynamic Psychiatry in Clinical Practice,* 3rd Edition. Washington, DC, American Psychiatric Press, 2000, pp 517–545. Used with permission.

symptoms that are replaced by new symptoms each visit).

The appearance and behavior of people with this condition are often inappropriately sexually provocative or seductive. This behavior is directed toward persons in whom the individual has a sexual or romantic interest but also occurs in a wide variety of social, occupational, and professional relationships beyond what is appropriate for the social context. Emotional expression may be shallow and rapidly shifting. These individuals consistently use their physical appearance to draw attention to themselves and are overly concerned with impressing others by their appearance. They expend an excessive amount of time, energy, and money on fashion and grooming. They may fish for compliments regarding their appearance and may be easily and excessively upset by a critical comment about how they look or by a photograph that they regard as unflattering.

People with histrionic personality disorder often have a style of speech and a form of logic that are excessively impressionistic and lacking in detail. Strong opinions are expressed with dramatic flair, but underlying reasons are usually vague and diffuse, without supporting facts and details. For example, a person with this personality disorder may comment that a certain individual is "the most wonderful human being I have ever met" yet be unable to provide any specific examples of good qualities to support this opinion. People with this condition are characterized by self-dramatization, theatricality, and an exaggerated expression of emotion. They may embarrass friends and acquaintances by excessive public displays of emotion (e.g., embracing casual acquaintances with excessive ardor, sobbing uncontrollably on minor sentimental occasions, or having temper tantrums). However, their emotions often seem to be turned on and off too quickly to be deeply felt, which may lead others to accuse them of being insincere about these feelings. They also have a high degree of suggestibility, as their opinions and feelings are easily influenced by others and by current fads. They may be too trusting of authority figures, whom they see as capable of magically solving their problems. They have a tendency to play hunches and to adopt convictions quickly. Individuals with this disorder often consider relationships more intimate than they actually are. For example, they may call almost every acquaintance "my dear, dear friend" or refer to professionals whom they have met only once or twice by their first names. They often make decisions based on emotionality rather than rationality and are frequently bored with facts and details. Flights into romantic fantasy are commonplace.

Epidemiology

According to DSM-IV-TR, the prevalence of histrionic personality disorder is between 2% and 3% of the general population and between 15% and 20% of people in inpatient and outpatient mental health settings. Given the long history of hysteria being conceptualized as a women's disease caused by misalignment of their uteri, it is not surprising that both hysterical personality disorder and histrionic personality disorder are diagnosed in the clinical setting far more commonly in women than in men. This might be changing, however. Although approximately 85% of the people diagnosed with these conditions in the past have been women (Millon 1986), more recent and better-designed epidemiological studies that utilize structured interviews for making diagnoses have found nearly equal rates among men and women (Nestadt et al. 1990). Even though researchers are now more able to diagnose histrionic personality disorder in men, I remain concerned that cultural and gender biases will persist in the clinical setting. I believe that DSM criteria for histrionic personality disorder such as "sexually seductive or provocative behavior"; "excessively dramatic, theatrical, and emotional"; and using "physical appearances to draw attention to self" will still be recognized in women more than in men.

Psychology of Hysterical Personality Disorder

Psychodynamics of Hysterical Personality Disorder

Unstable Family Triangle

Based on the early clinical observations and inferences of Josef Breuer and Sigmund Freud and the work over the ensuing years by successions of psychoanalytic theoreticians, hysterical personality disorder is thought to be the result of troubled relationships that occur early in the childhood of the person so affected (Blacker and Tupin 1977). The mothers of little girls who develop this condition are thought to be neglectful and emotionally unavailable to their daughters. The little girls compensate by seeking out the attention of their fathers. This leads to rivalry with the mother and fear of retaliation. Freud and others believed that ultimately the daughters wish to replace their mothers in all ways, including becoming the sexual partners of their fathers. These latter wishes and feelings are unsettling and unacceptable to the young girls and are therefore relegated to their unconscious minds and are expressed later in their lives as the signs, symptoms, and personality features subsumed under hysterical personality disorder. For example, self-dramatization, excessive emotionality, and sexual provocations are conceptualized to be derivations of the child's efforts to distract her father's attention from her mother. Similarly, competition with and devaluation of other women are thought to stem from the daughter's rivalry with her mother for her father. Symptoms such as overdependencies, underachieving, and childlike behaviors are thought to be the result of the failure of the child to form an identification with her mother as a mature and strong female figure. In addition, remaining "the little girl" is also understood as an unconscious response designed to avoid the hostile retribution of the mother for stealing away her husband: "How could an innocent little child be capable of winning away a grown man from a grown woman?"

Sexual symptoms and syndromes.   The sexual symptomatology of adult women with hysterical personality disorder is also theorized to be the result of their early-life sexual longings for their fathers and their having won their fathers away from their mothers. As the child grows older, she becomes drawn to engaging in forbidden relationships with older, married men (father figures), which encompass the exciting elements of danger and incest associated with her paternal longings. She also becomes attracted to being taken care of by an all-knowing, all-providing father figure. In such a relationship, she can remain the innocent, helpless, and dependent little girl. On the other hand, she has problems forming mature and intimate attachments with available and appropriate males of her own age. Frequently a pattern develops in which a woman with this condition is flirtatious and seductive with men of her own age to capture their attention and adoration. She particularly enjoys the courtship stage, in which she feels pursued and—until she makes a commitment—is in a position of power and control. As the relationship develops, however, her interest begins to wane, in part because her suitor becomes more familiar and "real" to her and can no longer compete with her idealized image of her father. She may have trouble experiencing fulfilling sexual intimacies with an eligible man of her own age for several reasons. First of all, it will be more difficult for her to remain the helpless, nonthreatening little girl in a mature relationship. She will be perceived by others and expected by her partner to engage in and enjoy adult sexual relationships. Second, adult sexual pleasure and fulfillment may also cause unconscious distress, because it evokes feelings of responsibility and guilt related to her repressed sexual feelings for her father. Third, with a suitor who is available, appropriate, and acceptable there is the real possibility and potential for a prolonged, mature, committed relationship. Unconsciously she might feel guilt associated with betrayal and abandonment of her father, which is partially tempered by her failure to experience sexual fulfillment with another man. Finally, many women with hysterical personality disorder harbor anger and deep resentment toward men. These potent feelings are the result of *unconscious* feelings associated with being "led on" and exploited by their fathers. They believe that their fathers, while doting on them and being generous, never fully came through for them by leaving their mothers and gratifying their sexual longings. This anger and resentment can manifest itself in later relationships with appropriate males by the woman's not giving them the pleasure of giving her pleasure.

Psychodynamics of men with hysterical personality disorder. The psychodynamics of men who meet criteria for histrionic (or hysterical) personality disorder are postulated to be similar to those of women with this condition. In this circumstance, however, the young male child develops an intense and eroticized relationship with his mother, with whom he closely identifies. For a variety of reasons—paternal absence, abuse, disinterest, extreme competitiveness—the son does not feel supported, safe, or close with his father. Freud and many other psychoanalysts believe that males who have this childhood experience also develop deep-seated feelings of genital inadequacy as a result. The adult consequences are myriad. Some men with this childhood experience develop a strong female identity, whereas others become hypermasculine. For example, a man with this condition may remain intensely involved with and feel a great responsibility to take care of his mother in the absence of an involved father/husband. As an adult, this man may not marry and he might live in the same house with his mother, travel on holidays with her, and take care of her devotedly through her old age. In addition, he may not manifest any interest whatsoever in adult sexuality with either women or men, or he may have several superficial, noncommitted sexual relationships over his lifetime. In seeming contrast, another man with similar family dynamics in childhood might, as an adult, assume a hypermasculine identity. Such a person might become a body builder, be obsessed with martial arts, and take risks—such as rock climbing—to demonstrate his strength and bravery. He might pursue many women and have many sexual encounters. He might even marry several times, often to a "trophy wife." However, this man will not develop a sustained, fulfilling sexual relationship with any one woman. He seems far more interested in being admired by women (and men) than in experiencing or giving sexual pleasure. As the women with whom he is involved get to know him better, they will realize that he is unfaithful, insecure, and not truly involved with them or interested in them as individuals. Rather, they will recognize him to be insecure, particularly about his masculinity, which drives his competitive, exhibitionistic, self-involved, and selfish behaviors. Like women with this condition, men with hysterical personality disorder, as children, are overinvolved with the parent of the opposite sex and have not been able to identify with—but rather fear retaliation from—the parent of their own gender.

Cognitive style of people with hysterical personality disorder.   In their thinking and communications, people with hysterical personality disorder tend to be impressionistic, diffuse, imprecise, and deficient in the detail and factual information required to be clearly understood. This cognitive style is best demonstrated by example. The following is a dialogue between Mrs. Heather Montrose, a wealthy Midwestern socialite, and Lewis Miller, a successful restaurateur and caterer. The conversation involves the preparations for the annual charity ball in support of a large hospital system in Chicago.

Mrs. Heather Montrose: I am so delighted to meet you, Lewis. All of my friends tell me that you are absolutely *the* best caterer in the entire world. I simply will not take on the crushing responsibility of chairing the Hospital Ball without you.

Mr. Lewis Miller: I am honored, Mrs. Montrose, that you have chosen my company to cater such an important event.

Mrs. Montrose: Please, please, please! Call me Heather. I have heard so much about you Lewis, I feel as if I have known you all of my life. I can tell already that we will work fabulously together. Now, how do we get started?

Mr. Miller: I'll start by telling you what little I know so far about the event. I understand that it will be held on Saturday, June 5th, in the Continental Ball Room of the Hyatt Regency Hotel. Do I have that right?

Mrs. Montrose: Lewis, darling. I know it is going to be held at the Hyatt, but don't hold me to anything else.

Mr. Miller: I realize that at this point you can't know exactly how many are expected to attend, but can you give me some ballpark figure?

Mrs. Montrose: I can tell you this. I expect everybody who is anybody in Chicago to be there.

Mr. Miller: Can you put a number to that?

Mrs. Montrose: Well, since you are pressing me, I would say, "Thousands upon thousands."

Mr. Miller: With your permission, I will check on how many attended last year's event and how many tables the Continental Ball Room can hold, and start my planning based on that number. Now let's get to the fun part, Mrs. Montrose. What would you like to serve?

Mrs. Montrose: Please, Lewis. I feel so old when you address me by my last name. Call me Heather. Well, I want the evening to be unique and special. A heavenly experience that will live forever in everyone's hearts and minds—and stomachs! That's where you come in. I do know what I don't want. What I don't want is to serve the same old boring things that they have at every one of these charity events!

Mr. Miller: Would you give me an example of what you might be thinking?

Mrs. Montrose: I'm not quite sure at this point what to think, Lewis. Give me some suggestions.

> **Mr. Miller:** Well, striped bass will just be in season by early June. That is rarely served at social events, can be most delicious, and would be in keeping with the hospital's theme of healthful living.
>
> **Mrs. Montrose:** No, no, no, Lewis. Much, much too boring. All fish tastes the same to me. And it looks so pale and pathetic beached on white china. However, you might be on the right trail. I am envisioning an ocean theme, bringing together the two coasts of America—right in our glorious Chicago. What about an ensemble of whole Maine lobsters and Alaskan king crab?
>
> **Mr. Miller:** That certainly could be done, but it would be extremely expensive and difficult to prepare for so many people. I fear that the cost would take a huge hunk out of the proceeds for the charity. What budget did you have in mind for the food portion of the evening?
>
> **Mrs. Montrose:** Budget, schmudget, Lewis! I haven't given one moment's thought to a budget. I don't even know if there is a budget. I do know that I want this to be the event of the year. If it costs a little bit more, so be it. Well, I think we have accomplished an absolutely enormous amount for one day. We are well on our way. Now, you go to work on our plans, and I will check with you in a month or so.

As the reader might imagine, Mrs. Montrose's lack of interest in quantifying the likely number of guests for the charity ball or in setting a budget combined with her enthusiastic and unrealistic expectations left Mr. Miller uninformed and very uneasy. Her cognitive style could be explained by psychodynamics. For example, her effusive, theatrical, too-personal manner of engaging authority could stem from behavioral patterns established in childhood, when she sought to capture the exclusive attention of her idealized father. Her imprecise, sparsely detailed style of thinking and communicating could be related to her hostile and competitive relationship with her mother. Specifically, Mrs. Montrose assumed an innocent, childlike manner to dodge the responsibility of winning away the father from the mother and to avoid the retaliation of her jilted parent. It is also possible that her cognitive style is the result of brain-based biological factors affecting thinking and temperament. What is currently known about these factors is reviewed in the next section below.

Biological Factors in Hysterical (Histrionic) Personality Disorder

As discussed above (see "Hysterical Personality Disorder Versus Histrionic Personality Disorder"), controversies about official nomenclature and diagnostic criteria for hysterical (histrionic) personality disorder have resulted in an extreme paucity of credible research related to the genetic and biological aspects of this disorder, more so than for any other commonly diagnosed personality disorder. Specifically, no valid adoption studies or epidemiological research have been conducted to determine whether or not this condition has prominent hereditary or genetic components. In addition, no valid laboratory or functional brain imaging research has been performed on people with this diagnosis to explore whether or not there are important underlying endocrinological or central nervous system factors. In the absence of dedicated research, any discussion of the biological aspects of hysterical (histrionic) personality disorder must be entirely inferential and speculative, not evidence-based as I would prefer. Nevertheless, the history of other psychiatric conditions—including schizophrenia, bipolar illness, depression, obsessive-compulsive personality disorder, and panic disorder—demonstrates that the psychological dimensions were originally overemphasized at the expense of the biological dimensions. Relatively recent research has proved the key role of the biological aspects of these conditions, and these findings have also been consistent with new and effective biological treatments. Therefore, I believe that in the future, key dimensions of hysterical (histrionic) personality disorder will also be proved to be biological. From my perspective, the most likely biologically based dysfunctions will be found to be related to cognitive style, suggestibility, and extroversion.

Cognitive Style

As discussed above (see "Cognitive Style of People With Hysterical Personality Disorder"), people with this personality disorder tend to be imprecise in their thinking and not particularly concerned about substantiating their assertions and opinions with details or facts. In the same way that people have brain-based capacities in mathematics, physics, and engineering, it is very possible that predilections and abilities for precise, fact-based thinking also have biological bases and variability. Perception, attention, concentration, and recall are critical components in cognitive functioning, and all of these functions have been shown to be disabled in brain-based illnesses such as Alzheimer's disease, traumatic brain injury, and depression. The bottom line is that the brain is certainly the organ that mediates cognitive functioning, and disorders of and differences in brain function could be responsible for the diffuse cognitive style of people with hysterical personality disorder. It is also not unlikely that these brain differences and dysfunction are in part hereditary.

Suggestibility

Individuals who are *suggestible* are too easily influenced by others, accept direction from others without sufficient critical examination, and therefore tend to be too compliant. Suggestible people have difficulties distinguishing between ideas and instructions that are their own and those that are being advanced by others. With their vivid imaginations and trusting natures, children can be highly suggestible. People who are highly hypnotizable tend to be more suggestible than most others, and they are even more suggestible when they are in the actual state of hypnotic trance. Interestingly, Jean-Martin Charcot utilized hypnosis in his pioneer work on understanding and treating women thought to have hysteria (Veith 1970, 1977). Many contemporary experts believe that there are brain-based predispositions to and epiphenomena of both suggestibility and hypnotizability (Barabasz et al. 1999; Maldonado and Spiegel 2003). When I was a psychiatry resident at Columbia University, I was privileged to study medical hypnosis with the noted authority Herbert Spiegel, M.D., who was certain that people who are the most highly hypnotizable are also the most suggestible. He believed that just like the ability to carry a tune or to be a gifted artist, suggestibility and hypnotizability are innate neurological capacities that are variable among individuals across a broad spectrum. He cautioned psychiatrists about unwittingly "implanting ideas and beliefs" in their most suggestible patients and thereby mistaking their patient's compliance with these suggestions for insight and therapeutic change (Spiegel and Spiegel 1987). Therefore, if suggestibility is a brain-based predisposition with a variable presence in the population, it is possible that this is a heritable trait that in part predisposes certain individuals to develop hysterical personality disorder.

Extroversion

People who meet criteria for either hysterical personality disorder or histrionic personality disorder are unlikely to have shy and retiring demeanors. Adjectives such as *colorful, enthusiastic, impulsive, exhibitionistic, dramatic, flamboyant, extravagant,* and *emotional* are frequently used to describe individuals with the two conditions. Their temperaments would most appropriately be considered *extroverted,* or outwardly turned, as opposed to *introverted* or inwardly directed. Such temperamental traits are thought by many experts to have strong genetic contributions (Yager and Gitlin 2000). Nonetheless, it is most likely (but unproven) that these personality disorders are the result of a combination of genetic predispositions, life experiences, and cultural factors. For example, a child who is genetically predisposed to have an extroverted temperament and who is fortunate enough to have parents who are nurturing, protective, mature, respectful of boundaries, and committed to one another would not be likely to develop hysterical or histrionic personality disorder as an adult. Rather, that child might grow up to be self-assured and gregarious and to have a personality that is well suited for leadership positions and for many professions such as broadcast journalism, politics, and theatre. Although people with hysterical personality disorder may also have talents and temperaments that enable achievement in such professions, their emotional and interpersonal difficulties often undermine their success.

Key principles in the diagnosis of hysterical personality disorder as exemplified by the case of Shelby Fairmont are summarized in Table 4–4.

The Case of Shelby Fairmont, Part 2: Trials and Treatment

Treatment of Shelby Fairmont

Initial Treatment Plan

Biweekly insight-oriented psychotherapy.   When Shelby Fairmont began psychiatric treatment at age 24, she was no longer the healthy, confident, successful person whom she had appeared to be to others throughout her childhood, school, and college years. Rather, she was gaunt, solemn, and noticeably anxious. As discussed above (see "Treatment Begins"), Ms. Fairmont clearly met DSM-IV-TR criteria for three serious psychiatric conditions: major depression, bulimia nervosa, and alcohol dependence. Although she did not fully meet criteria for histrionic personality disorder, I believed that her family history, psychodynamic profile, and interpersonal patterns were consistent with hysterical personality disorder, as defined in Table 4–2. Therefore, her treatment plan was tailored to reverse each of the four disabling disorders. I communicated to Ms. Fairmont my belief that although there would be many components to her treatment plan, the linchpin of her care would be her psychotherapy, which would be scheduled twice weekly for a minimum of 6 months. I believed that her initial response would likely be to the antidepressant, which would reduce her symptoms of depression and anxiety and even some of the compulsive components of her eating disorder. At the time of my initial evaluation, these symptoms were more apparent and bothersome to Ms. Fairmont than the subtleties of her self-destructive interpersonal relationships

TABLE 4–4. Key principles in the diagnosis of hysterical personality disorder as exemplified by the case of Shelby Fairmont

Historical fact	Key principle	Interpretation
Shelby had a hostile and competitive relationship with her mother.	Women with hysterical personality disorder often have distant, distrusting, and/or hostile relationships with their mothers.	Not having a loving, caring, nurturing role model for a mother made it difficult for Shelby herself to exhibit these qualities to others as she grew up.
Shelby adored her father, who felt closer to his daughter than he did to his wife.	Winning the oedipal struggle is a common dynamic that contributes to the development of hysterical personality disorder.	Shelby's competitive and distrusting feelings for women and her seductive behavior with older men stemmed from her family dynamics.
Shelby was a tomboy.	Women with hysterical personality disorder often devalue and eschew roles that are conventionally considered feminine.	Shelby's devaluation of her mother and idealization of and identification with her father led her to value and emulate traits that are conventionally considered masculine.
Shelby was outgoing and confident and enjoyed taking risks.	People with hysterical personality disorder often have extroverted temperaments.	The combination of Shelby's genetics (extroverted temperament) and life experience (her relationships with her parents) led to her development of hysterical personality disorder.

TABLE 4–4. Key principles in the diagnosis of hysterical personality disorder as exemplified by the case of Shelby Fairmont (*continued*)

Historical fact	Key principle	Interpretation
Shelby was an excellent student, a gifted dancer, and a fine athlete.	People with hysterical personality disorder can be competent and successful in important realms of their lives.	In addition to her extroverted temperament, Shelby also inherited from her parents many other positive traits that she developed, through hard work, into solid achievements.
Shelby competed to be the center of attention of her peers, dressed seductively, and spoke in hyperbolic terms.	People with hysterical personality disorder are often dramatic and theatrical and enjoy being the center of attention.	With a disinterested mother and a father who was preoccupied with business and travel, Shelby had to work hard to capture parental attention.
Shelby's first prolonged sexual relationship was with a man who was married, much older than she, and a friend of her father's.	People with hysterical personality disorder often replicate the oedipal dynamics of their childhoods in their adult sexual relationships.	By choosing her father's closest friend as her first sexual partner, Shelby experienced incestuous excitement and danger without committing incest.
Shelby's second prolonged sexual relationship was with a British rock star.	People with hysterical personality disorder often choose sexual partners who are emotionally unavailable or for whom they can not establish sustained intimate feelings.	Shelby felt unstimulated, unsafe, and uncomfortable having intimacy with a mature, appropriate, and available sexual partner.

TABLE 4–4. Key principles in the diagnosis of hysterical personality disorder as exemplified by the case of Shelby Fairmont (*continued*)

Historical fact	Key principle	Interpretation
Despite hard work and intelligence, Shelby did not fulfill her potential in college or in her career.	Over the long run, people with hysterical personality disorder are frequently underachievers in school and in the workplace.	Shelby's initiative and ambition were driven more by competitive drives and attention-seeking behavior than by mature interests and involvements.
Shelby had major depression, generalized anxiety, and bulimia nervosa.	People with hysterical personality disorder are also vulnerable to other serious psychiatric disorders.	The same life experiences, psychodynamics, and stresses that led to her hysterical personality disorder also contributed to Shelby's other psychiatric illnesses.

and her diffuse cognitive style. I was therefore concerned that she would consider herself to be cured by the antidepressant early in treatment and would leave therapy before identifying, understanding, and changing her psychological problems that were most amenable to insight-oriented psychotherapy. Thus, *the first component of Shelby Fairmont's treatment plan was to secure her commitment to engage in psychotherapy for a minimum of 6 months,* the period of time that I thought would be required for her to gain an initial appreciation for the role of her unconscious conflicts in her dysfunctional relationships and other self-defeating behaviors. Many uninformed critics of psychology and psychiatry believe that such advice for extended, intensive treatment is self-serving by professionals, whom they accuse of trying to increase their fees. Rather, similar to dosage and duration requirements for all antidepressants to be effective, the psychotherapy of people with hysterical personality disorder necessitates an adequate frequency of therapeutic meetings and period of time for the fundamental problems to be identified and the approach to treatment to be understood by the patient. I believe that undertreatment of people with personality disorders is mistreatment.

Psychiatric medications.   For the second component of Ms. Fairmont's treatment, I prescribed a selective serotonin reuptake inhibitor (SSRI) antidepressant as well as clonazepam (Klonopin), a long-acting benzodiazepine. I explained to Ms. Fairmont that the clonazepam would prevent potentially dangerous withdrawal symptoms from her discontinuation of alcohol and would immediately help attenuate her symptoms of anxiety before the several weeks that would be required for the SSRI antidepressant to become active. Given Ms. Fairmont's history of alcohol dependence and the fact that for some people benzodiazepines can be habit-forming and can aggravate depression, I clearly indicated to my patient that I would begin to taper and eventually discontinue that medication after a maximum of 6 weeks of treatment. Many professionals who specialize in the treatment of people with alcoholism and other types of addictive disorders do not believe that psychiatric medications of any sort should be prescribed for people with these conditions. They believe that the doctor is giving their patient the message that a "magic pill," as opposed to the self-discipline, is the basis of abstinence. Although there might be occasions when this is correct, for the most part this is another example of how a little bit of knowledge about medicine can be dangerous—and even deadly—to patients. Like pneumococcal pneumonia, major depression is in part a biological illness that can be life-threatening without the use of the appropriate medication. The mortality and morbidity rates of people with major depression are dramatically reduced by the administration of antidepressants. On the other hand, it is certainly true that many people with alcoholism are also addicted to prescribed pain medications and antianxiety medications. However, these patients are largely unmonitored on an intensive basis by psychiatric physicians; rather, their physicians generally see them briefly and infrequently while refilling their prescriptions on a recurrent basis. Before prescribing the medication, I fully informed Ms. Fairmont of the addictive properties and risks of clonazepam as well as its potential benefits to her. This discussion introduced my communication to her of what I considered to be the serious nature of her alcohol use, about which she expressed surprise and disagreement. Nevertheless, she understood the purposes of the antianxiety medication and that it would be discontinued in 6 weeks.

Diet, exercise, and the process of psychotherapy.   As with *every* patient whom it is my privilege and responsibility to care for, an important part of the treatment plan addresses nutrition, diet, and exercise. Psychiatric disorders and psychiatric medications almost always affect appetite and eating patterns. For example, many people with major depression lose the enjoyment associated with eating. When depressed, they no longer have to exercise the restraint that most of the rest of us must exert to refrain from eating the panoply of delicious, highly caloric foods that we regularly encounter in our lives. Their appetite and enjoyment of food return on recovering from their depression, along with the inevitable gaining of weight. Often they will attribute their weight gain to the antidepressant medication, which they will say makes them so hungry that they cannot resist sweets and other foods. This may or may not be true of some psychiatric medications, such as mood stabilizers and antipsychotics, which are indeed associated with significant increases in hunger and weight gain. With most of the newer-generation antidepressants, however, I have found that weight gain is usually a component of the return of the patient's regular appetite with the lifting of the depression. Early in treatment, and before I prescribe any psychiatric medication, I carefully review with my patients the effects of their psychiatric illnesses, medications, and recoveries on appetite and weight gain. I thoroughly review with them their eating habits, as well as their exercise regimens—if they have such. Because healthful exercise regimens and diets are key components in facilitating the recovery from most psychiatric conditions, my patients and I come to agreement about menus and exercise routines. As treatment progresses, I monitor the weight of all my patients closely, and if there are problems with weight gain or weight loss I make this an important topic and goal of treatment. I am certain that many of my professional colleagues would regard my careful attention to diet and exercise in *all* my patients as excessive, even fanatical. However, over my many years of consultative practice, I have been told the following by so many patients with recurrences of the psychiatric symptoms: "I discontinued my medication because I thought it was making me gain too much weight. I would rather be depressed or psychotic than obese."

There does not usually have to be a choice between recovery from a psychiatric illness and excessive weight gain. Addressing the problem at the very beginning of treatment with a clear diet and exercise plan and careful monitoring of weight during and after recovery will almost always obviate this Hobson's choice. Eating patterns, ideals of weight, and body image vary among different cultures, societies, families, and individuals. Each of these influences has variable meaning and importance in understanding a person's psychological development and, if applicable, dysfunction. In the life of Shelby Fairmont, diet and body image were of primary significance. As far back as she could remember, she was preoccupied with food while being fearful of getting fat. In her second session with me she communicated this concern as follows:

Shelby Fairmont: It is no wonder I am so obsessed with my weight. The only thing my mother cared about was the way she looked; and the most important part of her looks was how thin she was. She was constantly on a diet, and she worked out for hours every day with her personal trainer.

Dr. Y.: Was your mother concerned with your weight or eating habits?

Shelby: She tried to monitor everything that went into my mouth. From the time I was 3 years old until I was too big to let her do it to me, she would weigh me every day and record my weight on a chart. She didn't allow me to eat any sweets whatsoever: no candy, no ice cream, no donuts, and no snack foods were ever in our house. When we went out to eat, she would not let me order any desserts other than fruit. Of course I became the world's greatest sneak and cheat. When I would go to my friends' homes, I would sneak into their kitchen cabinets and steal whole bags of cookies. I would then make some excuse to go outside, where I would gobble down the entire bag. I was so active with sports and dancing that I didn't seem to gain weight until I was about 11. At that point I was old enough to buy my own junk food from vending machines, the school cafeteria, and even from other kids. Although I tried to hide it and wouldn't let my mother weigh me any more, she noticed I was getting chubby.

Dr. Y.: How did she react?

Shelby: She went insane. She would search my bedroom and all my stuff for any traces of food. Once, when she found an empty M&M

bag in the pocket of my jeans, she didn't let me eat dinner or have any meals for the entire next day. She told me that she was cutting down on my calories for my own good; otherwise, I would become obese and ruin my dancing career. At the time, I was about 12 years old, was about 5 feet 6 inches tall, and weighed less than 90 pounds.

Shelby did not require therapy to experience and accept ownership of her angry feelings for her mother. However, in treatment she was slow to recognize and reluctant to accept the psychological roots and complex significance of her defiant, secretive, self-destructive behaviors such as bingeing on cookies followed by self-induced vomiting. The following brief exchange is an example of the relatively superficial level of Shelby's psychological understanding when she began psychotherapy:

Shelby: I don't think that there is any deep psychological significance to my eating problems. I binge on sweets because I love the way they taste. I make myself vomit because I don't want to get fat. It's as simple as that.

Dr. Y.: What are you feeling when you binge and purge?

Shelby: I feel hungry, then I feel nauseated.

Dr. Y.: How do you feel about yourself on those occasions?

Shelby: I'll have to think about that for a few minutes....I hate myself when I binge and feel guilty when I make myself vomit.

Dr. Y.: Do you feel anything else?

Shelby: No, just intense guilt and self-loathing.

Over the next 6 months of treatment, Shelby began to make slow progress in understanding the many ramifications of her mother's concern with Shelby's weight. Two key issues emerged from our discussions:

Issue 1: *Although she was preoccupied with Shelby's weight, Colleen Fairmont was experienced by her daughter to be non-nurturing and insensitive to her feelings.*

Ramifications: Even as a child, Shelby Fairmont realized that the main reasons that her mother was so interested in her weight and physical appearance were to attract the attention and gain the admiration of other people. Colleen Fairmont was not attentive to her daughter's emotional life, nor to her many assets such as high intelligence, great energy, and leadership abilities. The result was that Shelby also overvalued her physical appearance and undervalued her other assets. As a young adult, Shelby felt secure only when she was very thin, was dressed in the most fashionable clothing, and was being admired by people whom she believed to be important. During college and after graduation she became involved and identified with people and groups who emphasized appearance and public attention and who demonstrated superficial values. Shelby came to recognize that often her bingeing and purging would occur when she felt unappreciated or let down by her friends—feelings that resembled how she felt after being mistreated or misunderstood by her mother. Shelby eventually discovered that she had unconsciously identified with her mother by being so intensely focused on her appearance and by her choice of superficial, self-centered people as her friends. This startling (for her) recognition intensified Shelby's incentive to understand herself better and to change: "The last person on earth whom I want to be like is my monster of a mother!"

Issue 2: *Colleen Fairmont prohibited her daughter from eating sweets or snack foods.*

Ramifications: Mrs. Fairmont exhibited the confusing combination of not being attentive to or in touch with Shelby's inner life while at the same time being preoccupied with her external appearance. Fixated on her daughter's having an ultrathin, model-like physique, Colleen Fairmont violated many of Shelby's personal boundaries as she militaristically monitored her food intake. Mrs. Fairmont forbade her daughter to eat high-calorie foods such as cookies, ice cream, and hamburgers—fare that all of Shelby's friends enjoyed on a regular basis. Colleen Fairmont would not permit such products in their home, and she also tried to prevent her daughter from sampling and enjoying these foods when she was outside the home. For example, Mrs. Fairmont would lie to the mothers of Shelby's friends and to the employees in the school cafeteria, saying that Shelby had allergies and intolerances to foods with sugar, flour, and high fat content. Shelby countered by also being deceptive, dishonest, and preoccupied with food, weight, and body image. She secretly defied her mother's will by bingeing on forbidden foods and thereby gained pseudoindividuation from her mother: "I exist because mother doesn't know I am stealing food and because she can't stop me from eating the stuff."

Through her treatment, Shelby slowly began to understand that true individuation from her mother required emotional self-sufficiency. Self-understanding, application of her intellectual assets, and actualization of her personal potential in relevant vocational pursuits and mature relationships would help with her self-definition far more than defiance and her many secretive, self-destructive behaviors.

This prolonged discussion of my therapeutic approach to Shelby Fairmont's eating disorder is intended to provide the reader with some flavor of the initial phases of psychiatric treatment, especially insight-oriented psychotherapy. Manifestly, Ms. Fairmont entered treatment with many other disabling symptoms and dysfunctional behavioral patterns that were also identified and dealt with in a similar fashion during the first 6 months of her treatment.

Two Years of Treatment of Shelby Fairmont

"Take care".   During Shelby's seventh month of treatment, her father, Roy Fairmont, contacted my office and indicated that he wished to speak to me, without the presence of his daughter, about his estate planning. I communicated this request to Shelby and my preference that the three of us meet together. Ms. Fairmont encouraged me to meet with her father on his terms. I agreed.

> **Roy Fairmont:** I want to thank you for your care of my daughter. I believe that she has needed psychiatric help for a long while, perhaps since she was a child. I understand that it is a long process, but I already see some signs of progress.
>
> **Dr. Y.:** It is my privilege and pleasure to care for your daughter.
>
> **Mr. Fairmont:** I know that you are a busy man, so let me get right to the point. My doctors have told me that I don't have much longer to live, and I am tidying up my estate. The bulk of my estate, which is substantial, will go to Shelby. I recognize that, at this point, she does not have the mental stability to manage her affairs. I fear that she would be taken advantage of by many people, including her greedy family and frivolous friends. I have two questions for you, Doctor: Do you foresee some point when Shelby can be trusted to have sole authority over her finances? If so, when will this be?
>
> **Dr. Y.:** I am sorry that you are in poor health, Mr. Fairmont. As you know, Shelby is highly intelligent and has many other assets. At the present time, however, she exhibits poor judgment in her personal relationships, is suggestible, is easily influenced by others, and behaves irresponsibly. These are all the necessary ingredients for financial exploitation, or for her just wasting her money. If she remains committed to her treatment and makes the necessary changes and decisions in her personal life, I believe that she has the potential, by age 30, to make sound financial determinations in her own behalf. There are so many unknowns and contingencies, however, that such predictions are practically without value.
>
> **Mr. Fairmont:** I am not at all surprised by your response, Dr. Y. I now want to run something by you for your input. I would like to place Shelby's inheritance into a trust that will be managed by the estates division of our family bank. I would also like to appoint you as one of two trustees who will have the authority to allocate

to Shelby funds from that trust. You will have the best sense of her mental capacity to make sound financial decisions; and you will also know what is going on in her life. You will be well compensated for this work.

Dr. Y.: I know you to be a man of great vision and integrity. I admire you immensely for your service to our nation and generosity to our community. However, I believe that the structure that you have outlined is not in the best interests of your daughter. The type of psychiatric care that Shelby requires will be disrupted by her psychiatrist's having authority over her finances. Try to find another model that will provide the required oversight, but one that does not involve her psychiatrist.

Mr. Fairmont: That can be done. I confess that I am disappointed with your response, but I also trust you to know your own business better than do I. I doubt that we will ever again speak to one another, Dr. Y. Please take good care of my daughter.

Two months after this conversation, Roy Fairmont died, leaving the bulk of his extensive estate in a trust for his daughter Shelby. The executor of his estate and sole trustee of Shelby's trust was one of his close friends and business associates. I was relieved when I learned that he did not designate as trustee and executor his lifelong friend Wallace Merritt.

Transference

During the initial phase of treatment, a therapeutic tightrope must be traversed by the clinician caring for a person with hysterical or histrionic personality disorder. The therapist must be sufficiently supportive, forthcoming, and directive—so that the patient does not feel frustrated, abandoned, and lost—without becoming a glorified, omniscient personal manager who takes over organizing the life of the patient and making decisions for him or her. So long as an appropriate balance is maintained between patient support and self-direction, there are significant opportunities for insight related to each tack taken. In the early phases of treatment of people with this condition (who generally are not insightful, data-based, or particularly interested in cause and effect), in general it is wise for the therapist to be more supportive and active. If too much emphasis is placed too early in treatment on patients' taking charge of their therapy, they will paradoxically feel out of control and highly anxious. Rather, in the initial phases of treatment, the clinician is more active in treatment, willing to provide specific advice and encouragement, and may take the initiative in identifying and addressing specific problems and target symptoms. This initial supportive phase helps engage the patient in treatment while providing the clinician sufficient opportunity to educate the patient about how psychotherapy works in conceptualizing and solving problems and in effecting change. Although this therapeutic tack prevents the patients from becoming so anxious and frustrated that they leave treatment, there are also important transference consequences. (Please refer to "Psychotherapeutic Techniques" in Chapter 6, "Narcissistic Personality Disorder, Part II: Treated Narcissism," for a review of the concept of transference.) The more active and directive posture of clinicians may foster regression in their patients, with the therapist being experienced by the patient as fulfilling a parental role. Powerful feelings about their actual parents will be unconsciously transferred to the therapist, and this provides the opportunity for interpretation and analysis.

Shelby Fairmont was devastated by the death of her father. Not only was he the only member of her family with whom she had a close relationship, but also, for as far back as she could remember, he had been the orienting force in her life. Before making important decisions in her life she would ask herself, "What would Daddy want me to do, and how will he react when I have done it?" In her treatment she began to realize that much of her motivation and ambition involved seeking her idealized father's approval. She also began to understand that her self-defeating behavior was linked, in part, to her conflicted feelings about her father. She felt constrained by him and angry toward him, because she believed that his approval—although essential to her—was so hard won. Ms. Fairmont also felt that their relationship was unfair. Although she knew that her father loved her very much, he was also a highly independent person. "He didn't revolve his life around me and my needs in the same way that I did for him. I really don't think that Daddy ever needed anyone—including me." Thus, in a paradoxical way she felt liberated by the loss of her father, while at the same time she felt lost and alone in the world. Given these circumstances, Ms. Fairmont felt increasingly dependent on me—both for support and for insight. Not surprisingly, she also experienced intense, diverse, and conflicted feelings for me that I endeavored to utilize therapeutically. An example occurred in a session about 2 months after her father's death.

Shelby Fairmont: Do you know what's my main problem in life, Dr. Y.?
Dr. Y.: I am not sure that I do. What do you think it is?
Shelby: That's the problem. You know me better than anyone else in the world. You are supposed to be a famous psychiatrist. Nevertheless, you never tell me anything that really helps me. It's enormously frustrating for me!
Dr. Y.: What makes you think that I would withhold something from you that I thought might help you?

Shelby: I know that you think that it's better for me if I figure things out for myself. But you are very wrong. I really don't know how to do that. It is so frustrating. You're so frustrating. I believe that my biggest problem is that I don't have a clue about what to do with my life, and I wanted to ask you for some suggestions. I know you won't give me any advice, and it makes me furious!

Dr. Y.: Are you saying that you are furious at me for not offering you the help that you need?

Shelby: That's exactly what I am saying. I am saying that this whole process is sadistic and perverse. You're sadistic and perverse!

Dr. Y.: Perhaps so. But I don't agree with your premise. You are suggesting that I know—better than you—what is best for you; what will give you pleasure and satisfaction. I am sorry that I am neither that smart nor that presumptuous. You are the world's authority on what is in your own best interest, on what will make you happy.

Shelby: You have no idea how angry that makes me. I am wondering why I am even coming to see you.

Over the next year, Ms. Fairmont experienced and expressed many intense feelings toward me, and we worked in treatment to understand the sources and meaning of these potent feelings, as outlined below.

Idealization.   When Shelby Fairmont began treatment, she was seriously ill with depression, bulimia nervosa, and alcohol dependence. Her clinical condition necessitated active and directive care on my part, including my prescribing medications and monitoring her withdrawal from alcohol. Within 2 months she experienced significant relief from her symptoms of depression and anxiety, was able to abstain from alcohol, and felt much better physically as a result of her improved sleep patterns and exercise and diet regimen. She soon began to communicate to me her belief that I had unique, extraordinary, and almost superhuman powers to understand her and to meet her needs. Recognizing that Ms. Fairmont was having a regressive response to my supportive care while perceiving me as the omniscient, omnipotent, and all-loving father, I tried to minimize her adulation:

Shelby Fairmont: I feel like a new person. I am so lucky to have you for my psychiatrist. All of my friends in New York complain to me about their doctors, those analyst-types, who won't say one word to them or do anything for them.

Dr. Y.: You are giving me way too much credit. I believe that your progress is due—almost entirely—to your hard work, both in and out of this office. The care that I have been providing is standard psychiatric treatment.

Shelby: You are being much too modest. I feel that you have the ability to see right through me. It's almost like you can read my mind.

> **Dr. Y.:** I can assure you that I cannot read your mind, and I am not even sure what it means to "see right through you." I only know that I have no ability to do any such thing. Rather, my help is totally dependent upon your willingness to communicate what you feel and your efforts to understand yourself and to change.

Novice clinicians are often too willing to accept the idealization of their patients. Unfortunately, this will engender unrealistic expectations on the part of their patients for perfect results and preferential treatment. Among the important principles of treatment are the following:

- The higher the pedestal on which the clinician allows himself or herself to be placed, the harder he or she will fall.
- The clinician who accepts the credit for a patient's improvement must be ready to accept the blame when things go wrong. And things always go wrong.

In the case of Shelby Fairmont, it was clear that she wished me to become the powerful father on whom she depended for almost everything as a child. There would be no way that I could meet such an expectation. Therefore I worked hard in her treatment to reduce her idealization of me and the attendant unrealistic expectations.

Rivalry.   Notwithstanding my efforts to deflect Ms. Fairmont's regression in treatment and idealization of me, a variety of feelings and behaviors accompanied this distortion. Although she had a brother and sister from her father's first marriage, she had almost no interaction with them. Shelby was essentially an only child who was doted on by her adoring father. After 6 months of treatment, my patient expressed great interest in the other people in my life and concern about whether or not she was special to me:

> **Shelby:** I ran into one of my high school friends yesterday. Cynthia Alcorn. We started to talk and catch up, and she told me that she is one of your patients. She told me that she got depressed after having her baby. How is she doing?
>
> **Dr. Y.:** You know very well that I do not discuss any of my patients.
>
> **Shelby:** I never really understood what the big deal was about this confidentiality business. You can learn more about people from magazines than you can from any psychiatrist. She told me that you are married and have three daughters who go to the same private school that we went to. She also told me that your wife is also a doctor and is very pretty. How come you never shared any of this with me?
>
> **Dr. Y.:** Before I answer this question, I would like to know how you feel about this information and about how you learned it.

Shelby: I really don't feel anything. It's probably a waste of time to talk about it. I don't feel that it is right for you to play favorites with your patients and tell some of them about yourself, and not tell others. That kind of makes me mad.

Dr. Y.: Are you saying that I care about some of my patients more than I care about you?

Shelby: I believe that what you say is probably true. You are so formal with me. I am certain that you don't think of me as a friend. I'm just a patient to you. It's totally a business relationship. Obviously, you feel much closer to some of your other patients.

Dr. Y.: How is that obvious?

Shelby: You talk about your personal life with your other patients; but certainly not with me.

Dr. Y.: Did your friend tell you how she came by this information?

Shelby: I'm not sure she mentioned it. How else would she have found out these things if you didn't tell her? I'll tell you something about Cynthia that you probably don't know. She has always been a terrible bigot. When we were in high school, she constantly complained about the influx of Jewish and Asian students to the school. She believed that the only thing they cared about was getting high grades. She really hated the minority students.

Since childhood, Shelby had been highly competitive with her mother and her female peers. Two related components of her paternal transference to me were her desire to be the most important woman in my life and her rivalry with any woman whom she thought might challenge her for that role. As indicated in the above dialogue, she regarded my other patients and the females in my immediate family as particularly threatening. Her belief that she had won her father's attention and affection from her mother led her to feel vulnerable that another woman would have the power to steal away all of my interest in her. The more she trusted me and the more she felt dependent on me in her treatment, the more apprehensive she was that she would lose me to another woman. This conflict was reflected in her other close relationships with men and led her to become involved with men who were either unavailable to her (e.g., older, married men) or men who were not capable of intimacy or commitment. Such men felt safer to her: "you can't take something away from me that I never really had."

Treatment involved encouraging Ms. Fairmont to express her full range of feelings for me and providing her with sensitive and respectful interpretations of the experiential and unconscious sources and life implications of these feelings.

Disappointment and anger. Embedded in Shelby Fairmont's paternal transference to me was the unconscious disappointment that she felt as a result of her father's not reciprocating, in kind, her intense involvement with him. As a young child, Shelby was preoccupied with capturing the approval and attention of Roy Fairmont. Without exaggeration, he was the absolute center of her life. Although he certainly did not neglect his daughter, he also was involved with other important interests, including his demanding law practice and the business deals that took him far away from home much of the time. In treatment, Ms. Fairmont became furious with me because she believed that I did not prioritize her over my other patients and members of my family. As we probed the bases for these feelings over many months, we came to understand that she felt worthless if she was not the center of my attention. Ultimately, Ms. Fairmont discovered that she had long believed that there must be something innately deficient or defective about her; otherwise, why was her intense love for her father not reciprocated? One long-term result was that she developed a sense of insecurity about her attractiveness to men, for which she tried to compensate by becoming the femme fatale with the power to capture the heart of almost any man. She also learned in treatment that she had great resentment toward her father for her unrequited feelings—anger that she generalized to all men who might have a romantic interest in her. Her usual pattern with young men who were interested in and capable of having a mature, intimate relationship with her would be to lead them on, build up their hopes, and then reject them and break their hearts. Through expressing her angry feelings toward me and examining their subtle and buried sources, she was eventually able to trust me more and risk feeling closer to me.

Lust and love.   Ms. Fairmont had been in treatment with me for more than 18 months before she felt sufficiently safe and comfortable to discuss her past sexual experiences and her current sexual feelings. Such reticence might not have been expected in a woman who could dress provocatively and behave seductively and who had had regular sexual experience since she was in her early teens. The understanding of her psychodynamics brings clarity to this seeming contradiction. Throughout her childhood, Shelby fought openly and ferociously with her mother while at the same time idealizing and adoring her father. Roy Fairmont had very little in common with his wife, Colleen, whom he tolerated but did not respect. The absolute triumph over her mother in the competition for her father had many long-term repercussions for Shelby beyond her distrust of and disrespect for other women. Young Shelby reveled in the understanding that her father loved her more than any other person, and she was especially delighted when he confided in her about significant personal matters or chose her to accompany him to important public events. Reinforced by the high regard in which Roy Fairmont was held by nearly everybody, Shelby believed her father to be perfect in almost every way.

With puberty, however, her monomaniacal adoration of and passionate relationship with her father assumed an unsettling new dimension. Her father was the exclusive object of her most passionate longings and strivings for as long as she could remember; but what about her budding sexual feelings? Ms. Fairmont discovered in treatment that her unconscious response to this quandary was to deny her sexual feelings and personal potency. First, although she appeared to be sensuous, she was more interested in the trappings of sexuality—such as flirtation and appearing attractive—than in achieving sexual gratification. Ms. Fairmont admitted that she didn't particularly enjoy sexual intercourse, nor did she care about experiencing orgasm. For her, sex was more a means of feeling secure—a test proving to herself and others that she could attract and control men. Second, Shelby Fairmont did not apply her considerable intelligence and energy to achieving her full potential as a formidable woman. Why? Such a woman could get what she wanted. She would have both the wherewithal to win over a man of the stature of her father and the confidence to accept and act on her potent sexual feelings for him.

Because Shelby's childhood and adolescent sexual longings for her father were morally and socially unacceptable and would evoke even greater hostility and retaliation from her mother, these powerful feelings were repressed. According to Freudian theory, repressed conflicted feelings are unconsciously expressed in symptoms such as anxiety and in dysfunctional thought patterns, feelings, and behavior. Shelby Fairmont's sexual relationship with Wallace Merritt, her father's close friend, can be best understood as the acting out of her unconscious sexual strivings for her father. Her later choices of relationships with inappropriate men such as rock musicians and married athletes who were unreliable and incapable of mature intimacy reflected the risk-laden, dangerous, and forbidden aspects of her incestuous feelings. Through her treatment, Ms. Fairmont began to appreciate her repetitive, unfulfilling relationship patterns with men in which she would be most excited during the courtship phase (which she described as "the chase") but would become progressively uninterested and turned off sexually as the liaison moved toward intimacy. "I always seem most interested in the man who is the most unavailable."

The psychotherapeutic relationship encompasses many of the ingredients that would elicit the sexual feelings of a person with the life experience and psychology of Shelby Fairmont: 1) an age difference approximating that between parent and child; 2) an authority-novice power differentiation; 3) the patient's lack of universal access to the therapist; and 4) a strict prohibition against sexual contact. However, the psychotherapeutic relationship was very different from Ms. Fairmont's previous relationships in the following two ways: 1) she was encouraged to express exactly what she was currently thinking, feeling, and experiencing about the psychiatrist *at all times* during the therapy meetings; and 2) her thoughts and feelings regarding me would be discussed and interpreted rather than acted on.

During her first 2 years of treatment, Ms. Fairmont disclosed and discussed many feelings toward me, most of which were negative. I tried to discourage her idealization of me by being clear and emphatic about my limited abilities and power. I avoided becoming her prescient advisor, because this would lead to her regressing and becoming increasingly dependent on me. I assiduously monitored therapeutic boundaries and resisted her expectations—and solicitations—that I be exclusively and universally available to her. All of these responses on my part engendered in my patient feelings of abandonment, frustration, and anger. I encouraged her to express these feelings, as well as to be deliberate, factual, and rational in their justification.

Ms. Fairmont became more practiced in being logical and forming conclusions based on evidence and rationality, and she applied this new skill to tracing the roots of her psychiatric symptoms and maladaptive behavior to experiences and relationships that took place in her childhood. Through this process she gradually began to feel more secure with making her own decisions and choices rather than trying to please others and respond to the expectations of father figures. She also began to experience me more as a real, individuated person, as opposed to a unidimensional repository of disparate, distorted transference feelings and perceptions. Her trust in me also grew, in step with her increased self-confidence and emerging sense of self-definition.

It was only after she began to understand herself better and to take positive actions toward fulfilling her potential that she began to experience me as a person beyond her personal needs and unconscious projections. At that point in her treatment she also began to become much more interested in what I could help her discover about herself than in what I thought about her worth and how she happened to look that day. In her third year of treatment, Ms. Fairmont began to talk about many of the thoughts and feelings about which she had previously been too embarrassed or ashamed to share.

Shelby Fairmont: This is very hard for me to tell you and to admit to myself. As you know, I like to be the one who is chased. After about the first month of my treatment with you, I thought that I was madly in love with you.

Dr. Y.: What made you think that?

Shelby: I am so, so embarrassed to tell you this. But here goes. I began to think about you all of the time. At first, I was mostly obsessed with what you thought of me. If you thought I was pretty; if you thought I was smart. I would spend hours at night just deciding what I was going to wear to the treatment session the next day. I was dying to know what you thought about how I looked each session, but I would never dare to ask you. Each session, I left feeling frustrated and angry because you never seemed to notice or care how I looked. After that I wanted to impress you with how smart I was. Before sessions, I rehearsed what I was going to say—and you could be sure I would never tell you anything that I thought might make you dislike me or disrespect me. I then became preoccupied with your personal life—where you live, what your house is like, what your wife is like, what your children look like, where you go on vacations, and everything else about you.

Dr. Y.: What do you mean by "everything"?

Shelby: What you are really like outside of your professional role. How you like to spend your free time, and how I might fit into your life. I began to fantasize about our being together all of the time. I began to create elaborate scenarios in my head about your leaving your wife and children and running away to France with me. It was truly nuts. I would spend my days lost in this fantasy about being with you in every way. My fantasy seemed real. But then I would see you in sessions in which you would want me to talk about my father or mother or some other topic, and that whole thing seemed unreal to me. All I cared about was if you thought I was beautiful that day and were attracted to me.

Dr. Y.: Attracted?

Shelby: That was the main part. I knew for certain that the only way that I could get you for myself was through sex. That's the way it has always worked for me. Don't get me wrong. I enjoy sex—for the most part—and thought a lot about what it would be like to have sex with you. But that's never been the biggest deal for me. Sex with you would have been a means to an end. And that end was to have you all to myself.

Ms. Fairmont's ability to probe and discuss her sexual feelings for me and others constituted a breakthrough in her treatment. She came to understand that her sexual preoccupations with me early in treatment had more to do with her sense of low self-worth and need to control than it had to do with me or with sex. The replication of the basic elements of her relationship with her father in her feelings for and behavior with me and other men became clear to her. A fundamental change occurred in the pattern of her relationship with me: she began to communicate openly about what she was thinking, feeling, and experiencing—something that she had never really done before with another person. This openness also permitted her to have, for the first time, an objective, informed partner as she worked to better understand herself and to change.

Long-Term Treatment

By her third year in treatment, the disabling and unsettling symptoms for which Ms. Fairmont had originally sought psychiatric care had, for the most part, been resolved. She was no longer depressed or plagued with chronic anxiety, she did not abuse alcohol, and she no longer experienced cycles of anorexia and bulimia. To her surprise, I recommended that she consider psychoanalytic treatment, which I believed would best help her to attain the following long-range goals: 1) developing the ability to forge trusting friendships and noncompetitive working relationships both with other women and with men; 2) developing the capability to sustain a mature, stable relationship with an appropriate man that could lead to greater intimacy and sexual gratification; and 3) developing the capacity to become a nurturing, supportive mother who derives gratification from the maternal role. The latter became an unanticipated long-range goal of Ms. Fairmont's—certainly it was not *my* goal for her—during her third year of treatment with me. She would not have considered motherhood to be an interest or a priority when she first sought psychiatric care. After many long discussions with me about the process and rationale of psychoanalysis and the implications of her leaving treatment with me, Shelby agreed to accept referral to a female psychoanalyst in New York City. One reason that she chose to return to New York was to be able to attend a 2-year course at Columbia University for college graduates who want to apply to medical school but who do not have the prerequisite courses in science and mathematics. Ms. Fairmont also stated that for the first time since she had abandoned her dream to become a professional ballet dancer, her life had direction and purpose.

Key principles in the treatment of people with hysterical personality disorder as exemplified by the case of Shelby Fairmont are summarized in Table 4–5.

Long-Term Progress of Shelby Fairmont

After leaving Houston to take premedical courses and to enter psychoanalysis in New York City, Ms. Fairmont regularly corresponded with

TABLE 4–5. Key principles in the treatment of people with hysterical personality disorder as exemplified by the case of Shelby Fairmont

Historical fact	Key principle	Interpretation
Early in his treatment of Ms. Fairmont, Dr. Y. prescribed her a selective serotonin reuptake inhibitor antidepressant.	The treatment of people with hysterical personality disorder often begins with the pharmacological treatment of comorbid psychiatric conditions.	Until her major depression, bulimia nervosa, and alcohol dependence had resolved, Shelby Fairmont was not able to benefit from psychotherapeutic treatment of her personality disorder.
Dr. Y. took an active, directive, and supportive tack early in his treatment of Ms. Fairmont.	In the initial phases of their treatment, people with hysterical personality disorder are often unable to think independently and rationally. Learning how to do so is a fundamental part of their treatment.	Dr. Y.'s directive treatment in the early phases of Shelby Fairmont's treatment prevented her from feeling confused, frustrated, and abandoned by the process of psychotherapy.
Dr. Y. prescribed a rigorous regimen of diet and exercise for Ms. Fairmont.	Treatment for hysterical personality disorder should not be limited to insight-oriented psychotherapy.	Shelby Fairmont would have left treatment had she gained weight as a side effect of her pharmacological treatment or as an untoward effect of her recovery from depression and anorexia.

TABLE 4–5. Key principles in the treatment of people with hysterical personality disorder as exemplified by the case of Shelby Fairmont (*continued*)

Historical fact	Key principle	Interpretation
Dr. Y. declined Roy Fairmont's request that he become a trustee/executor of his daughter's trust.	The therapist must establish and maintain strict therapeutic boundaries in all spheres of treatment of people with hysterical personality disorder for there to be a successful therapeutic outcome.	Had Dr. Y. assumed control over Ms. Fairmont's finances, her dependence on him would have increased, she would have regressed in treatment, and her idealized paternal transference to him would have intensified.
Dr. Y. resisted Ms. Fairmont's idealization of him.	A key to the treatment of people with hysterical personality disorder is interpreting the parental transferences.	Accepting the idealization of him by Ms. Fairmont would have led to a steep, slippery, and dangerous slope of unrealistic expectations that Dr. Y. be able to meet all of her needs and solve all of her problems.
Ms. Fairmont spoke disparagingly of one of Dr. Y.'s other patients.	Low self-esteem from not feeling special to parental figures is at the root of the competitive feelings and actions of many people with hysterical personality disorder.	Ms. Fairmont did not believe that Dr. Y. could care for other people and still care about her.
Ms. Fairmont experienced and expressed great anger toward Dr. Y.	The freedom and safety for patients to express negative feelings toward their therapists is essential in the treatment of people with hysterical personality disorder.	Ms. Fairmont unconsciously transferred feelings of anger and resentment toward both parents to Dr. Y.

TABLE 4–5. Key principles in the treatment of people with hysterical personality disorder as exemplified by the case of Shelby Fairmont (*continued*)

Historical fact	Key principle	Interpretation
Early in her treatment, Ms. Fairmont felt a strong sexual attraction to Dr. Y.	People with hysterical personality disorder transfer powerful and conflicted sexual feelings from their childhoods to their therapists.	Ms. Fairmont's intense and conflicted feelings for her father were manifested in her irresponsible and ungratifying adolescent and postadolescent sexual relationships with men.
Two years of treatment had passed before Ms. Fairmont was able to reveal or discuss her sexual feelings.	People with hysterical personality disorder have difficulties with sexual expression and gratification.	Ms. Fairmont's unconscious erotic longings for her father were manifested by repressed and suppressed sexual feelings and secretive behaviors.
After 3 years of treating Ms. Fairmont, Dr. Y. referred her for psychoanalytic treatment.	Psychoanalysis is often needed to help people with hysterical personality disorder achieve their full potential in their personal lives and vocations.	Psychoanalytic treatment helped Shelby Fairmont to reach her goal of becoming an accomplished physician and experiencing fulfillment as a wife and mother.

me by letter and e-mail. I received the following letter from her 8 years after she had moved to New York.

Dear Dr. Y.,

First of all, please accept my apology for not writing to you for such a long time. I hope that all is well with you and yours. So much has transpired in my life since we last communicated. Most important to me, Roy is now two years old, and he is thriving. He is bright and stubborn like his grandfather, and also has the artistic temperament of his wonderful father. There are two things related to Roy that I have never told you. First, I will be forever grateful to you for your faith in me during my treatment with you when I proclaimed that I never wanted to have children. I believe the reasons I gave you were that kids are "noisy, messy, and boring." You insisted that we explore this further, and I later discovered that I was fearful that I would be a terrible mother, as my mother was to me. When you asked me whether I thought I had any control over the type of mother that I might become, a whole new world of possibility opened to me. Like so many things in treatment, I have no idea how your simple question led to change. However, for the first time I was able to get in touch with my desperation to have a family of my own; and to have my own children. I now have a husband whom I cherish and adore and a son who is the center of my universe. I also never told you that I considered naming him after you, Dr. Y. Fortunately, I realized that you would have gone berserk if I had done that, and would have insisted that I get back into treatment. Naming him after my beloved, if imperfect, father is more appropriate and, ironically, less incestuous.

Now to catch you up on my career. I am about to complete my Ph.D. thesis in neuroscience, and will graduate this June with my M.D., Ph.D. degrees. It seems that it has taken forever, but I have loved every minute. I have never been so happy and excited about the future. I have decided to take the joint offer from Cornell Medical School, Sloan Kettering, and the Rockefeller Institute. It is the perfect job for me, as I can take care of cancer patients, teach medical students and graduate students, and do research on neural tumors. Although this is an ambitious plan, I do not have to take night call or emergency call. This will permit me to spend all my late afternoons, evenings, and weekends with my family. (I just love saying "my family"). Be certain, I will not revisit the sins of my parents on my son, Roy.

I know better than to ask anything about your life, you never tell me anything. You are such a stiff. Doesn't matter, anyway. I find everything I need to know about you from all your old New York buddies and Google. I still get a kick from violating your boundaries.

One last thing, Dear Doctor. As my father once told you concerning me, "Take care."

Shelby Fairmont, M.D., Ph.D. (almost)

Afterword

If you happened to catch sight of 22-year-old Shelby Fairmont dancing with a famous athlete at a chic New York City nightclub, you could not help but take notice. The tall, lithe, provocatively attired young woman was strikingly beautiful, and she could dance like a professional. Had you later learned that she was an heiress of one of America's most wealthy and politically influential families and was a recent honors graduate of a prestigious Ivy League college, you might have become even more captivated and intrigued. However, should you somehow have been granted the opportunity to be welcomed into her highly vetted inner circle and be permitted to know her better, Ms. Fairmont's dazzling glitter and sparkle would have gradually lost its luster. Eventually, you would have come to realize that her dazzle was more surface reflection than inner illumination. Although enticing, that surface would be revealed as an impenetrable barricade that kept you from getting closer to Shelby Fairmont, while it filtered out any feeling that she might have for you. You would have sensed that her interest in you had little to do with you but was all about her. However, if you happened to attend a lecture 10 years later that Dr. Fairmont was delivering to a class of Cornell medical students about the cell biology of cancer formation, you again would have taken notice. The fact that her figure was obscured beneath her billowing white lab coat, that she wore no makeup or jewelry, and that she spoke in the soft, understated tones of a scientist still would not disguise her great beauty and allure. Nonetheless, her appearance would not be what captivated you. Your attention would be drawn almost immediately from her person to the subject and substance of her lecture. As she spoke earnestly, compassionately, and movingly about the potential of basic science to reduce the suffering of the host of people with brain tumors, you would have been carried away to her subject. Shelby Fairmont's arresting persona was no longer defined by her great beauty, personal wealth, or fearsome competitiveness. Rather, her knowledge as a scientist and physician, her dedication to her patients and profession, and her compassionate focus on others somehow deflected your attention from Shelby as an individual to her scientific ideas and professional values. And the more time that you were able to spend with Dr. Fairmont, the better you would be able to know her, respect her, and like her. You would have come to know her as a dedicated wife, mother, physician, scientist, and friend. You would come to realize that she was, for the most part, content and fulfilled. You would come to realize that your relationship with Dr. Fairmont was as much about you as it was about her. Although this transformation would mostly be the result of the motivation, intelligence, hard work, and bravery of Dr. Shelby Fairmont, it would never—and could never—have occurred without her treatment.

References and Suggested Readings

American Psychiatric Association: Diagnostic and Statistical Manual: Mental Disorders. Washington, DC, American Psychiatric Association, 1952

American Psychiatric Association: Diagnostic and Statistical Manual of Mental Disorders, 2nd Edition. Washington, DC, American Psychiatric Association, 1968

American Psychiatric Association: Diagnostic and Statistical Manual of Mental Disorders, 3rd Edition. Washington, DC, American Psychiatric Association, 1980

American Psychiatric Association: Diagnostic and Statistical Manual of Mental Disorders, 4th Edition. Washington, DC, American Psychiatric Association, 1994

American Psychiatric Association: Diagnostic and Statistical Manual of Mental Disorders, 4th Edition, Text Revision. Washington DC, American Psychiatric Association, 2000

Barabasz A, Barabasz M, Jensen S, et al: Cortical event-related potentials show the structure of hypnotic suggestion is crucial. Int J Clin Exp Hypn 47:5–22, 1999

Blacker KH, Tupin JP: Hysteria and hysterical structures: developmental and social theories, in Hysterical Personality. Edited by Horowitz MJ. New York, Jason Aronson, 1977, pp 97–141

Gabbard GO: Cluster B personality disorders: hysterical and histrionic, in Psychodynamic Psychiatry in Clinical Practice, 3rd Edition. Washington, DC, American Psychiatric Press, 2000, pp 517–545

Maldonado JR, Spiegel D: Hypnosis, in American Psychiatric Publishing Textbook of Clinical Psychiatry, 4th Edition. Edited by Hales RE, Yudofsky SC. Arlington, VA, American Psychiatric Publishing, 2003, pp 1285–1331

Millon T: A theoretical derivation of pathological personalities, in Contemporary Directions in Psychopathology: Toward the DSM-IV. Edited by Millon T, Klerman G. New York, Guilford, 1986, pp 639–669

Nestadt G, Romanoski AJ, Chahal R, et al: An epidemiological study of histrionic personality disorder. Psychol Med 20:413–422, 1990

Spiegel H, Spiegel D: Trance and Treatment: Clinical Uses of Hypnosis. Washington, DC, American Psychiatric Press, 1987

Veith I: Hysteria: The History of a Disease. Chicago, IL, University of Chicago Press, 1970

Veith I: Four thousand years of hysteria, in Hysterical Personality. Edited by Horowitz MJ. New York, Jason Aronson, 1977, pp 9–93

Yager J, Gitlin MH: Clinical manifestations of psychiatric disorders, in Comprehensive Textbook of Psychiatry, 7th Edition. Edited by Sadock BJ, Sadock VA. Philadelphia, PA, Lippincott Williams & Wilkins, 2000, pp 789–823

NARCISSISTIC PERSONALITY DISORDER

Part I: Untreated Narcissism

You had one eye in the mirror
As you watched yourself gavotte
And all the girls dreamed that they'd be your
    partner...
You're so vain
You probably think this song is about you

—Carly Simon, "You're So Vain"

Essence

Have you ever worked for or had an important personal relationship with someone whom you *initially* believed to have unique talents, remarkable accomplishments, and exceptional personal qualities? Based on this individual's captivating persona and your belief in his superior abilities, did you place great trust in him on important matters affecting your life and your future? Did you gradually begin to realize that he overstated his accomplishments and was self-centered? Did this person seem to be preoccupied with "important" people but demonstrate little interest in others who were not in a position to advance his career or social status? Did you begin to perceive that he exploited you and took advantage of other people in order to get ahead? Over time, did you tire of his constant need to be admired by you and others, his overstating his personal accomplishments, and his constant bragging? Did you notice that the person seemed to feel special and entitled to privileges that he neither earned nor deserved? Was he incapable of owning up to his faults, mistakes, or deficiencies? In fact, did he cover over and lie about mistakes and mishaps? Did you finally recognize that he really did not appreciate your contributions or those of other people who had been devoted to him and had served him well? Did you detect that although he would feign interest in and concern for others, he was in fact not capable of true altruism or empathy? When you questioned him about his exaggerations and arrogance, did he withdraw from you? When you confronted him about being dishonest or not meeting commitments, did he devalue you, discredit you, threaten you, or even try to harm you? If you answer "yes" to many of these questions, it is very possible that this person may have narcissistic personality disorder. If so, this chapter should be helpful to you in gaining a realistic understanding of this person and how best to assess the implications of your relationship with him.

The Case of Congressman Dennis Smythe

Sources of Information

I met with Congressman Dennis Smythe on only four occasions. Congressman Smythe is the father of Reverend Martin Smythe, whose psychiatric disorder and treatment are described in Chapter 6, "Narcissistic Personality Disorder, Part II: Treated Narcissism." As a component of my assessment and care of Reverend Smythe, his parents participated in three extended-family sessions, which Reverend Smythe's wife also attended. I also met with each family member individually for 90 minutes. Years later, long after I had transferred Reverend Smythe to a psychoanalyst, he asked that I treat his mother, Mrs. June Smythe, for severe depression that had emerged subsequent to a stroke in the right side of her brain. Given his urging and the fact that my subspecialty concentration is neuropsychiatry, I agreed. Once she had recovered from her depression, Mrs. Smythe continued with me for several years in supportive treatment related to ongoing issues in her life. Thus my knowledge about Congressman Smythe derives from three sources: the direct observations and information that he provided during his four clinical visits with me, my treatment of his former wife and his son, and the extensive historical reports that they both provided about the congressman's background history and relationships with them. The reports Congressman Smythe's family gave about him were highly consistent with my clinical assessment.

History of Congressman Dennis Smythe

The Early Years: Home on the Farm and College

Dennis Smythe was the oldest son in a large, poor family that struggled bitterly to keep the weeds and grasses of the Illinois prairie from reclaiming their rightful home in the wind-battered fields of their small farm. As hard and unyielding as the dry, crop-spent soil in the hot August sun, Dennis's father expected his first-born son to "pull his own weight" from the time he was 7 years old. The family, which eventually included his seven younger siblings, depended on Dennis's hard work to survive. Dennis's mother did not have much time to devote to him. Rather, she was preoccupied with caring for her newborns that, like the red-winged blackbirds, seemed to arrive each September just in time to share the Smythes' meager harvest of matured corn. Not only did young Dennis have a grown man's menu of responsibilities on the farm, he also supplemented the family income by working, during summers and after school, as a hand for other farmers in his county.

One farm on which Dennis worked was owned by a wealthy Chicago businessman, Mr. Martin Greer. In time, the tall, handsome, and outgoing farm boy caught Mr. Greer's attention. Of particular interest to Mr. Greer was the fact that Dennis was an outstanding high school athlete, with state commendations in track, baseball, and basketball. Although Dennis's grades and test scores were not at all competitive, the businessman pulled some strings so that Dennis received a full athletic scholarship to play baseball at his alma mater, a highly regarded Midwestern university. Dennis was the first person from either side of his family to attend college. Dennis's father was not supportive of his going to college. Congressman Smythe recalls his father saying on the day that he left for college, "I reckon that you don't need your family no more—now that you're a big shot off to play baseball and drink beer with rich folks' kids." As it turned out, the father was pretty much on target, because no one in the family ever visited him at college, and only one brother was interested in how Dennis fared on the baseball team. For his part, Dennis rarely called home from college and usually spent his holidays at the homes of friends and his summers working in Chicago for his sponsor, Mr. Greer.

Getting Started: Marriage and Business

In the summer before his senior year of college, Dennis met June Gallagher. The occasion was an elegant party that was held in Winnetka, Illinois, an affluent suburb north of Chicago on Lake Michigan. The party was held to celebrate the merger of Mr. Greer's manufacturing company with another industrial giant owned by Mr. Spencer Gallagher, who resided in Winnetka. At that time, June was 19 years old and she had just completed her sophomore year at Smith College in Northampton, Massachusetts. June had grown up and attended high school in Winnetka and therefore knew many of the young people and adults who were at the party. She was nonetheless uncomfortable in most social settings, including at this party. June had always been shy and studious by temperament and was self-conscious about being overweight. Although she was quite surprised that the handsome and outgoing young man was paying so much attention to her that evening, June was not particularly interested in Dennis when they first met. To her great surprise, Dennis, having procured her mailing address from Mr. Greer, wrote to her the next fall in college. Moreover, Dennis invited her to be his date at an important winter formal event for seniors at his college. June's reserved nature and instincts told her not to accept the invitation. She had rarely been asked out by anyone and certainly had never been invited to a college ball. Her parents, however, encouraged her to attend the event. They reasoned that it would be a good opportunity for their daughter try to come out of her shell and to improve her social skills. Besides, their business associate, Mr. Greer, spoke very highly of Dennis Smythe.

June's visit to Dennis's college for his winter formal was overwhelming. Although she had been born and raised in an affluent family, she had never before been treated with such forethought, consideration, and attention to the details involved in her physical and social comfort. First, she was picked up at the airport in a limousine, which was most unusual for a college student in the early 1940s, particularly in the Midwest. Dennis had done his homework by finding out the two or three coeds from Winnetka whom June knew, and he arranged for her to stay with the one young woman with whom she had the closest relationship. Every aspect of her weekend was thoughtfully and sensitively planned. To her great surprise (she had been dreading the trip), June had a wonderful time. Dennis was the perfect gentleman, tried to get to know her well as a person, and brought out in her an undeveloped capacity to relax and have some fun. In truth, June had very limited experience with boys and men. She had attended a girls' private school through high school and had then gone to Smith College, an all-woman school with a mostly female faculty. Her father, Mr. Gallagher, was an active and successful businessman, and the little time that he spent with the family was primarily devoted to attending the sports activities of June's younger brother, Alex. Concerning that point in her life, June told me the following:

> **June Smythe:** I was completely inexperienced and naïve about men and dating. Given my bookishness and shyness, I was vulnerable and in way over my head when it came to Dennis's interest in me. Dennis began to send me letters on, at minimum, a weekly basis. On some weeks I received a letter from him every day. He showed a deep interest in everything that I was doing. For example, at the time, I was writing my honors English thesis on Emily Dickinson. Dennis read several biographies of the poet and studied her poetry. He asked me for the early drafts of my paper, which he read carefully and made constructive and intelligent suggestions for its improvement. He made me feel like I was the most important person in his life. In fact, for the first time in my life, I began to feel important.

Dennis invited June to his college graduation. Again he crafted "the perfect weekend." On that trip it became clear to June that her beau was highly regarded on campus. As the president of his senior class, Dennis spoke during the graduation ceremony. June noticed that although Mr. Greer attended Dennis's graduation, no one from Dennis's family was there. When Dennis kissed her the evening of the prom, it was the first time that June had ever been kissed by a young man.

After being graduated from college, Dennis began to work in the financial department of the merged business of Mr. Greer (who became president of the company) and June's father, Mr. Gallagher (who was chief executive officer and chairman of the board of directors). Intelligent, willing to work hard, and trusted by the senior leadership, Dennis soon became recognized as an up-and-comer. The business was expanding rapidly, primarily through the purchase of related industries around the globe. Dennis was in a fine inside position to learn how such purchases and takeovers were conceptualized, financed, and actualized. He had little spare time, and most of it was spent pursuing June. Dennis proposed to June during her last semester of college, and she accepted with great joy. On looking back many years later on her decision to marry Dennis, June said the following:

> **June Smythe:** Other than being a good student, I didn't really have much of an identity at that time. My family had discouraged me from going to graduate school in English literature, as, in my era, that was considered to be a "default decision" for girls who couldn't land a husband. Most of my classmates at Smith College were either married or engaged by graduation. I had never dated anyone else, had no alternative paths, and very little self-confidence. Of course I accepted his offer.

June saw very little of her husband during the first 5 years of their marriage. Dennis Smythe worked nearly around the clock, and his job took him to all parts of the world. She noted that he was far less attentive to her than he had been during the year that he courted her, and she was lonely. In their third year of marriage, Dennis was given the responsibility to manage and turn around a large steel mill that their business had purchased in Brazil, and he was away for months at a time. During that time, he never wrote to her and would phone her only on rare occasions. On the other hand, he maintained almost daily contact with Mr. Greer and Mr. Gallagher about the status of the new business.

Even though June desperately wanted a child, they almost never had sex. Dennis was either too busy with work and social engagements or too tired from work and social engagements. June was much too inhibited and insecure to initiate sexual relations, but she always kept count. During their third year of marriage they had sex only six times. What disturbed June was that on four of those occasions, Dennis was intoxicated. She began to worry that there was something terribly wrong and unattractive about her, a fear that was heightened by her husband's escalating criticism of her. Dennis seemed to be preoccupied with June's physical appearance—including how she dressed. When they were preparing to be in the company of wealthy and successful people, Dennis could be vicious in his criticism of June. He would scold her about her weight and tell her that she dressed like a "65-year-old librarian." Even worse, Dennis treated her as if she were stupid. In therapy, June told me the following:

> **June Smythe:** It seemed to me that the more confident that Dennis became as the result of his business success, the more embarrassed he became about me. The truth is that before I had the children, I did little other than read books and see a few close friends. When we were out with his important business acquaintances, I was terrified that I would not know something that was going on in the world or would say something wrong. When I did make a mistake, he would flash a hate-filled look at me and correct me in public using most condescending and disdainful tone. I would turn red as a beet and wish I could climb under the table. My self-esteem was lower than when I was in high school.

In their fourth year of marriage, June's father asked her if she and Dennis were having problems conceiving a child. June summoned up her courage and told her father that, as she understood it, it was necessary to have sexual relations to have children (and grandchildren). She also indicated to her father that Dennis did not seem that interested in having "relations" with her. Mr. Gallagher told his daughter that he thought he had been working Dennis too hard and that he would speak to him about cutting back so that he could have "some family life." That very night, Dennis, in a rage, confronted June as follows:

Dennis Smythe: How dare you sneak behind my back and discuss our personal lives with your father! Exactly what did you say to him?

June Smythe: When he asked me if we were having problems conceiving a child, I told him we rarely had relations.

Dennis: You little Benedict Arnold. Your father probably thinks that there is something wrong with me. He probably thinks that I am impotent or sterile, or something like that. Not that you are a fat, unresponsive sow! I will never, never trust you again. I can't believe that you would stab me in the back like that!

To June's astonishment, that night Dennis had sex with her. In fact, over the next 2 months they had more sex than they had had, cumulatively, during their 4-year marriage. June was well aware that Dennis did not show her affection or communicate intimate feelings during their intercourse, nor at other times. Ground down by his constant criticism and belittling of her, June accepted what she received. She did not feel that she deserved more. June was thus overjoyed when she became pregnant, at which point sexual relations with her husband stopped. Nevertheless, June held out the hope that a child would bring them closer together. However, the only aspect of her pregnancy and planning for the new baby about which Dennis showed interest was in the naming: if the baby turned out to be a boy, Dennis insisted that he be named Martin, after Mr. Greer. When Martin was born, Dennis was in New York City on business. He did not return home to see his wife and new son for three weeks. Rather, he sent a large bouquet of flowers to June at the hospital, but there was no accompanying note. Nor did he call June to ask her how she and the baby were faring. Dennis did not participate in caring for his new son: he never changed a diaper, never helped with a feeding, never arose at night when the baby was crying. The only times that Dennis would hold infant Martin was when there was company at the home, particularly his in-laws.

Success in Business

If Dennis had deficiencies in his family relationships, no such problems were perceived with regard to his effort and accomplishments in the family business. He concentrated all of his waking hours on his work. Highly personable, facile with words, handsome, and a fine athlete (he became excellent at golf), Dennis was rapidly recognized as a "natural" in sales and public relations for the gigantic corporation. Both of them being engineers, Mr. Greer and Mr. Gallagher were responsible for the technical operations of their expanding mining, milling, and manufacturing empire, and Dennis steadily assumed the leadership and control over marketing and promoting their products and the acquisition of new businesses. The aging founders of the company were considered "Misters Inside," and Dennis Smythe became known as "Mr. Outside." Through leadership in charities and community service, he represented the company in the many cities across America in which they had mines or factories and did business. Dennis was particularly adept in establishing positive relations with prominent elected government officials, and this resulted in lucrative contracts with the government and reduced the interference from costly environmental and labor regulations. During the initial 15 years that Dennis was involved in the family business, its net worth and profits increased more than fivefold; much of this success was attributed to Dennis Smythe's promotional efforts and business skills. By the time he was in his early thirties, Dennis was widely known and acknowledged as one of the America's most powerful young businessmen.

One aspect of Dennis's business activities that was of great concern to June was his relationship with her younger brother, Alex. Like his father, Alex was gifted in mathematics and science. He was graduated valedictorian of his class from Nutrier High School, a highly regarded and competitive public school that serves Chicago's affluent northern suburbs. At the Massachusetts Institute of Technology, Alex continued to distinguish himself in his dual major in chemistry and physics. In light of the highly technical nature of the family business, Alex would have been an extraordinary asset. However, Dennis discouraged Alex from working in any of the many industries that the family business owned.

> **Dennis Smythe (to Alex Gallagher):** Don't make the same mistake that I did by getting involved from the very beginning in a business owned by your family. By nature, people are envious and competitive. Throughout the company, I'm given a hard time by all the middle level and senior management who are jealous of my access to your father and Mr. Greer. It has been an uphill struggle for me the whole time that I've been here. The outside world discredits all of my accomplishments by saying that I owe my success to being the son-in-law of the boss. It would be even worse for you. I think you will have a much better life if you take a Ph.D. in physics and pursue an academic life. You certainly don't have to worry about money.

Dennis had different advice for Mr. Greer and Mr. Gallagher:

> **Dennis Smythe:** I have spoken with Alex, and he doesn't seem to have a passion for business. I think all those eggheads at MIT got to him, and he thinks that the practical work that we do here is be-

neath him. Because he lacks a real interest in business and a "fire in his belly" to succeed here, I think we would be making a mistake to encourage Alex to join the business. His working for us would be bad for the morale of our workforce, especially at the leadership levels. They respect me because of how hard I work and what I have accomplished. With Alex, they would worry that the company is getting too inbred and that there is a glass ceiling of opportunity for everybody but family members.

Alex was not offered a position in the family business. On the advice of his father and brother-in-law, Alex pursued a Ph.D. in theoretical physics at Cal Tech, where he excelled and was later granted a position on the faculty. June Gallagher Smythe, who was privy to these interchanges from conversations with her father and her brother, believed that her husband deliberately discouraged Alex to eliminate the competition of a family member with vastly superior intellect and integrity. Although she chose not to confront her husband or her father on the decision to exclude her brother from the business (and ultimately from leadership of the business), her eyes became opened to the deviousness and dishonesty of her husband.

Found Out

June Smythe's willingness and motivation to consider and confront the deficiencies of her husband developed gradually. First, she was horrified that Dennis had manipulated her father and brother to advance his own ambitions in business. Second, her self-confidence and self-esteem improved in her new role as mother. Three years after the birth of their son, Martin, June and Dennis were blessed with a daughter, Millie. Dennis Smythe was no more involved with his new daughter than he had been his son. On the other hand, June was wholly devoted to her children and to other children who were less advantaged than her own. She became involved—through personal service and through directing her family's substantial charitable foundation—in a variety of community activities: school boards, libraries, reading programs, cultural enrichment programs, medical services for pregnant women and children, and many other philanthropies. Coincident with June's accomplishments and recognition in the Chicago region as a selfless, intelligent, reliable, and effective public servant was the emergence of a sense of purpose and self-regard. To protect her children's interests and her philanthropic involvements, June, for the first time, became interested in her family's finances. Because Dennis would never discuss business issues with her, June arranged meetings with her father and the family attorneys and accountants. With dogged persistence she was alarmed to discover that Dennis was gradually assuming control, not only of the business, but also of the family's immense fortune. On the death of her father, Dennis was to assume control over the family trusts, including the powerful charitable foundation of which June had become administrative director. Realizing that her husband was too important to the family business for her to confront without cause, June began to collect data about what she considered her husband's deficiencies of character and honesty. The following is a summary of the data that she collected and *recollected* about Dennis over the 16 years of their relationship.

Dennis Smythe overstated his accomplishments.   **Exaggerated academic accomplishments.**   June had long recognized that her husband stretched the truth about his background and achievements. For example, when she first met him, Dennis had told her that he was the captain of his college baseball team, that he was an all-conference player, and that he had received Academic All-American honors as a baseball player. At the time, June had no reason to doubt Dennis, because many of his other striking accomplishments—such as being president of his senior class— turned out to be true. In retrospect she noted many inconsistencies between what he told her he had achieved and objective confirmation. She recalled sending him a letter when she was junior at Smith College in which she mentioned that she had been elected to Phi Beta Kappa. In his next letter, he told her that he was also a member of Phi Beta Kappa and that he had been told that he would be graduated summa cum laude. But at Dennis's graduation, June saw no indication in the graduation program that he had been awarded either Phi Beta Kappa membership or any academic honors (as there was for others so honored). At the time, she just assumed that these were typographical omissions in the program, and she didn't mention the matter to Dennis or think about it further. She had a copy of Dennis's formal résumé that he had submitted to the family foundation when he was made a member of its board of trustees—a résumé that had also been used for his successful candidacy for the prestigious Chicago chapter of the Young Presidents' Organization. In his résumé Dennis indicated that he had been graduated summa cum laude, but there was no mention of his being a member of Phi Beta Kappa. June theorized that Dennis knew that it was far easier to check out membership in Phi Beta Kappa, which publishes lists of members in local regions, than to find out about honors bestowed in college. Among the other college honors that Dennis mentioned was serving as captain of the college baseball team and being named Academic All-American in baseball. Through her library connections June was able to obtain a copy of the college yearbook for the year that Dennis graduated. The yearbook revealed many inconsistencies with his résumé and with what June had heard him say to her and others over the years. He did not appear in the group photograph of members of Phi Beta Kappa, nor was his name among the list of members. He was in fact included in the photograph of the baseball team; however, the captain and co-captain of the team were designated, and he was neither. The statement accompanying his senior picture was very long, and it included both significant ("president of senior class") and less significant ("pledge master of fraternity") accomplishments. The write-up was notable for what it did *not* include: no mention of any academic honors.

Exaggerated business accomplishments.   Over the years June had realized that Dennis bragged about his contributions to the family business. She first noticed that he changed the title of his position according to whom he was speaking with. When he first began working in the finance office he had no official title, but he would tell people whom he wished to impress that he functioned in the role of "special assistant to the vice president for finance." At the time, he was 22 years old. As the years went by and as Dennis rose through the ranks, June would bridle when he would take complete credit for the success of the company and belittle the contributions of coworkers; of her father, Mr. Gallagher; and even of his faithful sponsor, Mr. Greer. Although he was respectful and subservient to the point of obsequiousness when dealing face-to-face with the two founders of the business, on occasions when he was around prominent businessmen of his own generation, Dennis would refer to the founders as "antiques" or "conservative dinosaurs." On such occasions he would refer to June's family business as "my company."

Although June's father and Mr. Greer always kept a low profile, Dennis persuaded them to invest in extravagant perks such as private airplanes, elaborate corporate suites in professional sports stadia, and plush executive apartments in luxury resort condominiums. He delighted hosting, at great expense, important people such as famous professional athletes, well-known entertainers, and influential politicians. However, he rarely invited his wife or children to join him at ball games or concerts, or even on the lavish trips and vacations that he took. At the same time, he was not at all charitable, and he would become enraged when he learned that June had donated large sums of her family foundation money for college scholarships for inner-city students or to support medical care and research for children with severe and persistent medical and psychiatric illnesses such as cancer and schizophrenia. Dennis's charitable donations mostly constituted of large donations to politicians, with the bulk of the funds coming from Gallagher Industries or from money that he raised on their behalf from other people.

Dennis Smythe feigned humility.   When June first met Dennis when they were in college, she believed him to be modest and humble. Although he was excessive in his efforts to take care of her (e.g., picking her up at the airport in a limousine, making sure that she was served the types of food that she preferred), he seemed to go out of his way to minimize his own efforts and achievements. Often using expressions like "it was nothing" or "it was the least that I could do," Dennis would never accept her expressions of appreciation for the great pains he took to take care of her or to make her feel special. When discussing his election to the presidency of his senior class in college, he would say such things as "I won because of a sympathy vote for a poor farm boy," or "I was just lucky," or "I think everyone checked the wrong box on the voting form." When others would compliment him on the completion of a project or product that clearly took great time and effort, he would deflect their praise by saying things such as "Just part of my job," or "you are thanking the wrong guy. The staff did all of the work." The net result was that Dennis was undeniably charming and made a powerful and positive first impression. As she got to know him better over the years, however, June began to notice behaviors—and particularly *the absence of behaviors*—that raised her doubts about his humility and genuineness. Although he almost never praised his wife or children, he would fish for compliments for himself. For example, when getting dressed up for an important social event, he would say, "Don't you think this suit makes me look old and fat?" Because Dennis was tall, handsome, in great physical shape, and had his suits custom made from the finest fabrics by the best tailor in Chicago, June and the children would honestly respond with comments as "You look wonderful. You could be a leading man in the movies." As he rose in the business, every year he would deliberate over the choice of photographs of him that would appear in the company's annual report. He would personally see to it that pictures of him with famous people would be inserted in prominent places in the report and was careful to ensure that his photograph was of equal size and on the same level as those of Mr. Gallagher and Mr. Greer. He loved having his name and picture in business magazines and newspapers. He was so self-promoting that an inside joke in the very large public relations department of the business was that their department's official name should be changed to "private relations."

Dennis Smythe was dependent, but he espoused self-sufficiency.   Although June did almost everything in the household (including taking care of all child-related responsibilities, maintaining the home, paying the bills, and planning vacations), Dennis believed himself to be entirely self-sufficient and low maintenance. Never at a loss for gratuitous self-effacing comments (e.g., "Don't worry about me;" "Take care of yourselves, I'll be fine"), he nonetheless expected that his needs be taken care of before those of others. Although he would not come home for dinner at a designated time (and often would eat elsewhere without notifying June that he would not be home), he would be petulant and angry if his meal were not ready to be served the moment he arrived. June became an expert in preparing gourmet-quality meals for Dennis that could be reheated quickly without diminishing their tastiness. He would never compliment his wife on a great meal that he obviously enjoyed, but on the occasions that he did not care for the culinary fare, he would be highly critical of June. He would say, "I work like a dog all day and can't expect to come home to a decent meal. You don't work, have all the help in the world, and can't get it together to have a good dinner for me."

From the very start of their marriage, all of the family purchases and living expenses came from June's personal trust funds. This included the large expenses such as paying for their fine new house, their automobiles, and their vacation home, as well as smaller sums such as the costs of going out to dinner or buying gasoline. Funds placed in savings for their children's future needs—college tuitions, weddings, and the like—all came from June's accounts. Dennis deposited the entirety of his salary and investment income into his personal accounts, to which June had no access. Between his expense account from work and June's paying for all family-related costs, Dennis literally had no expenses other than paying taxes. He even tried to persuade June to pay his taxes, but June's accountant countermanded this scheme. He expressed envy and antipathy for June's great wealth and would say, "Other than being born to the right parents, what did you ever do to deserve all your money? I have to slave for every penny that I make, and all you have to worry about is how to spend it."

Dennis Smythe wished to be regarded by others as brilliant and principled, but he lacked intellectual depth and a social conscience. Almost from the time that she first learned to read, one of June Smythe's great passions in life was reading great literature. Well aware of her love for the well-written word when he was courting June in college, Dennis presented himself as if he were also an enthusiastic and dedicated reader. He immersed himself in the works of the poet Emily Dickinson, the subject of June Smythe's honors English thesis. June recalled that many of his ideas about Dickinson's work and his critiques of her thesis were thoughtful and creative. Once they were married, however, June never again saw him read a poem or work of fiction. In fact, Dennis rarely read anything other than the sports, business, and society sections of the local newspapers and business magazines. On occasion, he would read parts of biographies written by contemporary scions of industry, but he rarely completed these. He liked movies and watched what June considered to be a great deal of television. He was particularly interested in shows about entertainment and celebrities. With intended irony, June disclosed that a show that he never missed was called "Lifestyles of the Rich and Famous." June marveled, however, about how well-read Dennis sounded. She could not recall anyone ever asking him if he had read a certain book or a play when her husband did not reply, "Yes." Dennis would then ask that person several questions about the book before expressing his own opinions and insights. For the first years of their marriage, Dennis was so convincing in his responses that many times June would ask him, "Do you recommend that I read the book?" or "May I have the book when you are finished reading it?" Only much later did she understand that Dennis was prevaricating about his reading to appear as if he were a well-informed intellectual. A summary of what June recognized as deficiencies in her husband's personality, character, and behavior is presented in Table 5–1.

Dennis Smythe was self-centered and lacked compassion and empathy.   One evening during her pregnancy with their second child, June had the sudden onset of copious vaginal bleeding. Her hemorrhaging began just when Dennis was about to leave their home in the suburbs to attend his first meeting of the Young Presidents' Organization, which was being held in downtown Chicago. He had arranged for the company limousine to pick him up and take him to the meeting. When June told Dennis that she was bleeding and needed to go to the hospital right away, the following conversation ensued:

> **Dennis Smythe:** Are you telling me that you want me to take you to the hospital? That will mean that I will be late for the most important meeting in my life.
> **June Smythe:** All I am asking is that you have the car take me to Evanston General Hospital. I am hemorrhaging and am afraid that I will lose our baby.
> **Dennis:** Dropping you off at the hospital will take us at least 20 minutes out of our way, if we are lucky with the traffic. You are overreacting again. You are so neurotic when you are pregnant. There is no real need to make me late for my meeting. You can either drive yourself or call a cab. I really don't have time for your selfish, hysterical nonsense. Are you too dumb to realize how important this meeting is for us?

TABLE 5–1. Dennis Smythe's deficiencies in character, personality, and behavior as recognized over time by his wife, June Gallagher Smythe

1. Dennis was preoccupied with appearances and constantly strove to impress people.

2. Dennis would change information and tell lies to appear knowledgeable and to gain people's admiration.

3. Dennis was such an excellent and convincing extemporaneous speaker that by lying and changing facts he was able to appear as if he knew a great deal more about nearly every subject than was truly the case.

4. Dennis wished to be thought of as "cultured," but he was not interested in perusing Chicago's many great art and science museums or attending performances of its outstanding opera and fine symphony orchestra.

5. In public Dennis would act as if he were deeply concerned about helping people who were downtrodden or who had experienced discrimination. However, among his closest friends he would be dismissive of people who were disadvantaged, whom he termed "the dregs of society" and "parasitic drains on my tax dollars."

6. In business presentations and public addresses, Dennis would emphasize the importance of values, particularly honesty; respect for others; prioritization of family; and the importance of spirituality, self-reliance, and community service. Dennis evidenced none of these values in business or in his personal life. He rarely attended church and never prayed at home, and all family charity contributions came from June's personal foundation money.

Dennis left for his important meeting in the company limousine. June called her next-door neighbor, who dropped what she was doing and drove her to Evanston General Hospital. June recalled hoping, for a brief moment on the trip to the hospital, that something was seriously wrong with her so that, somehow, she could get through to the feelings, empathy, and compassion of her husband. Instantly, June recoiled in horror as she realized that such a wish would jeopardize the viability of her unborn child. (Importantly, she did not even consider her own safety and value until my discussion of this event with her some 40 years later.) That moment was a turning point in June's life, because she accepted for the first time the probability that her husband was incapable of true empathy or altruism. Precipitated by her deep love for her unborn child, June became nauseated as a wave of recognition of the depths and intractability of Dennis's self-centered exploitation, entitlement, and emotional coldness flooded over her. June then made a vow to herself that if she survived this medical emergency, she would take direct steps to change her relationship with Dennis or leave him.

It turned out that the bleeding, although of considerable medical concern, did not immediately threaten June or her fetus. After her emergency hospital evaluation she was sent home for 2 weeks' bed rest. Dennis did not call June or the hospital to find out if she was safe. When he returned from his meeting late that night and learned that June was in no acute danger, he said the following to her: "See, I told you that you were overreacting and that there was nothing to worry about. If you had listened to me in the first place, you could have avoided all of this hassle." Dennis did not ask his wife how she was feeling or if the fetus had been endangered by the bleeding.

June Gallagher Smythe Makes Efforts to Improve Her Relationship With Dennis Smythe

Making Changes

For more than 10 years June Smythe had been trying hard to please her husband. She reasoned that if they were to relate better to each other, it was important for her to respond to Dennis's many criticisms of her. Because he constantly criticized her about her weight and appearance, she went on a strict diet and began a vigorous exercise program. Even though June reduced her weight to its lowest level since she was in junior high school, Dennis never once complimented her on how much better she looked. Rather, he began to criticize how she fixed her hair and how she dressed. June responded by working with consultants to help her improve her makeup, hairdo, and wardrobe. Although June was pleased with the changes she had made in her appearance, Dennis did not seem to notice.

Sharing Interests

June had long recognized that Dennis did not share her avocational passions for reading, music, the fine arts, and charitable activities. Dennis was very active and involved with politics at the state and national levels. However, the political issues, philosophy, and party that Dennis championed were at the very opposite end of the political spectrum from those supported by June. She chose to look at recreational activities as a source of common ground in their marriage. She also reasoned that if she were to spend recreational time with her husband it had to be on his terms. Dennis loved to hunt exotic animals in Africa, to race cars, and to play golf and tennis. Although June was not a natural athlete, she tried to take up golf and tennis. She read voluminously about the fundamentals of both sports, took daily lessons from expert coaches, and practiced, practiced, practiced. After several years of hard work, to her great surprise, she not only began to enjoy the sports but also to became proficient at the games. At first, Dennis belittled her efforts and told her that it was a waste of his time to play golf or tennis with someone at her low level. Over time, however, June became better in golf than most of the wives of his golf partners. Highly competitive and an excellent athlete, Dennis loved beating his friends in couples golf. However, when June would hit a bad shot, he would become enraged with her and belittle her publicly. It was at tennis that June particularly came to excel. On one occasion, June actually beat Dennis in a singles match comprising three sets. Rather than being happy for her, he threw down his racket, sulked off the tennis court, and refused to play tennis with her again.

Communicating

Shortly after the birth of their daughter, June disclosed to her husband that she was not happy in their marriage:

> **June Smythe:** Dennis, I would like to schedule some time with you on an ongoing basis so that we can work on our marriage.
>
> **Dennis Smythe:** If you are talking about going to see shrinks, I have never met one who isn't weird or flat-out crazy. Most of them are Jews and communists. There is nothing whatsoever wrong with me, and I would never even consider going to see one of those guys.
>
> **June:** At this point I just want to talk with you about what I perceive to be the problems in our relationship. I want to discuss with you why I am not very happy. We can decide later about how to fix the problems.
>
> **Dennis:** I don't have a problem with the relationship. If you're not happy, you're the one with the problem. If you ask me, I think you have too much time on your hands. You have nothing else to do, so you make problems for yourself.

June chose not to respond defensively to her husband's devaluation of her responsibilities for caring for the children and running the household but instead replied,

> **June:** Aren't you even interested in what I think are the problems in our marriage?

> **Dennis:** Not really, June. I am too busy a man to listen to your pointless whining. If you have a problem, just fix it. If you're not happy, find some way to make yourself happy. As I said before, I don't have any problem with our relationship. And I really don't want to discuss this any further.

June Gallagher Smythe Faces Reality

After 15 years with her husband, June finally came to accept the following facts about her marriage and about Dennis:

- Dennis had little meaningful involvement with her or their children.
- She was unhappy in her marriage.
- Her many efforts to improve herself did not benefit her relationship with Dennis.
- Dennis had no intention to work with her to improve their relationship or marriage.
- She no longer trusted, respected, or loved Dennis.

For the second time during the course of her marriage, June spoke with her father about her marital problems and what she had come to learn over the years about her husband's personality and character. She was shocked by how her father responded to her:

> **Mr. Gallagher:** June, I am terribly upset but not at all surprised by what you have just told me. In fact, I was looking for the right opportunity to speak with you about your husband. As you were, Mr. Greer and I were also taken in by Dennis, and at this very time we are in the process of trying to repair the damage that he has caused to our business.
>
> **June Smythe:** What do you mean, Daddy? I always thought that Dennis was a great asset to the business.
>
> **Mr. Gallagher:** At first he seemed to be a hard worker and a responsible person. When Dennis first joined the company, our business had many opportunities to expand through mergers with and purchase of similar industries. Dennis proved to be excellent in the marketing, selling, and public relations work that was associated with this growth. However, as he assumed more responsibility and authority, he became increasingly reckless with his accounting and accountability. We are just now learning that he has overstated the profitability of many of the companies and products that are in his line of responsibility. Worse, he has utilized accounting methodologies that he terms "innovative and progressive" but that we believe might be unlawful. Initially, we used a large accounting firm to audit the entire company. Based on the concerns raised by the auditors about Dennis's areas of responsi-

bility, we called in another group of consultants to conduct a second, more intensive review of that part of our business that is under his management authority.

A summary of the principal conclusions of the initial audit by the accounting firm, as June recalled them, was as follows:

- The 14 divisions of Gallagher Industries that were under the authority of Dennis Smythe had, over the past 10 years, overstated their earnings by more than $500 million.
- A variety of unconventional accounting practices and legal transactions were used by Dennis to overestimate earnings, transfer expenses, and hide losses.
- Several dummy corporations had been set up by Dennis Smythe that had not been reported to Mr. Gallagher or to Mr. Greer. These corporations evidenced "self-dealing" at best—with the possibility of Dennis receiving illegal off-the-books kickbacks for granting construction contracts and for special inventory purchases.

Mr. Gallagher told June that when Dennis learned that a second audit would be conducted concentrating on the areas of Gallagher Industries under his administrative responsibility, he became angry and uncooperative. He hired his own attorneys and threatened to sue Gallagher Industries "if my reputation is in any way tarnished by this witch hunt." This second audit confirmed the findings of the previous consultants and also uncovered numerous other areas of "malfeasance and serious concern." In the course of their investigation, the consultants spoke with Gallagher employees at all levels and concluded that Dennis was an ineffective manager and a poor leader. The behaviors and values that I believe characterize managers and leaders with narcissistic personality disorder are summarized in Table 5–2; most of these behaviors and values were exhibited by Dennis Smythe.

Mr. Gallagher told June that he and Mr. Greer had informed Dennis that they would terminate his employment with Gallagher Industries. Her father indicated that Dennis at first responded by approaching their business competitors in search of a prestigious job. Dennis told them that he could lure large and lucrative contracts away from Gallagher Industries to their companies. What Dennis did not realize is that the leadership and boards of the competitive companies whom he had approached had long, respectful, and trusting relationships with Mr. Gallagher and Mr. Greer. However, they did not trust Dennis Smythe nor did they appreciate his many years of putting down their compa-

TABLE 5–2. Twenty common characteristics of narcissistic managers

1. They value loyalty in their subordinates more than competence or productivity.

2. They overestimate their own knowledge about nearly every area of the business or organization.

3. They do not appreciate the important contributions of others.

4. They take personal credit for the accomplishments of others.

5. They are competitive with and threatened by peers and competent managers.

6. They micromanage competent subordinates in areas in which they themselves have little expertise.

7. They insist on making all decisions—even minor ones—themselves, often with insufficient information about and understanding of the relevant issues.

8. They overstate their own and the organization's successes—to the point of bragging.

9. They never admit to making mistakes.

10. They blame others for their own mistakes and failures.

11. They distrust, intimidate, or fire subordinates who make independent decisions or raise concerns about their questionable decisions or business practices.

12. They surround themselves with "insiders" who constantly praise and never disagree with them.

13. They do not mentor their subordinates or advance their careers.

14. They pursue highly visible (i.e., flashy) short-term successes at the expense of supporting solid, long-range strategic plans.

15. They misappropriate the organization's resources for their personal benefit and self-aggrandizement.

16. They devalue and underestimate the achievements of competitors in similar businesses or enterprises.

17. They miss out on important opportunities by not recognizing their own lack of knowledge in some areas.

18. They display great deference toward and respect for their superiors to their faces yet criticize, devalue, and undermine them behind their backs.

19. They respond to constructive criticism of their work with anger, defensiveness, and thoughts or acts of retribution.

20. They prioritize their own ambitions for advancement over the needs of the organization.

nies when competing for business. Finally, Dennis accepted a termination agreement with a modest compensation package. Mr. Gallagher and Mr. Greer agreed not to prosecute Dennis for or attempt to recoup the personal fortune that he had accumulated as a result of his illegal activities at Gallagher Industries.

For the first time, June confided to her father that Dennis was not an involved, dependable, or trustworthy husband or father. She revealed to Mr. Gallagher that she had concluded that she was not able to please her husband and that long ago she had ceased blaming herself for all of the problems in their relationship. Mr. Gallagher told June that he would understand and support her if she decided to divorce her husband. He also advised his daughter on the selection of an attorney who would help protect her considerable financial assets from Dennis, whom he now considered to be avaricious and dishonest.

The Divorce

Dennis Smythe's Demands

Before June had an opportunity to consult an attorney, Dennis Smythe filed for a divorce and moved out of their house. He gave June no advance warning of his taking such an action and would communicate with June only through his attorney after she had been served with the divorce action. June soon learned that Dennis had hired a lawyer who was notorious in Chicago for seeking outrageously inflated settlements for his clients and for using the most unsavory tactics to prevail. In his filing, Dennis accused June of "mental cruelty" that included depriving him of emotional support and refusing to engage in a sexual relationship with him. In the suit, he blamed June for "poisoning" his relationships with Mr. Greer and Mr. Gallagher, and he demanded millions of dollars in compensation and penalties for the termination of his employment with Gallagher Industries and "for damaging my reputation in the industry at large." Furthermore, he sued for the substantial increase in the value of June's estate during the years of their marriage, his rationale being that his financial advice and unique contributions in her family business accounted for the bulk of the growth in the estate. In reality, June's estate was managed by a large trust company, and Dennis had no role whatsoever in investing her personal funds or managing her trusts. What shocked June the most, however, was Dennis's contention that she was "a neglectful and unfit mother," and his suit for sole custody of their children. He cited her consultation with a child psychiatrist to help with her shyness and social anxiety during her adolescence as evidence of June's "deep-rooted psychological problems." On learning of this aspect of Dennis's divorce suit, June became panicked that she would lose her children. At that point she realized that she had long been afraid of her husband and that she believed him to be capable of nearly any cruelty or dishonesty.

June Gallagher Smythe Takes Control

After being served with divorce papers by her husband, June met with Frederick Loomis, the attorney recommended by her father.

> **June Smythe:** I know you will try to convince me to contest Dennis's financial proposals in the divorce, but I am willing to concede these in order to get custody of the children.
>
> **Mr. Loomis:** It is not so simple, Mrs. Smythe. I know the modus operandi of your husband's attorney very well. He is a dangerous man. First answer this question: Do you really think that Dennis is really interested in gaining full custody of the children? Or is this a tactic to get more of your money?
>
> **June:** Dennis has never shown any tangible interest in our children or in being with them. He doesn't attend their school performances, their parent-teacher meetings, or their birthday parties or even ask about them when he has been away for months on business trips. He has never made any effort to take care of them in any way. He does not join us on vacations, and he spends very little time with them when he is at home.
>
> **Mr. Loomis:** That answers my question. He is using the children for leverage to get at your assets. Once his attorney realizes that this strategy is working—that you will agree to almost anything in order to gain custody of your children—there will be no end to the demands.
>
> **June:** I don't care about the money. The only thing I care about is my children. I must protect them from their father.
>
> **Mr. Loomis:** If you want to protect your children and yourself, you will have to listen to me and follow my advice. And the very first thing that I want to do is to find out everything I can about the extra-familial, personal life of your husband. In my experience, husbands don't just walk away from their families without other things going on.

At the urging of her father, June agreed to follow the counsel of Mr. Loomis, who hired a team of private detectives to learn anything they could about Dennis's personal life when he was away from his family. Toward that purpose, Mr. Loomis subpoenaed Dennis's credit card records going back 15 years, records of his cell phone calls going back 10 years (all of which were Gallagher Industries property, since his cell phone was paid for by them), bank account statements, personal investments, and real estate holdings. What was learned about Dennis was shocking. The private detectives uncovered that from the first year of their marriage, Dennis had been unfaithful to June. He had many affairs, including with several female employees of Gallagher Industries who were under his administrative authority, acts in direct violation of company policy. The detectives also discovered that he had set up domestic relations with one of these employees—a lobbyist living in Washington, D.C.—and they had two young children together. Furthermore, this relationship had not stopped Dennis from having affairs with other women. Dennis had also amassed a personal fortune, far more than could be accounted for by his generous salary from Gallagher Industries. Mr. Loomis's team uncovered firm evidence of what the consultants to Gallagher Industries had suspected: that Dennis had committed many illegal acts involving bribes and kickbacks in exchange for lucrative contracts from suppliers to and service contractors of Gallagher Industries.

When confronted by Mr. Loomis with the detailed documentation of his infidelity, illegal behavior, and illegal acquisition of his personal assets, Dennis was enraged. He stormed over to June's home and confronted her. Although she had been instructed by Mr. Loomis to communicate with Dennis only through him, the following exchange occurred:

> **Dennis Smythe:** What are you doing? Are you trying to ruin the father of your children? Do you know what it will do to *them* if you try to have me prosecuted? I can assure you that nothing will happen to me, and I will see to it that the children are dragged into the middle of all of this. Can you imagine what it will do to them if they learn that they have a brother and sister whom they have never met? Are they are old enough to understand that? Given your mental instability, I have no choice but to fight you on all of this, unless you back down.
>
> **June Smythe:** Finally, Dennis, I am willing to stand up for myself and my children. I plan to fight you on every aspect of your divorce suit, using all the resources at my disposal. And these, as you know, are considerable. I also have every reason to believe that if the information that we have on you is made public in a divorce trial, you will be prosecuted criminally for tax evasion and racketeering. Now please leave my home, before I call my father and the police.

A few weeks later, Dennis revised the original divorce action that he brought against June. Six months later, she was awarded sole custody of their two children, and there was no financial settlement.

Dennis Smythe Goes to Congress

The Campaign

Dennis Smythe had long been active in state and federal politics. At the time of his leaving Gallagher Industries, he worked in his party to contest the incumbent congressman in his district who belonged to the competing political party. Dennis proved to be a gifted and formidable campaigner: he had appealing looks, was an excellent speaker, could connect with an audience, could think on his feet, and was charming in personal and group interactions. He had also made many powerful political allies over the years through generous financial contributions (mostly from Gallagher Industries) to his political party. In addition, he loved talking about himself and his business accomplishments and was comfortable making lofty promises about what he would do for the people in his district. He portrayed himself as follows to a crowd of voters during his first campaign for Congress:

> **Dennis Smythe:** I know, first hand, what it means to suffer hard times, not to know if you can find a job, not to be sure if there will be enough food on your table for the children. I am from a large, poor family with humble farm roots, so I also know what it means to work hard for everything you get. I remember working three jobs throughout high school in order that my family would have food on our table. Unlike my opponent, who was born rich and who attended fancy private schools, I had nothing handed to me. I know only too well what a dollar means. Having gone to a state school on a baseball scholarship, the first in my family to attend college, I appreciate what it means to have strong, well-supported state schools for the children in our state who are willing to work hard and make the best use of these tax dollars. By the way, I don't believe in wasting your tax dollars on kids who aren't willing to work as hard as you did when you earned that money. I know the manufacturing business inside out. I have a record of making money in the manufacturing business, and, personally, for creating thousands of new jobs for our region. Although I know how to make a dollar in business, inside and out, my opponent has never had a job other than in government, paid for by your hard-earned tax dollars. He has no understanding of the real world. I don't believe that he has ever really worked for a living, so he doesn't know what business is all about. He doesn't know what you are all about. Having never had a real job, my opponent doesn't have the first idea about what it means to be laid off from work. I have worked all of my life; and I have been out of work, too. I remember all too well how it feels to be hungry and not to know where my next dime is coming from. I will use this hunger

> and the vivid memory of being unemployed to spur me on to work tirelessly on your behalf to bring new jobs to our community.

As someone always concerned about what people thought of him and as a person who was not fearful about treating his opponent unfairly, Dennis Smythe turned out to be a natural at getting people to like him, to believe in him, and to support his candidacy. In his first election he defeated the incumbent by a large margin.

Dennis Smythe as a Congressman

Dennis did not arrive in Washington, D.C., without knowing many people in influential positions. At Gallagher Industries he had lobbied representatives and senators for large government contracts, and he had treated key people very generously at company expense. As he had done with June Gallagher two decades before, he courted the representatives who were in the best position to advance his career. By almost every measure, Dennis Smythe was a successful politician. He managed to get appointed to committees that enabled him to cut deals that further increased his power and influence. Dennis did many favors for his constituents (and for the local political leaders in his party), and he was skilled in using the local and national media to enhance his image. He never stopped campaigning, and he was reelected every 2 years by steadily increasing margins.

In tandem with his growing power and influence was his confidence and sense of entitlement. He viewed himself as having made great personal and financial sacrifices to serve the public. He once told his son, Martin, "I could have made much more money and had a much easier life as an executive in business; but instead, I have dedicated my life to help out my fellow man." However, very few business executives manage to amass a greater fortune than did Dennis Smythe. After he had been in Congress for many years, an investigative reporter for a local newspaper in Dennis's district wrote a series of articles on the financial holdings and investments of Congressman Smythe. First of all, his constituents who heard Dennis speak so frequently about his humble farm roots on the Illinois prairie were shocked that their congressman was one of the wealthiest people in their state. The vast proportion of his holdings were managed by a blind trust, but they were also in investments that could directly affected by decisions made by committees that he influenced or information to which he had access. The reporter also uncovered that Dennis led a lavish lifestyle, often traveling at government expense to resort areas of uncertain economic or strategic value to the United States. He also reported that Congressman Smythe was an inveterate womanizer who had made out-of-court settlements with several female government workers who had at one time been on his payroll. Not only was Congressman Smythe never prosecuted for any of the unsavory dealings and putative indiscretions revealed by the reporter, but he was reelected during the next congressional cycle by an even larger margin.

DSM Diagnosis of Congressman Dennis Smythe

My first knowledge of Dennis Smythe came from historical information offered by his son, Reverend Martin Smythe, whom I was evaluating and treating for sexual transgressions among his parishioners (see Chapter 6, "Narcissistic Personality Disorder, Part II: Treated Narcissism"). Many details from Reverend Martin Smythe's account of his relationship with his father raised my diagnostic suspicion that the congressman had narcissistic personality disorder. Among the most characteristic behaviors were Dennis Smythe's elevated sense of self-importance; his bottomless need for admiration—even from his children when they were very young; his lack of involvement with or empathy for his son or wife; his exaggeration of his accomplishments; and his exploitation of Martin's mother and other members of the Gallagher family. These suspicions were further confirmed by my direct observations during four sessions when he met with me during my care for his son. During those meetings, Congressman Smythe would not accept that his behavior—including the virtual abandonment of his wife and children—had any bearing on his son's psychological problems. He told me the following:

> **Congressman Smythe:** I do not subscribe to the psychiatric notion that all problems should be blamed on the parents. When Martin was growing up, I was working like a dog to support my family. I can tell you without reservation that the Gallagher family business would have gone under if it were not for my accomplishments there. In addition, Doctor, I will not apologize for working equally hard in the service of my country as a congressman. Martin had every conceivable advantage—most of it made possible by my generosity. If he has gotten himself into trouble he has no one but himself to blame. As a congressman, I have traveled to Third World countries, where children starve and have no access to education or medical care. I refuse to feel sorry or take the blame for my son, who had every conceivable advantage.

The extensive history provided by June Smythe helped to confirm that Congressman Smythe had narcissistic personality disorder. His self-serving behavior, his exploitation of June Smythe and her father, his feelings of entitlement, his pursuit of powerful people and personal power, his overestimation of his own accomplishments, his devaluation of other people, and his sense of being special and deserving special considerations are prototypical of people with this personality disorder. Summarized in Table 5–3 are the DSM-IV-TR diagnostic criteria for narcissistic personality disorder (American Psychiatric Association 2000); presented in Table 5–4 are key principles of narcissistic personality disorder as exemplified by the psychiatric history of Dennis Smythe.

TABLE 5–3. Diagnostic criteria for narcissistic personality disorder (slightly modified from DSM-IV-TR)

A pervasive pattern of grandiosity (in fantasy or behavior), need for admiration, and lack of empathy, beginning by early adulthood and present in a variety of contexts, as indicated by five (or more) of the following:

1. A grandiose sense of self-importance (e.g., exaggerates achievements and talents, expects to be recognized as superior without commensurate achievements)

2. A preoccupation with fantasies of unlimited success, power, brilliance, beauty, or ideal love

3. The belief that he or she is "special" and unique and can only be understood by, or should associate with, other special or high-status people (or institutions)

4. A requirement for excessive admiration

5. A sense of entitlement, that is, unreasonable expectations of especially favorable treatment or automatic compliance with his or her expectations

6. Interpersonal exploitiveness, that is, taking advantage of others to achieve his or her own ends

7. Lack of empathy: is unwilling to recognize or identify with the feelings and needs of others

8. Enviousness of others or belief that others are envious of him or her

9. Arrogant, haughty behaviors or attitudes

Source. Adapted from American Psychiatric Association: *Diagnostic and Statistical Manual of Mental Disorders,* 4th Edition, Text Revision. Washington, DC, American Psychiatric Association, 2000, p 717.

TABLE 5–4.   Key principles of narcissistic personality disorder as exemplified by the case of Dennis Smythe

Historical fact	Key principle	Interpretation
Dennis Smythe received little parental attention or emotional nurturing.	People with narcissistic personality disorder are often emotionally neglected by their parents.	A likely source of Dennis Smythe's low self-esteem was his parental neglect.
Dennis Smythe demonstrated neither gratitude nor loyalty to people who trusted him or advanced his career. Examples include Mr. Greer, June Gallagher, and Mr. Gallagher.	People with narcissistic personality disorder feel entitled to special consideration from others.	Dennis Smythe was fundamentally too insecure to acknowledge that he required or benefited from the help of others.
Dennis Smythe overstated his accomplishments in college, in business, and in his personal life.	People with narcissistic personality disorder persistently inflate the level of their abilities and achievements.	No personal achievement was sufficient to bolster Dennis Smythe's impaired self-worth.
Dennis Smythe was attracted to the wealth and power of June Gallagher and her family.	People with narcissistic personality disorder seek to align themselves with people and institutions of wealth and power.	Dennis Smythe tried to offset his deep-seated feelings of social insecurity and financial impotence though marrying June Gallagher.
During their courtship, Dennis Smythe treated June thoughtfully and respectfully.	People with narcissistic personality disorder are at their very best when selling themselves.	Dennis Smythe did not experience June Gallagher as a person but rather as a commodity that would advance his ambitions.

TABLE 5–4. Key principles of narcissistic personality disorder as exemplified by the case of Dennis Smythe *(continued)*

Historical fact	Key principle	Interpretation
As a young woman, June was naïve, inexperienced, and trusting.	People with narcissistic personality disorder characteristically seek out and exploit vulnerable people whom they believe can advance their needs and ambitions.	The combination of June Gallagher's great personal wealth and naïveté made her attractive prey for the predatory Dennis Smythe.
At work, Dennis Smythe was obsequious with and ingratiating to Mr. Greer and Mr. Gallagher while belittling the employees who reported to him.	People with narcissistic personality disorder experience people as objects to be exploited in gratification of their own needs and ambitions.	At an unconscious level, Dennis Smythe did not value himself; he thus was not capable of forming intimate and respectful relationships with others.
Dennis Smythe took the credit for the work and accomplishments of others.	People with narcissistic personality disorder are envious of others and feel entitled to their intellectual and material property.	Dennis Smythe's low self-esteem constituted a bottomless pit that he tried to fill through measurable accomplishments and material possessions that would lead to the admiration of others.
Dennis Smythe fired the employees who questioned his business decisions or caught on to his dishonesty.	People with narcissistic personality disorder are threatened by and become enraged with people who disagree with them or (especially) those who catch on to their dishonesty.	Because he had violated so many ethical standards, Dennis Smythe tried to devalue or destroy all those who understood his character flaws.

TABLE 5–4. Key principles of narcissistic personality disorder as exemplified by the case of Dennis Smythe (*continued*)

Historical fact	Key principle	Interpretation
Dennis Smythe had little interest in his wife, his children, cultural activities, or charities.	People with narcissistic personality disorder have little capacity for altruistic involvements, compassion, or empathy.	Dennis Smythe was devoted to taking care of himself. He displayed personal or social concerns only when it made him look better to others.
In public, Dennis Smythe made a point of appearing humble and deflecting praise.	People with narcissistic personality disorder try to hide—publicly, and often from themselves—their fathomless needs for praise and credit.	So deep-seated was his insecurity and desire for admiration that Dennis Smythe feigned discomfort and humility when he was favorably recognized.
Although he achieved material and social success through the exploitation of his wife, her family, and his employees, Dennis Smythe thought of himself as being independent and self-sufficient.	People with narcissistic personality disorder are threatened by being perceived as dependent or needy.	For Dennis Smythe to acknowledge his need for, dependency on, or benefit from others would resonate too closely with his unconscious feelings of emptiness and low self-worth.
June Gallagher Smythe's attempts to communicate better with her husband or improve their relationship were unsuccessful.	When people with narcissistic personality disorder have problems in relationships, they blame the other party. They do not see a need to change themselves in any way.	Honest communication, acknowledging the rights and values of others, and accepting that he had made mistakes would threaten Dennis Smythe's unconscious feelings of low self-worth and his behavioral compensations for them.

TABLE 5–4.   Key principles of narcissistic personality disorder as exemplified by the case of Dennis Smythe (*continued*)

Historical fact	Key principle	Interpretation
When confronted by June Gallagher, her father, and Mr. Greer with his pervasive lack of integrity, Dennis Smythe became enraged, combative, and desperate to preserve his material wealth.	There is nothing that people with narcissistic personality disorder dislike more than being found out and exposed as liars and cheats.	Since Dennis Smythe did not invest in intimate and honest relationships, he clutched at symbols of self-value—like money and material possessions—when exposed as a fraud.
Dennis Smythe used his children as pawns to gain financial advantage in his divorce proceedings with June.	People with narcissistic personality disorder will destroy friends and family to preserve their material possessions and public image.	Dennis Smythe showed no more substantive involvement with his own children than his parents did with him.
Dennis Smythe was defeated in his lawsuits with his wife and father-in-law.	People with narcissistic personality disorder often underestimate as opponents people whom they have previously deceived and exploited.	Dennis Smythe was not used to being in a confrontation with June Smythe or Mr. Gallagher where the playing field was level and the rules were fair.
By certain measures (reelections and political clout), Dennis Smythe was a successful congressman.	People with narcissistic personality disorder can have many personal assets that can lead to certain types of success.	Dennis Smythe was intelligent, hardworking, obsessed with power, ruthless, and dedicated to getting people to admire him. These traits led to a certain form of success as a politician.

Biological Aspects of Narcissistic Personality Disorder

Overview

By virtue of the work of brilliant psychoanalytically oriented clinicians and theoreticians, much has been learned about the psychological and interpersonal manifestations of narcissistic personality disorder. Far less, however, is known and understood about the biological dimensions of the disorder. In fact, much more is known about the neurobiology (i.e., the role of the brain, genetics, toxins, endocrinology, etc.) of most of the other personality disorders and psychiatric conditions considered in this book than is understood about these aspects of this personality disorder. This could mean the following:

1. The roles of life experience, stress, and psychology are more prominent in the development of narcissistic personality disorder than the biological factors.
2. At the present time, less valid research has been conducted about the biological aspects of narcissistic personality disorder than for many other personality disorders.

Although it is possible that both of the above explanations are true, I have great concern about the dearth of valid, contemporary research on the neurobiology of people with narcissistic personality disorder. Schizophrenia, panic disorder, obsessive-compulsive personality disorder, depression, and bipolar illness were all once thought to result from psychological and experiential stresses. As more was understood about the causative roles of biological factors, the treatment of people with these conditions improved dramatically. I believe that this process of discovery leading to more effective treatments will also, some day, apply to people with narcissistic personality disorder. Given the extraordinary psychological trauma that people with this condition inflict on their families and people in other important relationships with them, and given the incalculable societal costs associated with their behaviors (e.g., the large companies that fail because of the narcissism of their chief executive officers), it is hard for me to explain or understand the reasons for the relative lack of biological research on narcissistic personality disorder.

Epidemiology

Narcissistic personality disorder is diagnosed more commonly in men than in women. Approximately 1% of the general population has been found to have this disorder. Depending on the study, the condition can be found in about 10% of people with other psychiatric diagnoses. People with this disorder have exceptionally high risks of also having major depression, alcoholism, and other personality disorders such as antisocial personality disorder. It is possible that the low self-esteem commonly found in people with major depression can lead to compensatory feelings and behaviors associated with narcissistic personality disorder. It is also likely that the interpersonal and occupational failures that are common for people with this condition could, over time, lead to these other psychiatric conditions such as depression, alcoholism, and substance use disorders. Although adolescents frequently display the clinical features of narcissistic personality disorder, I do not believe that this condition should be diagnosed in people younger than age 25. The self-esteem and personality of many adolescents and young adults undergo rapid and extreme fluctuations during this period of their lives, and symptoms such as entitlement, grandiosity, and arrogance often attenuate with advancing age and maturity.

Genetics

There is an little valid research on the genetics of narcissistic personality disorder. Even though most clinicians who treat people with this disorder are struck by the tendency of the condition to run in the families of their patients, this does not necessarily mean that the disorder is inherited through genetic transmission. As was so evident in the cases of Congressman Dennis Smythe and his son, Reverend Martin Smythe (see Chapter 6, "Narcissistic Personality Disorder, Part II: Treated Narcissism"), the neglect and abuse of children by parents with narcissistic personality disorder can also lead to this disorder by a variety of means. First, for example, it is possible that a child could learn or model the dysfunctional behavior of his parent. Second, the deprivations and stress of having a parent with narcissistic personality disorder could lead to the low self-esteem that is thought by many mental health professionals to be at the root of this personality disorder. Third, several mental disorders that are known to have strong genetic predispositions (such as major depression) and are also recognized to be associated with narcissistic personality disorder could be genetically linked or inherited together. Carefully designed genetic research—such as twin studies and adoption studies—would certainly shed light on the heritability of narcissistic personality disorder, but unfortunately such studies have not yet been conducted.

The Misperception of Parental Neglect

Many people with narcissistic personality disorder have the *experience* of having been emotionally neglected by important caregivers, especially their parents, during infancy and childhood. Although this fact seems to implicate psychological and experiential dimensions in the causality of this condition, it could also be deceiving. It is possible that biological dimensions are importantly involved as well. For example, what if the parents of a child who, as an adult, develops narcissistic personality disorder are truly involved, loving, and nurturing, *but the child is unable to perceive their caring?* Is it not possible that in the same ways that certain people cannot perceive colors or are tone deaf, there are those among us who cannot register, and therefore do not benefit from, healthful parental involvement? From my clinical experience with patients with narcissistic personality disorder and their families, I believe not only that this phenomenon is possible but also that it is not rare. In addition, I believe that what I term *the misperception of parental neglect* is largely a brain-based condition. Although I could not uncover in the published literature solid research data to support this contention, it nonetheless does not seem to me to be far-fetched. Consider the symptoms of people with the common psychiatric disorder major depression—certainly an illness with fundamental biological underpinnings. People with major depression characteristically view their world through lenses that are dark, negative, and pessimistic. They feel great guilt over, experience shame about, and blame themselves for many ills of their world for which they bear little or no responsibility. If complimented by others for their real accomplishments, people with depression will neither experience satisfaction from their achievements nor accept the credit for them. Therefore, as a result of the cognitive and emotional distortions of their depression, they will deflect and not process the positive communications of others. In a recent paper Watson et al. (2002) explored the relationship between narcissistic personality disorder and depression. Their findings support a hypothesis of a psychological continuum involving narcissism and self-esteem in which certain symptoms of narcissistic personality disorder—such as grandiosity, arrogance, and entitlement—are the result of maladaptive psychological mechanisms to compensate for the low self-esteem associated with depression.

In summary, in my clinical experience many adults with narcissistic personality disorder have indeed been emotionally deprived and neglected by their parents. Many others have been loved deeply and nurtured by their parents. I believe that in the latter circumstances, brain-based disorders led to the patients being unable to experience and thereby benefit developmentally from their parents' love for and devotion to them. *I advise both therapists and others to be careful not to presume parental neglect as a causative factor for the symptomatologies of people with narcissistic personality disorder.* Do not be drawn by your patients into complicity in blaming their parents for the patients' perceptions of being unloved. Because just as mental health professionals were wrong and damaging in their blame of mothers for causing schizophrenia in their children—recall the so-called schizophrenogenic mother—we could be (and probably are) again wrong in blaming parents for causing narcissistic personality disorder. It is possible that in many cases narcissistic personality disorder is a brain-based illness that is entirely unrelated to the quality and degree of parental care. It remains the role of future research to confirm or refute this thesis.

Psychosocial Aspects of Narcissistic Personality Disorder

Much of the current understanding of the psychology of people with narcissistic personality disorder is based on psychoanalytic conceptualizations. The term *narcissism* is derived from the ancient Greek myth in which a handsome young man, Narcissus, becomes enamored of and obsessed with his own reflection in a spring. When the young man tries to embrace his reflection, he falls into the pool of water and is drowned. Sigmund Freud used the name of the subject of this myth for the process of the psychological acquisition of self-love and self-regard. In his essay "On Narcissism: An Introduction," Freud wrote, "The libido that has been drawn from the external world has been directed to the ego and thus gives rise to an attitude which may be called narcissism" (Freud 1914/1966, p. 75). In this essay Freud indicated that drawing pleasure from the external world to build a healthy self-concept is a healthful psychological process, but also that interference with the process can lead to significant psychological disorders. Freud believed that the newborn baby and infant are "narcissistic," in that they are entirely invested in the gratification of their own physical and psychological needs, as opposed to those of other people. Over time, through relationships with the mother and other important people in his or her life, the infant gradually recognizes that the sources of this gratification often come from other people, and thereby the child becomes less self-absorbed or egocentric. With this recognition comes the ability to experience the value and worth of others. However, if problems occur in the infant or young child's important nurturing relationships—such as neglect, abuse, or even a serious illness of the mother—the child will not receive sufficient attention and nurturing from the caregiver. To compensate for this deficiency, the infant or child will return to the more primitive state of self-investment and preoccupation with his or her own needs. According to certain psychoanalytic theories, this pattern persists into adulthood, with the resultant development of "pathological narcissism" with the features described in Table 5–3.

Over the nearly 100 years since the initial publication of Freud's essay on narcissism, many psychoanalysts have crafted useful refinements of his original concept. Should the reader wish an in-depth understanding of these conceptual advances, I recommend the reading of Chapter 10 of Otto Kernberg's (1975) classic text *Borderline Conditions and Pathological Narcissism,* in which the author traces the evolution of the linked concepts of "normal" and "pathological" narcissism. Other recommended works include those of Heinz Kohut (1971, 1977), Arnold Cooper (1998; Cooper and Ronningstam 1992), and Glen Gabbard (2000). Post-Freudian psychological conceptualizations of narcissism are well reviewed in an excellent book by Joseph Sandler, Ethel Person, and Peter Fonagy (Sandler et al. 1991).

Treatment of People with Narcissistic Personality Disorder

Overview: Impediments to Diagnosis and Treatment

Although Congressman Smythe participated briefly in the treatment of his son, Martin, he would not accept treatment for himself. Refusing to acknowledge having any type of psychiatric disorder is common for people with narcissistic personality disorder. Presented in Table 5–5 is a summary of why many people with this condition most often go undiagnosed and untreated.

Approaches to the Treatment of People With Narcissistic Personality Disorder

Engagement

As was the circumstance of Congressman Dennis Smythe's son, Reverend Martin Smythe (discussed in Chapter 6, "Narcissistic Personality Disorder, Part II: Treated Narcissism"), many people with narcissistic personality disorder who engage in treatment do so under duress or at the behest of others. During the assessment phase of treatment, the clinician endeavors to engage the patient and motivate him or her to participate actively in meaningful treatment. By showing respect for the

TABLE 5–5.   Reasons people with narcissistic personality disorder often refuse treatment

1. Many people with this condition will not accept that they have *any* personal problems, much less significant problems with their personality.

2. Many people with this condition are high achievers by conventional measurements, such as job-related prestige and personal wealth. Therefore they and *some* others who know them do not believe that they have significant problems.

3. The reality of societal stigmatization of people with mental illnesses is an additional impediment to people who wish to be regarded as superior to others.

4. People with this condition are grandiose and like to view themselves as being fiercely independent and not needing the help of others—certainly not of a psychotherapist.

5. Even when people with this personality disorder will acknowledge the need for *some* help, they do not feel that any therapist is sufficiently intelligent or skilled to treat a person with their special gifts, personal qualities, and qualifications.

6. People with narcissistic personality disorder desire the constant praise and admiration of others, so the thought of having a mental health professional point out their problems and deficiencies would not be appealing.

7. People with this disorder do not tend to pursue in great depth any challenges (such as psychiatric treatment) that by their nature will not garner public attention and admiration.

8. People with narcissistic personality disorder tell lies to enhance their self-esteem. Truthfulness with the therapist is a prerequisite for successful psychiatric treatment.

patient, by avoiding power struggles, by demonstrating patience with the patient's resistance to insight about psychological problems or interest in therapy, and by providing *different points of view* about key quality of life issues for the patient, the therapist can facilitate engagement. Many patients become disillusioned with psychotherapy when their clinician initially asks too many questions and doesn't tell them much that they don't already know. One of the highest compliments that I can receive from a patient is when he or she says, "I never looked at it that way before." Reverend Martin Smythe became engaged in treatment when he discovered how much responsibility he felt for the emotional life of his mother and the bottomless depths of his anger with his father for his abandonment of him.

Assessment

Because diagnosis needs to come before treatment, every person who enters treatment with a mental health professional requires a comprehensive and systematic evaluation. Among the important considerations in the assessment of people for narcissistic personality disorder is whether the individual has any other concurrent medical or psychiatric conditions. When their dishonest behaviors begin to be discovered, when their grandiose schemes unravel, and when they receive rebukes rather than adulation, people with this personality disorder frequently become anxious and depressed and abuse alcohol and other addictive substances. Therefore, people with narcissistic personality disorder must be assessed for anxiety disorders, depression, alcoholism and other chemical dependencies, and the many associated physical disorders associated with these conditions (such as anemia, duodenal ulcers, and traumatic brain injury).

Treatment

Careful assessment of people with narcissistic personality disorder frequently reveals the presence of other conditions that must be treated concurrently with the personality disorder. For example, if the person is depressed, treatment with antidepressants is often required before substantial progress can occur with psychotherapy. Psychiatrist and psychoanalyst Steven P. Roose (2001) wrote an outstanding review of the reasons for combining psychotherapy with psychiatric medications— an example of what can be termed *integrated treatment.* If the patient has significant marital problems, couples therapy or family treatment might be indicated and helpful. If the patient has difficulty appreciating how others perceive his bragging and his devaluation of other people, group therapy can be prescribed. Nonetheless, individual psychotherapy is by far the most commonly utilized treatment for people with narcissistic personality disorder, and many types of individual psychotherapy have been studied for this purpose. The treatment with insight-informed psychotherapy and psychoanalysis of Reverend Martin Smythe—who, like his father, met DSM criteria for narcissistic personality disorder—is described and explained in Chapter 6, "Narcissistic Personality Disorder, Part II: Treated Narcissism." (A brief review of other types of individual psychotherapy, couples treatment, and group treatments for patients with this condition can be found in Groopman and Cooper 2001.)

Special Issues Regarding Narcissistic Personality Disorder

Lying

It should not be surprising that people with narcissistic personality disorder tell lies. These are, after all, people who have low self-esteem at the core of their personality, who desire to be admired by everyone, who have grandiose fantasies of being perfect and all-powerful, who are intensely competitive with others, who exaggerate their achievements and take credit for the important accomplishments of others, and who will not admit to making mistakes or having failures. *All* people with narcissistic personality disorder misrepresent the truth about themselves to gain the admiration of others as well as to advance their personal ambitions. The characteristic pattern is to exaggerate their accomplishments to those whom they first meet and especially wish to impress. They will lie about events and achievements that are very difficult for the other person to substantiate—such as sports achievements in high school or success at a previous job in another city. Most often, people with the disorder will pepper their misrepresentations with pseudomodest understatements and false humility. The most intelligent among them can be quite convincing and, *at first,* can be successful in convincing others to believe and admire them. With the passage of time, however, *some* people will catch on to the pervasive mendacity. Dennis Smythe's pattern of lying was prototypical of that observed in people with narcissistic personality disorder. For example, when he first met June when they were both college students, Dennis did not tell her that he was president of his class. When she visited him on his campus, she was soon told by several other students that Dennis had been elected to the position. June thought it very modest of Dennis not even mention it to her. When she asked him about it, Dennis replied, "Oh, it's nothing. They couldn't find anybody else who was willing to take the job." In reality he had worked very hard to win election as class president, and for the rest of his life he made certain that the fact appeared prominently on all his résumés and biographical summaries. He also made certain that others would tell June about his election during her first visit to the campus. He specifically did not mention it to her before her first visit to the campus so that she would think him modest. On the other hand, over the subsequent years, Dennis lied to June about being the captain of the baseball team, about being an outstanding student who was elected to Phi Beta Kappa, and about many other nonexistent achievements during college. Modest, honest, and mature, June at first did not suspect her husband of telling lies. However, over the ensuing years she grew to understand that her husband was a habitual liar. When Dennis realized that June was catching on to his lying, he became enraged with her and devalued her even further for being disloyal to him by daring to doubt him.

Dennis evidenced the same pattern of dishonesty in his work-related activities. To his superiors, Mr. Gallagher and Mr. Greer, Dennis would take credit for the accomplishments of others, alter data to appear more successful, blame others for problems, and not disclose failures. He would exploit his subordinates, never share the limelight with them, and blame Mr. Gallagher and Mr. Greer for his own unpopular decisions and policies, such as reductions in wages and benefits. Dennis pressured others to change documents to cover up his own failed decisions and dishonest activities. On the occasions when he was challenged or opposed by an employee or auditor for being less than honest, Dennis would attack those individuals' abilities and credibility through lies about their job performance, work ethic, and intelligence. Over time he formed around him a group of insiders whom he would promote and reward for their willingness to cover for his dishonesty, and he would undermine those who tried to do the right thing for the corporation.

Sadly, the combination of burning ambition and a willingness to distort the truth in people with narcissistic personality disorder can lead them to acquire substantial power and high position. These individuals harm many innocent people along the route to their personal aggrandizement. On the frequent occasions when their deceptions and dishonesties lead to a collapse of the house of cards they have created, even larger numbers of others are damaged. It is also true that some people with this personality disorder—like Dennis Smythe in his career as a congressman—achieve great fame and power without their dishonesty ever being exposed.

Readers who are interested in learning more about the psychological aspects of lying may wish to refer to the excellent book on the subject by psychiatrist Charles V. Ford (1996) titled *Lies! Lies! Lies!: The Psychology of Deceit.*

Having a Parent with Narcissistic Personality Disorder

Neglect

The children of a parent (or parents) with this condition tend to describe one of two patterns of treatment. In the extreme scenario, parents with narcissistic personality disorder neglect or even abuse their children.

Their self-centeredness, their lack of empathy, and their need for constant praise do not fit well with the realities of caring for infants and raising children. Certainly, people with this condition have difficulties meeting the emotional needs of their children. Because this pattern of parenting is exemplified by Martin Smythe's experience with his father, Dennis Smythe, I will not expand on it further here.

Narcissistic Extension

In the second typical pattern, the parent exploits the children for the enhancement of his or her own self-esteem. In this type of behavior the child becomes the *narcissistic extension* of the parent, and the parent tries to mold, manipulate, and control his or her children in ways that will bring attention and admiration to the parent. Inherent in this relationship pattern is that the parent has little regard for the inner life, feelings, proclivities, and aspirations of his or her children. Rather, the parent tells the children what they should want, how they should feel, and how they should respond—all furthering the goal of aggrandizing the parent. An example is a child in a restaurant who chooses chocolate ice cream for dessert. Her mother is concerned that the ice cream might soil her daughter's new dress and is also hypervigilant about her daughter gaining weight (even though the daughter does not have a weight problem). The source of the mother's concerns is how the daughter's appearance to others will reflect on the mother. The mother will say to the waiter, "My daughter really doesn't really like ice cream. You can just slice an apple for us and bring us some Equal." To her daughter she will say, "An apple with Equal really tastes better than chocolate ice cream. And it will keep you thin and pretty, like Carol Norton's little girl." Clearly, no matter what the motivation, telling a child what she feels and prefers is both confusing and frustrating to that child.

Another example of using a child as a narcissistic extension is the father who compels his son to try out for the football team rather than competing on the swimming team, for which the son has a great passion. The son is a superior athlete, and his father wants the many parents who attend the high school football games—as opposed to the small handful who show up at swim meets—to be aware of his son's prowess. The father says to his son, "Swimming is for sissies who can't make it in a real man's sport. I can tell you that if you don't play on the team everyone will think you are chicken about getting hurt. Also, if you don't play football, you will let me down and make me ashamed. Think of how many hours I worked with you to get you ready for this opportunity. It would all go to waste if you choose a girls' sport like swimming. I could never face my friends."

TABLE 5–6.   Examples of parental narcissistic extension

1. The "tennis mom" whose entire life is devoted to advancing her daughter's professional tennis career.

2. The "ice hockey dad" who jumps onto the rink and shoves the referee, whom he feels made an unfair call against his son.

3. The "beauty pageant parents" who go into bankruptcy from buying clothes and paying professional coaches for their young daughter, who competes in Junior Miss contests.

4. The "cheerleader mom" who makes an anonymous death threat to a rival of her daughter's before tryouts for the cheerleading squad.

5. The "Ivy League dad" who hounds his son over school grades, has him tutored every summer beginning in the sixth grade in preparation for the Scholastic Aptitude Test, and tries to pull strings to get him accepted to an Ivy League university for which he is not academically qualified.

Parents with narcissistic personality disorder will overidentify with their children, especially during situations that involve public performances. They will live vicariously though the achievements of their children, especially those who have special talents, such as in the arts or in sports. Notorious examples of ways in which parents use their children as narcissistic extensions of themselves are illustrated in Table 5–6.

Not surprisingly, the children of parents with narcissistic personality disorder become confused about their feelings, develop pathological dependencies on their parents, grow up to have difficulties making important choices and independent decisions, and are unable to determine what they really want. As adults, the children of parents with narcissistic personality disorder are prone to develop close relationships with other controlling people who do not respect their personal boundaries or rights as individuals. They feel confused about their identities and often will say such things as "I don't feel like a complete person" or "I really don't know who I am." Depression and relationship problems with their spouses are often the reasons that adult children of people with narcissistic personality disorder seek treatment, where they often undergo positive and significant changes as the result of the insights offered them.

Having a Spouse With Narcissistic Personality Disorder

The course of June Gallagher Smythe's painful and destructive relationship with Dennis Smythe is characteristic of the experience of being married to a person with this condition. I have treated the spouses of many people with narcissistic personality disorder and have noted a common pattern in the course of their relationships, as indicated in Table 5–7.

Having an Employee or Subordinate With Narcissistic Personality Disorder

First Phase: Getting Off to a Good Start

In a pattern of behavior similar to that noted in their personal relationships, people with narcissistic personality disorder come on strong in the initial phases of their employment and fade into disfavor with the passage of time. When they start a new job, they will work longer hours and give more of themselves to the position than is expected. They are adept at learning about and responding to the special needs of their bosses, and they soon set themselves apart from their peers. They try to ingratiate themselves with their superiors by performing special favors that can exceed the expectations or even the boundaries of their jobs. An example is a legal aide who travels across town before work each day to purchase, at his own expense, the special pastry that his boss relishes. Such employees will look for opportunities to develop personal relationships with their bosses by doing such things as picking up the boss's children at school or at the airport when the children return from college. Although the real goal of these employees is to secure and advance their position at work, their special favors are disguised as supporting the organization by helping the boss use his or her time more efficiently. These employees portray themselves as being fiercely loyal to their employers, and their goal is to become indispensable. They develop intense rivalries with other workers at the same level, and they use their special relationship with the boss to intimidate those whom they view as competition. Over time, the most ambitious and capable of these employees will come to be regarded as fast risers and as uniquely valuable to the company or organization.

Employees with narcissistic personality disorder will next endeavor to consolidate their position and power by taking every advantage of the access and opportunities that their early success opens up for them. In this phase of their employment, their work is of benefit both to their organization and to their career, which is their prime interest. For example, the legal aide was asked by his employer to handle the logistics of a weekend retreat for the law firm's long-range planning. For months in advance of the retreat, the aide planned out every detail of the event.

TABLE 5–7.   Three phases of marriage for a person with narcissistic personality disorder

A. **Courtship phase**

Is attentive to and considerate of prospective partner

Idealizes prospective partner

Exaggerates, embellishes, and lies about personal accomplishments to appear unique and attractive

"Sells" himself or herself to family and close friends of prospective partner

B. **Marital phase**

Becomes progressively critical and devaluing of spouse and his or her immediate family

Is competitive with spouse for the attention and admiration of others, including the children

Tries to control spouse though psychological and emotional manipulation, such as by communicating anger and contempt when spouse acts independently or even expresses opinions that differ from his or her own

Tries to control the spouse by making all important family-related decisions, especially those related to finances

Becomes emotionally detached from spouse

Refuses to assume a fair and reasonable share of marital responsibilities

Either neglects his or her children or seeks to gain the attention and admiration of others through the children

Engages in secretive, dishonest, and unsavory relationships outside the marriage

Becomes emotionally and/or physically abusive to spouse

C. **Dissolution phase**

Becomes enraged and abusive when spouse challenges his or her exaggerations, embellishments, and dishonesties

Blames spouse for all the problems in the relationship and the marriage

Through lies and distortions, seeks to turn family members and mutual acquaintances against spouse

Transfers dependencies from spouse to other parties outside the marriage and family

Feels entitled to an undue proportion of the marital assets

Deploys distortion, coercion, and deceit to secure the material assets of the marriage

Wields children as a weapon to harm spouse and to leverage from spouse an undue share of marital assets

Once divorce is finalized, is hostile with spouse and reduces involvements with children

He called all the resort hotels in the region and located a luxurious hotel and spa that could give the law firm a special rate because a scheduled convention had been canceled. He devoted his weekends before the event to determining the best meeting room, selecting the optimal menus, and testing the appropriate audiovisual equipment. He made himself available to all the presenters and prepared the slides for their talks. Although it had not been done for previous retreats, he put together a comprehensive manual providing copies of the slides and background information for each speaker. He even arranged for the presentations to be videotaped and the relevant talks placed on the company's Web site so that all law partners, associates, and employees could be "on the same page" with regard to the long-range plan. When complimented by the attendees for the great success of the retreat, the aide affected a modest, self-effacing mien and ascribed all credit to his boss: "Anyone can handle the boring details and logistics of a retreat; it is my boss, who handled the programmatic content, who deserves all the credit." To the employee's boss and others at higher levels of the organization, the aide appeared to be a true treasure. However, because his motives were purely to gain attention and to advance his personal ambitions—as opposed to truly caring about the missions and success of the firm—problems arose with this employee over time.

Second Phase: Problems Arise (An Introduction to Lomax's Law)

As time passes, ambitious and capable employees with narcissistic personality disorder gain stature and security on the job. Their attitudes toward peers and those at lower ranks in the organization are at best indifferent and dismissive. If they feel threatened by other qualified peers, the employees with this disorder become competitive and hostile. Such employees will devalue their co-workers to their boss, who will then be placed in the uncomfortable position of having to arbitrate heated disputes. In these circumstances the supervisor, who has accepted many personal favors from the employee with narcissistic personality disorder and who has become dependent on this employee for his or her extra efforts and many accomplishments, has no choice but to take the side of this employee. Such a situation is often the first indication of the high cost of the special relationship with the employee with this condition.

With the passage of more time and with increased confidence and job security, employees with narcissistic personality disorder will come to expect and will try to extract special consideration and treatment from their employers. For example, they will not understand why the corporate limitations of annual salary increases for people at their level should apply to them—after all, who else is as competent and gives so much of themselves to the organization, or is as deserving? Often people with narcissistic personality disorder express their desire for special consideration indirectly, such as by being silent and moody and appearing resentful for long periods of time when they learn that they have been given a raise that is "only" at the top end of the permitted limit. On the other hand, if their employer goes to bat for them by petitioning for a raise in excess of the limit, they still do not indicate appreciation for being treated more favorably than others. The reason is twofold. First, an elevated sense of self-importance and entitlement leads them to believe that no level of remuneration could compensate them adequately for their extraordinary contributions. Second, if they communicate an appropriate level of appreciation for being well compensated, they believe they will expend some hard-earned "chips" that they could have used for their next entitlement.

Lomax's Law.   My close friend and colleague James Lomax, M.D., is associate chairman for education in the Menninger Department of Psychiatry and Behavioral Sciences of Baylor College of Medicine. Together we manage a very large department with psychiatrists, psychologists, and other mental health professionals and many invaluable support staff members. On rare occasions, we have been asked by certain gifted and highly productive junior faculty members to forgo the customary rules and protocols to help advance a research or educational project. For example, they may to be excused from required clinical and teaching duties to pursue a special research initiative. More often than not, the special consideration does not lead to a productive outcome. In addition, rather than being grateful for being given special accommodations, the faculty member is angry and resentful when we ask that they resume their usual duties, for which they have been hired and are being paid. Based on these and related experiences, Dr. Lomax came up with the following principle, which I have termed Lomax's Law:

> Once you acquiesce to a subordinate's request for special treatment, two things are certain:
> 1. It won't be enough.
> 2. He or she will hate you for it.

Based on this law, Dr. Lomax has suggested that such people should have a T-shirt on which the following is printed:

> (on the front of the shirt), *I Want More!*
> (on the back of the shirt), *More Is Not Enough!*

Third Phase: Parting of the Ways

People with narcissistic personality disorder have been shown to have motivations and involvements that are based on superficial, self-serving goals. Although in public these people may tout the importance of the mission and values of their organization, they are truly interested only in how others in the organization view them and in how they can use the organization to advance their own ambitions. As they become more secure in their jobs and overestimate their work-related contributions, their feelings of entitlement snowball. They devote progressively less time and energy to becoming recognized through their accomplishments on the job and instead work harder at extracting even more for themselves from their employers. They become embittered because they believe that they have not been treated fairly or remunerated commensurately with what they perceive to be their great value to the enterprise. Their supervisors, on the other hand, become disappointed with their diminishing productivity and angered by their endless requests for increased compensation and favored treatment. Eventually, the supervisor, who has been hesitant to confront the narcissistic employee because of all the special favors the supervisor has accepted, has no choice other than to speak to the employee about his or her deficiencies or submit an honest and accurate job performance appraisal. Like pulling the pin from a grenade, the boss's action detonates an explosive response from the employee. The employee, who is shocked by the negative aspects of the report, becomes precipitously enraged with the supervisor for what he or she believes to be a baseless betrayal and an unjustified attack. The employee is absolutely incapable of using the evaluation in ways that are constructive and that will lead to improved job performance.

Employees with narcissistic personality disorder are incapable of seeing a balanced picture and placing their deficiencies into the context of their positive contributions. On being reprimanded, their first thoughts are about how to negate or reverse their negative evaluation, and they quickly realize that this will entail undermining the credibility and authority of the supervisor who wrote the evaluation. Often these employees have engineered themselves into positions of great trust within the organization, where they have access to highly confidential information. If their superiors have comported themselves with integrity in both their job-related responsibilities and their personal conduct with their employees (i.e., no special favors), there is not much that an employee embittered by a negative but fair performance review can do. If, on the other hand, supervisors or bosses have accepted personal favors from such employees or if there are problems with the integrity of the organization, a power struggle will ensue, the outcome of which is difficult to predict. What is certain is that the special relationship the narcissistic employee has with the boss is now over. The reputation and career of the boss are usually damaged as well. Presented in Table 5–8 are some tips for avoiding or dealing with employees and subordinates with narcissistic personality disorder.

Afterword

People with narcissistic personality disorder may seem quite attractive and special in the initial phases of a relationship, but their self-centeredness, dishonesty, and exploitiveness will eventually harm those who depend on them. The most intelligent among those with this disorder may rise to positions of great importance, which may bolster their grandiosity and heighten the level of damage that they will ultimately cause. Many people with this disorder will eschew psychiatric or psychological treatment because they believe that such help is beneath them. They are also threatened by gaining access, through treatment, to the insecurities and low self-esteem that form the roots of their substantial problems, and therefore they avoid all honest and intimate relationships, including psychotherapeutic ones. The case of Congressman Dennis Smythe is an example of a bright and capable person who would not accept psychotherapeutic help, did not gain insight about his insecurities, would not change, and consequently hurt many people. However, the case of his son, Reverend Martin Smythe (Chapter 6, "Narcissistic Personality Disorder, Part II: Treated Narcissism"), provides an example of a person who engaged in productive psychotherapy and psychoanalysis, gained an understanding of the sources of his insecurities, and as a result made remarkable, positive changes in his behavior, relationships, and emotional life. Nonetheless, because so many people with narcissistic personality disorder do not feel the need to change, and because relationships with people with this condition are so fraught with frustration and devaluation, it is wise to be able to recognize them and avoid important associations with them where possible. This chapter should help you spot the characteristic personality and behavioral patterns that will facilitate this recognition and avoidance. For those who are currently in relationships with people with this personality disorder who will not accept treatment, the chapter should impart understandings that will enable you to end the relationship, should you deem it necessary. If for some reason you must remain involved with a person

TABLE 5–8.   Tips for avoiding or dealing with employees or subordinates with narcissistic personality disorder

1. **Do your homework before hiring new employees.** Call previous employers to ascertain how the candidate for the position performed in past jobs. Ask specific questions about his or her relationships with supervisors. Prevention is the best medicine. (If you are in the role of an administrator or supervisor, rereading this chapter may be worth your while).

2. **Interview candidates for new positions carefully.** Look for the characteristic behavioral and relationship patterns of people with narcissistic personality disorder during the interview. If, for example, the candidate makes assertions such as "I was indispensable to my previous boss" or "I handled everything in my previous employer's personal life," or "The company was a complete mess before I came, but I fixed most of the problems," or "I left my last job because my efforts and contributions were not appreciated," your index of suspicion should be heightened. The chances are high that you will be viewed by this person as the next incompetent leader that he or she props up.

3. **Do not accept personal favors or special treatment from any employee.** You will pay back these favors manifold at the cost of your professional reputation and perhaps your career.

4. **Maintain clear boundaries and separations between your vocational and your personal relationships.** Personal relationships with subordinates often confuse appropriate vocational lines of authority.

5. **Never make a business or personal decision related to any employee that cannot stand the bright light of public scrutiny.** If what you are planning to do has to remain a secret, you probably should not be doing it in the first place.

6. **Restrict access to confidential information (such as the medical records or salary information of other employees) to experienced personnel with mature personalities and good character.** An employee who is inexperienced or immature or whom you believe has a personality or character disorder should not have access to privileged information.

7. **Conduct and document regular and judicious performance reviews on all employees and subordinates.** Do not include only positive comments; every employee has areas that can benefit from improvement. Beware of employees or subordinates who cannot accept or who overreact to fair and constructive critiques. Such individuals cannot grow on the job and will become underproductive and embittered employees over time.

TABLE 5–8. Tips for avoiding or dealing with employees or subordinates with narcissistic personality disorder *(continued)*

8. **Beware of employees who require inordinate praise and demand special entitlements.** No matter how much they contribute to the organization at the time, they are most likely motivated by self-serving ambitions. Ultimately they will be disappointing and destructive workers.

9. **Beware of employees who compete with and devalue their peers (and previous employers).** People with narcissistic personality disorder have difficulties working as team members to achieve organizational goals.

10. **Beware of employees who overstate and overvalue their contributions to the organization.** These individuals often cut corners and make short-sighted decisions to appear better than they are and call attention to themselves.

11. **Beware of employees or subordinates who are not appreciative of or satisfied with fair and generous compensation.** These individuals will ultimately become bitter and are likely to undermine your authority and position.

who will not accept treatment for this condition, an understanding of his or her psychology and behavioral patterns should help you to have realistic expectations for the relationship and to protect yourself. Of one thing you can be certain: this person will not be looking out for *your* best interests!

References and Suggested Readings

American Psychiatric Association: Diagnostic and Statistical Manual of Mental Disorders, 4th Edition, Text Revision. Washington, DC, American Psychiatric Association, 2000

Cooper AM: Further developments in the clinical diagnosis of narcissistic personality disorder, in Disorders of Narcissism: Diagnostic, Clinical, and Empirical Implications. Edited by Ronningstam EF. Washington, DC, American Psychiatric Press, 1998, pp 53–74

Cooper AM, Ronningstam EF: Narcissistic personality disorder, in American Psychiatric Press Review of Psychiatry, Vol 11. Edited by Tasman A, Riba MB. Washington, DC, American Psychiatric Press, 1992, pp 80–97

Ford CV: Lies! Lies! Lies!: The Psychology of Deceit. Washington, DC, American Psychiatric Press, 1996

Freud S: On narcissism: an introduction (1914), in The Standard Edition of the Complete Psychological Works of Sigmund Freud, Vol 14. Translated and edited by Strachey J. London, Hogarth Press, 1966, pp 73–102

Gabbard GO: Cluster B personality disorders: narcissistic, in Psychody Psychiatry in Clinical Practice, 3rd Edition. Washington, DC, Ame ....t Psychiatric Press, 2000, pp 463–489

Groopman LC, Cooper AM: Narcissistic personality disorder, in Treatments of Psychiatric Disorders, 3rd Edition. Edited by Gabbard GO. American Psychiatric Publishing, Washington, DC, 2001, pp 2309–2326

Kernberg O: Borderline Conditions and Pathological Narcissism. New York, Jason Aronson, 1975

Kohut H: The Analysis of the Self. New York, International Universities Press, 1971

Kohut H: The Restoration of the Self. New York, International Universities Press, 1977

Roose SP: Psychodynamic therapy and medication, in Integrated Treatment of Psychiatric Disorders. Edited by Kay J (Review of Psychiatry Series; Oldham JM and Riba MB, series eds). Washington, DC, American Psychiatric Publishing, 2001, pp 31–50

Sandler J, Person ES, Fonagy P: Freud's "On Narcissism: An Introduction." New Haven, CT, Yale University Press, 1991

Watson PJ, Sawrie SM, Greene RL, et al: Narcissism and depression: MMPI-2 evidence for the continuum hypothesis in clinical samples. J Pers Assess 79:85–109, 2002

Chapter 6

NARCISSISTIC PERSONALITY DISORDER

Part II: Treated Narcissism

I CELEBRATE myself;
And what I assume you shall assume;
For every atom belonging to me, as good belongs
   to you.

> —Walt Whitman, *Leaves of Grass*

The Case of Reverend Martin Smythe

Background Information

Reverend Martin Smythe is the son of Congressman Dennis Smythe, whose case history is presented in Chapter 5, "Narcissistic Personality Disorder, Part I: Untreated Narcissism." Reverend Smythe, a 47-year-old married father of three children, was referred to me by the chairman of the board of trustees of a large local church for evaluation of his fitness to serve as the congregation's senior minister. Reverend Smythe did not seek my counsel voluntarily. Rather, he was told that if he did not submit to psychiatric evaluation and treatment, he would be fired from his job. I was informed by the board chairman that an employee of the church, a married woman, had filed a lawsuit charging Reverend Smythe with sexual misconduct and work-related exploitation. Subsequent to the publicity related to the lawsuit, three other women, all members of the church, came forward and reported that Reverend Smythe had engaged in sexual relationships with them. According to an internal report conducted by the church, each woman stated that she had been told by the reverend that having sex with him would be a test of her religious faith and a measure of her spiritual commitment to the church. One woman reported that she had had sexual intercourse with Reverend Smythe on numerous occasions while receiving individual counseling from him for stress related to her divorce proceedings.

Complicating this consultation were the facts that Reverend Smythe adamantly denied each allegation and that most of the members of his church appeared to believe him rather than his accusers. The graduate of a prestigious secular university and the valedictorian of his seminary class, Reverend Smythe was highly and widely regarded for his rhetorical skills on the pulpit as well as for several best-selling religious texts that he had written. He had hired one of the region's most renowned defense attorneys to represent him in the case brought by the church employee, and his legal fees were being paid by a prominent member of the church. Unique to my clinical experience, I had been chosen to evaluate Reverend Smythe as the result of a negotiation between the internal review committee of the reverend's church and his lawyer, probably because of my position as chairman of the department of psychiatry of the local medical school. With considerable trepidation, I acquiesced to this request.

Initial Consultation

In my office, Reverend Smythe appeared confident and assertive. Calling me by my first name, he began our initial meeting by detailing how well thought of I was by many of the important members of his church—all of whom were also his close personal friends. He complimented me on the specifics of my academic training, which he had also checked before our first meeting. He used this discussion as an opportunity to compare my training with his own. Although the reverend indicated that he had attended universities that are conventionally considered to be more prestigious than those from which I had graduated, he graciously acknowledged me to be a colleague and a peer on his level. He did not seem to mind at all when I carefully specified the dual nature of my consultation: in part to provide an opinion to his church regarding his fitness to return to work, and in part to recommend to him whatever psychiatric help might be indicated. Reverend Smythe quickly reassured me that both charges would be easily accomplished—"particularly for a professional of your excellent qualifications and skills." He also added that it was highly unlikely that he would require any psychiatric care. Reverend Smythe had agreed to my role of providing a professional consultation to his church related to the allegations of his sexual misconduct with an employee of the church and three other women in his congregation. He adamantly denied having such involvement and had no explanation of the motivations underlying their accusations other than that "they obviously have significant problems and wild imaginations. Don't you believe, Doctor, in a church with over 2,000 families, that there will be at least three or four women with serious psychological issues?"

Childhood and Adolescent History

Paternal Influences

I devoted a large portion of my second and third sessions with Reverend Smythe to reviewing his early life experiences with his father and mother. Initially, Reverend Smythe spoke of his father in idealized and global terms. For much of his childhood he did not spend much time with his father, who would work long hours and would frequently be away on business trips. When Martin was 13 years old, his father was elected to a position that took him away during most of the year to Washington, D.C., while the family remained home in the Midwest. From that time forward, Martin became the man of the household that consisted of Martin, his mother (whom he adored), and his younger sister (whom he tolerated). During our second meeting, Reverend Smythe also admitted that much later in life he had learned from his mother that during his parents' marriage his father had maintained a second family in Washington without his mother's knowledge. Eventually his mother and father were divorced, but his father never married the other woman, and Martin had never met his two half-siblings. Notwithstanding the stress and disappointments associated with his relationship with his father, Reverend Smythe would not acknowledge any anger or even hard feelings toward him. Rather, he would emphasize how his father would encourage his success, such as by sending him a congratulatory letter when he graduated from college at the top of his class. When I asked him if he was disappointed that his father did not attend his graduation ceremonies, Reverend Smythe maintained that he understood that his father was required to be in Washington at the time, "doing the important work of the nation." His mother also did not remarry, and it was clear that her only son became the center of her universe.

Maternal Influences

Two principal psychodynamic themes became evident: First, even though his father had essentially abandoned him when he was 13 years old, Reverend Smythe did not acknowledge feeling any anger toward his father. In fact, he would not even admit to being disappointed in his father. Second, after being abandoned by her husband, Reverend Smythe's mother devoted herself almost exclusively to caring for her two children. She was concerned that she had to be "both mother and father" to compensate for the absence of a father figure in their lives. She was particularly concerned about the welfare and academic development of her son, Martin, whom she recognized was gifted intellectually. A great reader, Mrs. Smythe personally chose books for Martin to read throughout his childhood and young adulthood. She would read the books along with her son, and they would spend many pleasant hours discussing what they were reading. Until he was almost 17 years old, Martin would join his mother in her bed to read and discuss books with her. Although Mrs. Smythe was also attentive to and affectionate with Martin's sister, the relationship of the mother with her daughter was not nearly so close as that with her son. In addition, after her husband left her, Mrs. Smythe never dated another man. She looked to her only son as her primary source of emotional support. At the close of our third meeting, I asked Reverend Smythe if his mother's intense involvement with him came with any cost. I was surprised by the authenticity of his response, "Yes, she has given so much of herself and her own life to me. I have always felt, therefore, that I was responsible for her happiness. That has been a heavy burden for me most of my life."

Psychodynamic Formulation

Among the tools available to psychotherapists is *parallel history*. What this means is that as the patient is providing a history of his or her conscious recollections of the significant events of his or her life, the therapist is putting together a pattern of the patient's unconscious responses to these events. The therapist's *psychodynamic formulation* comprises a hypothesis about how these unconscious responses lead to ("cause") the patient's psychological symptoms. In the case of Reverend Smythe, my parallel history encompassed the patient's repressed feelings of anger toward his father, about which he felt great guilt and confusion. Second, I believed that the patient had repressed sexual feelings for his adoring, emotionally dependent mother. In addition, I had suspicions that he unconsciously blamed himself for the abandonment by the father and also felt vulnerable to his father's retaliation as the result of his "winning" the mother. My preliminary psychodynamic formulation was as follows:

1. The patient harbored unconscious beliefs that his abandonment by his father was a result of his inadequacy as a son. This led to deep-seated problems with self-esteem, masked by bravado and preoccupations with close relationships with powerful people.
2. The patient unconsciously feared that his father would retaliate against him for winning away the wife/mother. Combined with his father's role model of dishonesty and betrayal, this led to the patient's fear of and defiance toward authority, including that of his own role as a leader/minister, as well as the authority of the church.
3. His mother's placing him in the role of the father and man of the house evoked his unconscious sexual feelings for her. This led to his inability to express mature intimacy toward his own wife while being drawn to and stimulated by "forbidden" sexual encounters with other women.

Although I certainly had no proof, I believed at that point that the patient's life history, his personality, and his psychology were consistent with the sexual misconduct of which he was accused. I also postulated the following, about which I planned to question him in our third meeting:

4. As a result of his anger toward and disappointment with his father, his distrust of and contempt for authority would extend to the "ultimate authority." I suspected that he would have problems with his religious faith.

Given Reverend Smythe's guardedness about acknowledging any issue that might reflect poorly on himself, I was uncertain about whether he would admit to having difficulties with religious faith, even if it were true. I reasoned that this topic was serious but far less threatening than sexual violations. His responses on the subject would be revealing: if he denied having a problem in this realm, his prognosis for true disclosure and therapeutic help would be remote. This would lead me to strongly suspect the diagnoses of antisocial personality disorder or pathological narcissism—both severe personality disorders that lead to fatal flaws. Should he acknowledge problems of religious faith or any similar difficulties, it was likely that he had a less severe form of narcissistic personality disorder, which, with his cooperation, might be amenable to therapeutic amelioration.

The Treatment of Reverend Martin Smythe

Initial Phase: Engagement

During the course of Reverend Smythe's third consultative visit, I asked him if he was experiencing difficulties with his religious faith. He inquired as to my reasons for the question, and I answered him in a forthright fashion: "I believe that your unresolved feelings that are a result of your abandonment by your father and his hurtful deceptions would lead to your pervasive distrust of authority." Somewhat to my surprise, Reverend Smythe admitted to what he termed "a crisis of faith." This acknowledgement constituted not only a turning point in my evaluation of Reverend Smythe but also, quite literally, a turning point in his life. The following dialogue ensued:

> **Reverend Smythe:** I never made a connection between my feelings for my father and my problems with religious faith.
>
> **Dr. Y.:** I don't believe that you ever had the opportunity to explore your feelings for your father. You were only 13 years old when he left the family.
>
> **Reverend Smythe:** What good would it have done, anyway? I would have felt terrible, and it wouldn't have changed anything.
>
> **Dr. Y.:** What do you recall of your feelings as you learned, over time, that your father would be unavailable to you?
>
> **Reverend Smythe:** I don't recall feeling anything. I do know that I became somewhat of a liar around that time. I told all my friends that my father came home on weekends and that he called me on the telephone every evening. I made up endless stories about his accomplishments in Washington. In truth, I don't remember him ever calling me or telling me about his job with the government.

At the conclusion of our third meeting, Reverend Smythe requested an additional session, which occurred 6 days later. The day before the meeting, he asked my permission to include his wife at that meeting. I readily acquiesced.

Second Phase: Treatment Plan

Reverend Smythe began our fourth meeting as follows:

> **Reverend Smythe:** This really hurts. I have already told my wife. The accusations that the women in my church have made against me are true. I want your professional help in dealing with this and in getting healed. This is so hard for me. I don't like asking for help.

In that session, the patient, his wife and I established a preliminary treatment plan:

1. Reverend Smythe would inform his attorney of the facts of his sexual misconduct and ask his lawyer's advice about how to inform the chairman of the board of trustees of his church of the true situation.
2. Cyndy Smythe expressed a willingness to remain married to her husband and to work with him in therapy on rebuilding their marriage. I referred Cyndy to a social worker who specialized in both individual and couples treatment to handle both aspects of this care.
3. I agreed to meet twice weekly with Reverend Smythe over the next 2 months to develop the goals of treatment and to structure a treatment plan.

A great deal was accomplished over the next 2 months and 16 therapeutic sessions. During that time I provided support and limited guidance to Reverend Smythe as he dealt with the legal and financial aspects of his personal life and job situation. His church and attorney made separate financial settlements with the four women on the contingency of their dropping their legal charges against the church and against Reverend Smythe. Reverend Smythe agreed to relinquish his position with the church, which generously agreed to pay his salary and his legal and medical bills for 1 year.

Believing that I would be much more valuable to Reverend Smythe in helping him understand the psychological origins of his emotional and behavioral problems, I deliberately avoided falling into the role of being an advisor to him about his abundant legal and financial problems. Nonetheless, through interpretation of the unconscious bases of his misbehavior and poor choices, Reverend Smythe was able to "self-correct." An example of this is a discussion he had with me about how to deal with one of the women with whom he had a sexual relationship.

> **Reverend Smythe:** I don't believe that the church should pay Mrs. X anything. I had no interest in her whatsoever until she "came on" to me. In fact, on the first two occasions that she came on to me, I rebuffed her. Finally, she wore down my defenses, and this led to my indiscretions.
>
> **Dr. Y.:** Are you saying that you, your mother, and your sister had some responsibility in your father's abandoning his family and taking up with another woman?
>
> **Reverend Smythe:** O.K., I think I get it. I believe what you are telling me is that, in my role of pastor, it was my responsibility to be sure that the rules were followed. It wasn't the responsibility of the flock.
>
> **Dr. Y.:** Not completely. What I am saying that it is always your responsibility to do the right thing. However, this is hard for you because your mistrust and enmity for authority is so great that you under-

mine and oppose your own authority. You unconsciously believe that if you permit yourself to be an admired authority figure—as was your father by most people—you will become like him.

Reverend Smythe (with intense feeling): My father is becoming the last person on earth whom I would want to emulate. I am beginning to understand how much I despise him! (Long pause.) I think I see what you mean. By my humiliating my own wife and children and by my trying to avoid responsibility for my own missteps, I have become pretty much like him.

Psychotherapeutic Techniques

Several key features and techniques of the psychotherapeutic process are illuminated by the interchange presented above under "Second Phase: Treatment Plan." A goal of psychoanalysis and psychoanalytically informed psychotherapy, which was my approach with Reverend Smythe, is *insight.* Insight has two different meanings in psychiatry. The first meaning refers to a person's recognition that he or she has a psychological problem and has a realistic understanding of how to go about getting help to solve the problem. Because Reverend Smythe entered treatment under some duress, he gained this level of insight after his third session. The second meaning refers to a patient's enlightenment about and understanding of the unconscious sources of his or her emotional symptoms and maladaptive behaviors. This type of insight would take far longer. The theory is that once a person brings to consciousness the unconscious determinants of painful affects and self-defeating behaviors, that person comes into a position for constructive change.

In the example above (under "Second Phase: Treatment Plan"), I was endeavoring to help Reverend Smythe make the connections between the unconscious feelings associated with his treatment by his father and how he treated other people. In this specific instance, his denial of his mistreatment by his father (and the associated feelings) led to a blind spot for his mistreatment of the female parishioners under his religious authority. As hard as it might be to imagine, it did not initially occur to Reverend Smythe that he was injuring and exploiting the four women in his church with whom he had had sexual relationships. He originally stated, "I thought that they were willing participants and that they enjoyed our encounters as much as I did." His conscious acknowledgment that he had been emotionally neglected and lied to by his father enabled Reverend Smythe to feel, for the first time, his deep-seated rage toward his father. This insight led to further insights, including an understanding of his pervasive conflicts with and undermining of almost all authority—including his own, his church's, and God's.

Transference is another potent tool of psychoanalysis and insight-oriented psychotherapy. This term refers to the unconscious displacement onto the therapist of unresolved feelings from significant relationships in the past. A representative and recurrent example of transference occurred during my treatment of Reverend Smythe. We had established a regular pattern of twice-weekly treatment sessions, which had been held unbroken for 2 months. This pattern was first disrupted by my being away for a week to attend the annual meeting of the American Neuropsychiatric Association. Reverend Smythe was first told about my travel about 7 weeks before my trip. On my return from the meeting, he was, for the first time, late for our appointment. In addition, he seemed depressed and was somewhat surly in his interactions with me. When I questioned him about his response to my being away, he stated, "I actually was quite happy to have the extra time to complete my applications for graduate school in theology." During the course of this session he recounted a dream that he had had the night before:

> **Reverend Smythe:** My dream was about you, Dr. Yudofsky. You were giving a paper at your meeting. It was a very complex and esoteric presentation about the brain and behavior. At the end you asked the audience questions to see if they understood your paper. No one could answer your questions. On the other hand, I knew the answers and kept raising my hand. Either you couldn't see me in the audience, or you refused to call on me.

I asked Reverend Smythe about his feelings that accompanied the dream. He admitted to feeling frustrated but did not disclose feelings of anger or being hurt. Eventually, on his request, I interpreted his dream.

> **Dr. Y.:** I believe your dream to be unconscious expressions of your feelings that were evoked by my being away and the canceling of our therapeutic sessions. I believe that you had been working hard during the previous sessions—in part to get better and in part to please me. In your dream, I appeared unaware of or unconcerned about your understanding, your efforts to please me, or, most importantly, about you. I believe that my trip to the meeting evoked unconscious feelings that are similar to those that you experienced on your father's many trips away from home when you were a boy. I also believe that the dream indicates that you feel that if only your father could have understood how smart you were and how hard you were trying, he would not have abandoned you and your family in the first place.

My point to Reverend Smythe was that he was *unconsciously*—as revealed in his behavior and his dream—*transferring* powerful feelings for his father onto me. He responded to this interpretation, in a highly ironic tone of voice, as follows:

> **Reverend Smythe:** What psychobabble! How trite and conventional! For once the "great doctor" is all wet. Trust me that I know you are a lot different from my father; and believe me that I am not at all interested in impressing you.

I responded that perhaps he was right and that I had overinterpreted his lateness and his dream. I further decided at this point not to call to his attention his high level of irritation with me on advancing this interpretation. I reasoned that if my interpretation was true, the angry and resistant response would recur with further separations, such as during vacations and public holidays. In due time he should feel sufficiently safe and should trust me to consciously recognize his pattern of response to my being away as a representation of the abandonment by his father. Indeed, Reverend Smythe "completely forgot" about his first appointment after my summer vacation. At his next appointment he recounted the following dream:

> **Reverend Smythe:** I was leading a memorial service in church. The parishioners were very upset. I wanted to say something personal about the deceased, but I couldn't remember who had died. I felt very unprepared and vulnerable. By the size of the crowd, I was sure that it was someone very important. I began to worry that they would blame me. I felt increasingly guilty and anxious. The more I tried to figure out who it was, the more anxious I became. I awakened suddenly in a cold sweat. My heart was racing.

After Reverend Smythe's presentation of his dream, he asked me what I thought it meant. I purposely did not respond directly. Instead, I asked him what he thought it might mean. He instantly lashed out at me for my "retentiveness":

> **Reverend Smythe:** You shrinks have the best racket in the world. You can make a good living by saying, "What do you think about this? What do you feel about that?" If you think that is helping me, you are very, very wrong.
> **Dr. Y.:** You seem to be angry with me.
> **Reverend Smythe (shouting):** I thought you were here to help me. You are damn right I am angry. Do you know what? I don't really need your help. I can interpret this dream better than you can.
> **Dr. Y.:** I think you are questioning my involvement with you and my commitment to you. This is more important to you than any other aspect of our relationship. I believe that my being away from you during my holiday precipitated both your dream and your "for-

getting" to keep your last appointment. Also, I am truly interested in how you would interpret your dream.

Reverend Smythe: O.K. I'll play your game. I'll be Dr. Yudofsky and interpret my own dream. The guy in the coffin represented both you and my father. My guilt represented my feelings of responsibility for his death. These feelings came from my murderous anger at your leaving me for a vacation, which represents my father's never being there for me.

Dr. Y.: That sounds right to me. I would also add that you are uncomfortable feeling dependent on me or anyone else. From the quality of your interpretation of your own dream, I believe that you are less dependent on me than you might think.

My reason for making the last comment was to indicate to Reverend Smythe that I was most comfortable with his identifying with me in ways that would lead to his own strength and independence. This aspect was certainly lacking in his relationship with his father.

Referral of Reverend Smythe for Psychoanalytic Treatment

The protected structure of the therapeutic setting and the firm rules limiting outside relationships between therapist and patient permits the transference and interpretation of unconscious feelings and behaviors. Over time, Reverend Smythe grew to trust the integrity of my interest and involvement with him. Eventually this trust enabled his increasing acceptance of some of my interpretations of his transference of feelings for his father onto me. With this insight he was able to understand and begin to change how he generalized such feelings far beyond the therapeutic setting to nearly every important aspect of his personal and professional life. Given the nature of his presenting problems (sexual misconduct), given the severity of his diagnosis (narcissistic personality disorder), and given his initial resistance to treatment, I was happily surprised by the degree and rate of his response to treatment. I attributed this unanticipated progress in treatment to his many other personal strengths, including his superior intelligence and his ability to access and understand the implications of his unconscious mental processes, which is another way of saying that he had an unusually high capacity for insight.

These strengths and attributes—combined with Reverend Smythe's motivation to work hard in psychotherapy and *outside* of psychotherapy to change his behavior and improve his relationships—resulted in my changing my preliminary belief that he exhibited fatal flaws of personality and character. From experiencing his efforts and progress in psychotherapy, I later believed that his psychiatric disorders were in fact amenable to significant improvement through psychotherapy.

After 18 months of treatment with me, Reverend Smythe was accepted as a Ph.D. candidate in theology at an outstanding university in a distant city. This provided an opportunity to consider a referral of Reverend Smythe to a female psychoanalyst in that city. Initially, his need for structure and support would have made such a referral untenable. In psychoanalytic treatment, the patient meets with the therapist four or five times a week. Psychoanalysts place even greater emphasis on revelation and interpretation of unconscious thoughts and feelings that lead to unsettling feelings and self-defeating behaviors. This is accomplished, in part, by the psychoanalyst's being less directive than are therapists in insight-oriented psychotherapy. When Reverend Smythe first entered treatment with me, he would not have been psychologically or motivationally ready for psychoanalysis. However, his personal life had stabilized, and he had become much less resistant to and gained more facility in exploring the unconscious bases of his interpersonal and emotional problems. Nonetheless, in Reverend Smythe's work with me, he had made insufficient progress in establishing mature, respectful, and trusting relationships with his wife and two daughters. I believed that the intense experience of psychoanalysis with a female therapist, combined with Reverend Smythe's superior intelligence and motivation to change, augured well for progress in this and other important dimensions of his life.

Treatment Outcome

Given the nature and seriousness of his initial symptoms and behavior, the psychoanalyst to whom I referred Reverend Smythe had significant reservations about his suitability for psychoanalytic treatment. She nonetheless agreed to devote several sessions to assessing his treatment capacity. Thereafter, she also expressed both surprise and enthusiasm for his progress to date in treatment, his motivation for further change, and his intellectual ability to benefit from the psychoanalytic process. She accepted him as a patient, and Reverend Smythe remained in intensive treatment with this clinician for 5 years. On occasion he would write to provide updates about his progress, which by all measures was remarkable. First, his relationships with his family improved significantly—both from his perspective and from theirs. He disclosed that for the first time, he was able to access his true feelings of love for his wife and children. Second, he changed his career path. He completed his Ph.D. in theological studies and accepted a position as an assistant professor in the prominent university that he had attended for undergraduate studies. Although employment as a college professor was far less remunerative and publicly prominent than his earlier role as pastor of a large church, Reverend Smythe gained a much higher level of satisfaction and contentment in his new position. Third, Professor Smythe disclosed that he achieved a "far higher and less conflicted level of spirituality and closeness with my Maker" than he had before entering psychoanalytic treatment.

Summarized in Table 6–1 are key principles in the treatment of patients with narcissistic personality disorder.

Lessons Learned From the Case of Reverend Smythe

Don't Rush To Judgment

After my first two meetings with Reverend Smythe, I was not optimistic about his capacity to engage in meaningful treatment that would lead to significant changes in his behavior and relationships. The disturbing nature of his alleged misconduct; the fact that his psychiatric consultation took place under duress; his denial of any serious psychological problems or symptoms; his self-centeredness; and his grandiose way of relating with me led me to believe that he had pathological narcissism and that he had little motivation to understand himself and little capacity to change his behavior. Thus, it initially appeared that Reverend Smythe had fatal flaws of personality and character. I must admit that my initial pessimistic impressions were not changed by his many strengths, which included his high intelligence, his superior communication skills, his strong track record for hard work and productivity, and his fine sense of humor. I would have balanced these strengths with the realization that it is common for people with fatal flaws of personality and character to have other attractive and admirable qualities. (It would be interesting to know how his wife, Cyndy, would have filled out the Fatal Flaw Scale [Appendix A in Chapter 2], but it had not been developed at the time of his initial consultation. Had she completed the scale, I would hope that her recognition of her husband's many strengths would have provided clues to his potential for constructive change through psychotherapy.) The fact that sufficient professional time—a minimum of three full-hour sessions—was allocated for his psychiatric evaluation permitted Reverend Smythe to learn about and to accept the psychotherapeutic process and permitted me to have a more positive view of his prognosis.

TABLE 6–1. Key principles in the treatment of a patient with narcissistic personality disorder as exemplified by the case of Reverend Martin Smythe

Historical fact	Key principle	Interpretation
Reverend Smythe did not voluntarily seek psychiatric assessment and treatment.	The stigma associated with mental illness deters many people who could benefit from psychotherapy from seeking or accepting such treatment.	Reverend Smythe's grandiosity and his pride in being self-sufficient combined to keep him from pursuing the psychiatric care he required.
Reverend Smythe lied about his sexual misconduct.	People with narcissistic personality disorder persistently tell lies.	Reverend Smythe lied both to impress and to exploit others.
Dr. Y. did not challenge or confront Reverend Smythe over his lies about his sexual misconduct.	Psychiatric care is an advocational relationship, not an adversarial one. There are important differences between psychiatrists and detectives.	Establishing a therapeutic relationship with Reverend Smythe was more important than pointing out inconsistencies in his account.
Before treatment, Martin Smythe was unaware of his deep-seated feelings of anger for his father.	The structure and protected safety of psychotherapy enables patients to explore important repressed feelings.	As a child, Martin Smythe learned, through experience, that his anger for his father got him in trouble with his father and did not change anything. Therefore, he repressed his rage.
Before his treatment, Reverend Smythe was self-defeating.	Important and powerful feelings that are repressed gain expression as symptoms, including impaired mood and dysfunctional behavior.	Internally directed anger led to Reverend Smythe's depressed mood and self-destructive behaviors.

TABLE 6–1. Key principles in the treatment of a patient with narcissistic personality disorder as exemplified by the case of Reverend Martin Smythe (*continued*)

Historical fact	Key principle	Interpretation
In treatment, Reverend Smythe became aware of his anger for his father and could feel it.	Insight involves both mind and body, both thinking and feeling.	In treatment, Reverend Smythe discovered the sources and profound implications of his low self-esteem.
Reverend Smythe's "crisis of faith" was not about religion.	Self-discovery holds many surprises.	Reverend Smythe's unresolved hatred for his father, whom he regarded as an authority figure, interfered with his ability to accept or trust an "ultimate authority."
Reverend Smythe overreacted when Dr. Y. was away on scheduled holidays or job-related trips.	Although the associated feelings are strong, transference is an unconscious process.	Unwittingly, Reverend Smythe transferred his feelings of paternal abandonment to Dr. Y. and to other perceived authority figures.
Reverend Smythe worked hard in psychotherapy, and later in psychoanalysis, for many years.	"Quick fixes" in the treatment of people with significant personality disorders do not happen.	As the direct result of his working diligently over many years of treatment, Reverend Smythe was able to make constructive changes in many important realms of his life.

TABLE 6–2.   Reasons why the potency of psychotherapy is often underestimated

---

1. The stigmatization of the mentally ill is often transposed to mental health professionals who practice psychotherapy.

2. Many improperly trained and incompetent people represent themselves as being psychotherapists.

3. Because of the stigma attached to mental illness, people do not talk about the beneficial results of their psychotherapy.

4. Our society values the tangible; therefore procedures such as surgery and medicinal treatments seem more potent than "talking cures."

5. When the biological dimensions of mental disorders are not addressed through medications, exercise, and proper diet, psychotherapy will fail.

Psychotherapy Is a Powerful Tool for Change

The efficacy of psychotherapy is often underestimated for the reasons summarized in Table 6–2.

Nonetheless, scientific data from over 1,000 controlled-outcome research projects consistently document that highly trained psychotherapists who adhere to strict professional guidelines produce profound results in treating motivated patients with the full range of mental illnesses, including those with biological components. Readers who are interested in psychotherapy research may wish to inquire about the Society for Psychotherapy Research (http://www.psychotherapy-research.org), an international organization that has more than 1,000 members and is the sponsor of the scientific journal *Psychotherapy Research*.

Reverend Smythe's dramatic improvement as the result of insight-oriented psychotherapy and psychoanalysis is not a rare event; rather, multitudes of people with challenging behavioral and emotional problems have received great benefit from the full range of ethical and enlightened psychotherapeutic modalities.

Never, Never, Never Give Up Hope[1]

Reverend Smythe had shamefully violated the trust of and had harmed vulnerable women in his church who were under his religious author-

---

[1]On people who are willing to accept help in changing themselves.

ity. Initially he was without insight and honesty about this exploitive behavior. He was coerced by the board of trustees of his church to seek psychiatric assessment and initially showed resistance to participating authentically in psychiatric treatment. By almost every measure, Martin Smythe would not be regarded as a promising candidate for insight-oriented psychotherapy. Nonetheless, he ultimately made significant and constructive changes in his personality and behavior as a direct result of his psychotherapeutic experience. An important lesson from the experience of Martin Smythe is that because no expert can determine in advance who will or will not benefit from psychiatric care, the opportunity for such care should be offered to all those who require it. So long as the psychotherapist has had excellent training, is experienced, and demonstrates consummate professionalism and integrity, the success or failure of the treatment to lead to meaningful change will be up to the patient. The good news is that many people surprise themselves and others by making fundamental changes in their personality and behavior as a result of psychotherapy.

Spirituality and Religion in Mental Illness and in Recovery

The case of Reverend Smythe provides an excellent opportunity to discuss the role of spirituality and religion in mental disorders and their treatment. Throughout history and in every known culture, spiritual beliefs and religious expression have been fundamental elements of the human condition and experience. Many mental health professionals now believe that spirituality and religious expression are, in general, protective factors that help prevent many types of mental illness. These elements also provide critical sources of support and hopefulness in the recovery from psychiatric disorders.

Spirituality and Religion as Components of Mental Illness

Given how important religion and spirituality are to the human experience, it should be expected that they represent common manifestations of psychiatric disorders. For example, patients with schizophrenia may have delusions that they are being persecuted by the devil, or they may experience hallucinations in which they hear the voice of God. Individuals who are in states of mania may believe that they themselves have special spiritual powers, such as the ability to heal illnesses in other people by placing their hands on the ill person. Conversely, people with depression often become alienated from their religious faith or feel that they are evil and deserving of divine retribution. People with obsessive-compulsive disorder may become preoccupied with religious rules and tormented by interminable ritualized observances. Religious expression can be distorted in many ways that lead to mental illness. An all-too-common example is the religious fanaticism in some cultures that institutionalizes the oppression and exploitation of women and thereby leads to their disillusionment and to many types of reactive mental illness.

Spirituality, Religion, and Flaws of Personality and Character

Insincerity: The Mask of Spirituality

As demonstrated by the case of Reverend Smythe, conflicts with authority that are the results of abuse in early life can be reflected in impaired trust in and abuse of religious authority. People with serious flaws of personality and character notoriously misuse religion and spirituality for narrow, self-centered purposes. Examples are legion—and on occasion lethal. The prototypical example is people who attend their church, temple, or mosque without fail, who are highly visible leaders in public charities, who promote religious and ethical values in their companies' mission statements, but who are also dishonest in their businesses, exploitive in their friendships, unfaithful in their marriages, and abusive to their employees and family dependents. For such people, religion is a mask behind which they hide the full face of their distorted thinking and antisocial behavior. Still others with flaws of character and personality take advantage of the religious faith of others to further their own selfish purposes.

Murderous Messengers Have No Messages

The worst distortions and abuses of religion and spirituality by people with fatal flaws of character and personality occur among political leaders, terrorists, charismatic leaders of cults, and members of the clergy. The pain, destruction, and death perpetrated over the centuries in the name of religion and spiritual causes are immeasurable. There are many kind, constructive, and charitable ways to effect societal change. Why do certain people choose violent coercion? The answer comes from within them: usually despots and terrorists have multiple fatal flaws of personality and character. Consider the paranoid and antisocial personality disorders of Hitler; Stalin; Saddam Hussein; David Koresh, the leader of the Branch Davidian cult; Timothy McVeigh, who bombed the federal building in Oklahoma City, Oklahoma; and John Allen Muhammad, the Washington, D.C.–area sniper. Consider the narcissistic and antisocial personality disorder of Osama Bin Laden and the schizotypal and antisocial personality of Theodore Kaczynski, the Unabomber. All these people killed innocent others in the name of some "higher cause." They claimed a higher spiritual authority than the rest of us to justify their exploitation and murder of many others—while they painstakingly protected and took very, very good care of themselves. *The truth lies in the personality and character disorders of the messengers, not in their messages.* Their vile actions are purely extensions of their fatal flaws of personality and character. To put it another way, their cruel and cowardly crimes are all about *them* and have *nothing whatsoever* to do with the so-called causes or issues that they espouse.

Finally, when unethical clerics exploit their positions of holiness and authority to prey on the young and vulnerable, they do double damage. Not only do they harm those whom they explicitly exploit, but they also diminish the faith and trust of the many others in their spiritual leaders, most of whom are honorable servants of their parishioners, their religions, and their Maker.

Spirituality and Religion in Psychotherapeutic Treatments

Why Religion and Spirituality Have Been Deemphasized in Psychotherapy

Mental health professionals have perennially underestimated the important role of religion and spirituality in preventing mental illnesses and have underutilized the clergy who could help support and inspire the recovery of their clients and patients. There are many reasons—historical and practical—that have led to this professional disservice. Much has been written about Freud and religion, and it is clear that both he and his most prominent disciples were wary of religion's "intrusion" into psychotherapeutic practice. Although many historians have attributed Freud's manifest distaste for the presence of religion in psychiatric practice to his personal conflicts with his own Jewish upbringing and heritage, I do not accept these theories. Rather, I believe that Freud's bitter experience with the institutionalized anti-Semitism that was pervasive in the European universities and hospitals where he studied and practiced led him to be concerned that religious prejudice and fanaticism might gain influence in psychoanalysis to harm vulnerable patients in psychotherapy. The consummate expression by the Nazis of this anti-Semitism in Austria, Germany, Italy, France, and Spain resulted in the murder of many psychoanalysts and their patients and Freud's flight with his family from Austria to Britain. For a detailed portrayal of the prejudice toward and vicious persecution of Jewish physicians and academicians in Germany, I recommend to interested readers *Unlocking the Golden Cage,* the biography of one of my esteemed mentors, psychoanalyst Hilde Bruch (1996). Dr. Bruch was a pioneer in understanding and treating people with anorexia nervosa and other eating disorders. If, after reading the biography of Dr. Bruch, your spirit, heart, and stomach can bear to go further, you may wish to read the recent biography of Rosalind Franklin (Maddox 2002). This biography documents how, even in the twentieth century, prominent English academicians and scientists in distinguished British universities wielded anti-Semitism and prejudice against women to humiliate and deny this brilliant woman her proper recognition for her important role in the discovery of DNA. I belabor the discussion of the sources of the underrepresentation of religion and spirituality in psychotherapy because I believe that—just as in psychiatric illnesses—we must first diagnose the true causes of problems before effecting meaningful cures.

The Proper Role of Religion and Spirituality in the Treatment of People With Psychiatric Disorders

I believe that *with the appropriate understanding and strict professional oversight,* mental health professionals must now include spirituality and religious faith in the treatment of the vast majority of their patients and clients who are so inclined. First and foremost, this must be accomplished without the introduction of bias of any sort—either against or in support of any particular approach to religion. Rather, the direction must come from the patient, and we must support the types and degree of religious expression that the patient believes are best suited to his or her recovery.

Even the best-intended referral of a person with a mental illness involving problems of faith to a spiritual counselor will often backfire. The manifest bias of the therapist can discourage the patient from expressing his or her feelings of antipathy related to religion, expressions that might be required before the patient approaches the underlying *sources* of these negative feelings. To emphasize the importance of this point, let us reconsider the case of Reverend Smythe. Given his shame over his transgressions as a pastor and his significant problems with his own faith, he was at first reluctant to introduce the topic of spirituality into his treatment. About 6 months into his treatment, he said, "I assume that you, like all psychiatrists and scientists, are an atheist; so I will not offend you with what I believe to be the basic hypocrisy and small-mindedness of organized religion." Although I never disclosed to Reverend Smythe my personal attitude toward religion, I listened, nonjudgmentally, for many weeks as he disclosed his cynicism about spirituality and religious practice. Given his inside knowledge, he presented endless examples of the hypocrisy and misdeeds of his superiors in the church hierarchy. Over time, however, he was able to recognize how his disappointing experiences with and unresolved rage at his father led him to be exquisitely sensitive to the relatively rare bad examples among church leadership, while ignoring the impressive good works of the majority of his leaders. Through his ensuing work in psychoanalysis, he came to accept his own powerful spiritual drives and became comfortable with his religious faith. I do not believe that this process or result would have been possible with a therapist, no matter how open and nonjudgmental, whom he believed to have a formal affiliation with organized religion. As a final note of caution, I believe that the utilization of the psychotherapeutic process as a vehicle for proselytizing to patients or clients about a particular religion constitutes malpractice.

Afterword

The case of Reverend Martin Smythe provides an example of how people with narcissistic personality disorder *who are motivated to change* can often derive far-reaching benefit from psychodynamically informed psychotherapy and psychoanalysis. Reverend Smythe's case also highlights the importance of spirituality in the biopsychosocial-spiritual model in understanding and treating people with mental disorders. For most patients, the biopsychosocial-spiritual approach to care is like a four-legged stool. If any one of the four components is missing, the stool will tip over and treatment will be incomplete or will even fail. Often in psychotherapy, the spiritual leg is missing. This is a potentially damaging omission that our professional fields must work hard to change as soon as possible. The bottom line is that I recommend that you choose for yourself or refer a person with a psychiatric disorder to an experienced, gifted, and *impartial* psychotherapist who is *open* to including— if you so choose—religion and spirituality in treatment and recovery.

The case of Reverend Smythe also raises an important question: What is the role of genetic heritability and biological factors in narcissistic personality disorder? As presented in Chapter 5 ("Narcissistic Personality Disorder, Part I: Untreated Narcissism"), Reverend Smythe's father, Congressman Dennis Smythe, also met DSM criteria for this condition. In medicine, when serious disorders are present in families, our indices of suspicion about genetic predispositions and protective factors are raised. Very little valid research has been conducted about the genetics and neurobiology of narcissistic personality disorder. Consequently, most of the focus on the conceptualization of the condition and its treatment is based on psychodynamic models. Many other psychiatric disorders, including schizophrenia and bipolar disorder, were originally understood to be the result of experiential and psychological factors (e.g., the "schizophrenogenic mother") but later proved to have profound genetic and neurobiological bases. This understanding dramatically improved diagnosis and treatment. Many people with narcissistic personality disorder will not accept treatment or will not benefit from psychotherapeutic treatment. Perhaps one leg of the stool is too short.

References and Selected Readings

Bruch JH: Unlocking the Golden Cage: An Intimate Biography of Hilde Bruch, M.D. Carlsbad, CA, Gürze Books, 1996

Frattaroli E: Healing the Soul in the Age of the Brain: Becoming Conscious in an Unconscious World. New York, Viking, 2001

Fromm-Reichmann F: Principles of Intensive Psychotherapy. Chicago, IL, University of Chicago Press, 1950

Gabbard GO: Sexual Exploitation in Professional Relationships. Washington, DC, American Psychiatric Press, 1989

Gabbard GO: Psychoanalysis and psychoanalytic psychotherapy, in Comprehensive Textbook of Psychiatry, 7th Edition. Edited by Sadock BJ, Sadock VA. Philadelphia, PA, Lippincott Williams & Wilkins, 2000, pp 2056–2079

MacKinnon RA, Yudofsky SC: Principles of the Psychiatric Evaluation. Philadelphia, PA, JB Lippincott, 1991

Maddox B: Rosalind Franklin: The Dark Lady of DNA. New York, HarperCollins, 2002

Sulloway FJ: Freud, Biologist of the Mind: Beyond the Psychoanalytic Legend. New York, Basic Books, 1979

Chapter

7

ANTISOCIAL PERSONALITY DISORDER

The man who hath no music in himself,…
Let no such man be trusted.

—William Shakespeare,
The Merchant of Venice

"I take because nobody gives" (Exploitation)
"I won't give what I never got" (Lack of empathy)
"If it doesn't hurt me, it doesn't hurt" (Deficient
   conscience)

—Stuart Yudofsky, The Three
Laws of Sociopathy

Essence

Most of us go about our lives with the belief that we are practically invulnerable. Although we recognize that modern life is fraught with dangers, we have faith that we can maintain our safety by taking reasonable and appropriate precautions. We avoid dangerous metropolitan areas, live in safe neighborhoods, and put alarms in our cars and in our houses. We cannot, however, lead isolated lives or put alarms on ourselves and on our loved ones. We assume that the people who become part of our personal or professional lives share our values about the rights of others and the sanctity of human life. We are very naïve. They look and know how to act just like you and me. They know how to gain our trust, how to make us feel safe and comfortable with them, and how to gain access to our personal lives and to our person. However, they are very different from what they seem, very different from you and from me. Even though they are aware of society's rules, they do not believe that its laws should apply to them. Their guiding principle is not doing what is right, but doing what they believe is right for themselves. They take what they want and what they can get away with. They want a great deal from us, and they are very good at getting what they want. If you have a problem with that, *you* become "the problem." And they have no compunctions about doing whatever it takes to get rid of "the problem." At that point you had better understand with whom you are dealing. You had better know how to protect yourself.

The Case of Andrew Kramer: Infancy Through Adolescence

Early Years

Over the years, Melissa Kramer often said, "No child was ever more wanted than Andrew." Melissa and Greg Kramer had been married for 14 years before they adopted Andrew as a newborn baby. Before that time, the Kramers had tried unsuccessfully to conceive a child. For 9 years they had worked intensively with a fertility center that was associated with the obstetrics and gynecology department of an excellent medical school. Although no specific anatomical or physiological problem was identified for either Melissa or Greg that prevented them from conceiving a child, a broad range of remedies—from fertility medications to in vitro fertilization—was attempted, to no avail. The only information that was shared with the Kramers about Andrew's biological parents was that they were both teenagers in good physical health when their baby was born and that the baby was born out of wedlock.

At the time that Andrew was adopted, both Melissa and Greg were engaged in successful careers in law. Greg was a partner in a large urban law firm, and he specialized in corporate law. Melissa was a well-known and highly regarded judge in family court. She had special expertise in child custody cases. On the adoption of Andrew, Melissa relinquished her position on the bench to devote her full time to caring for her son. She thought him to be a "marvelous baby and toddler." As an infant, Andrew was happy, hungry, and calm and would sleep through most of the night. He reached all of the developmental milestones on time as he grew older. He seemed to be intelligent, was adept with language, was well coordinated, and was gifted mechanically. Because most of Melissa and Greg's close friends had children who were older than Andrew, and because the couple lived in a luxury condominium with mostly older adults, Andrew did not have the opportunity to spend much of his time during his early years with children of his own age. He seemed more than content to engage primarily with his doting mother, who introduced him to books, music, and nature.

Pre-Kindergarten

When he was 3 years old, Andrew's parents enrolled him in a pre-kindergarten program. They were shocked by the feedback that they soon received from his teacher, Miss Kirkland.

> **Miss Kirkland:** There is no question that Andrew is a very intelligent little boy, and his motor skills are superior. However, we believe that he has a problem getting along with other children.
>
> **Melissa Kramer:** Specifically, what problem does he have?
>
> **Miss Kirkland:** He seems to want his way all of the time. He bullies the other children, and they are all afraid of him.
>
> **Melissa (with some irritability and impatience):** I asked you to be specific. All I hear now are undocumented allegations!
>
> **Miss Kirkland:** I know that it is not easy to hear unflattering comments about your son, whom I know you just adore. To be specific, today another child was playing with a toy cash register. Andrew pushed the little boy away from the toy and started playing with it himself. The little boy started crying, and I tried to help Andrew learn to play together with the other child. Andrew would have no part of sharing. He pushed the little boy again, very hard; and he also hit me on my hand.
>
> **Greg Kramer:** This is most unusual behavior for Andrew. I cannot recall a single incident when he has been physical with another child, or anybody for that matter. Perhaps the two children just don't get along, or perhaps one of them is just having a bad day.
>
> **Miss Kirkland:** You are right about all children having bad days and about some children who have personalities that clash with specific other children. But this is not the case here. We have observed Andrew for over 3 weeks, and he just does not do well with any of the other children. He always wants his own way. When he doesn't get his way, he threatens, intimidates, or physically attacks the other children. We have been unsuccessful at changing this pattern of behavior. I have spoken about this with Mrs. North, our school psychologist. She came in today especially to observe Andrew's behavior. She concluded that Andrew is not yet ready for preschool. She also asked that I recommend that he be evaluated by a child psychologist or psychiatrist. We can give you some names of professionals if you like.
>
> **Melissa (with obvious rage):** I can't believe what I am hearing. Andrew is only 3 years old, and you are speaking of him as if he is a psychotic criminal! You are way, way out of line! First of all, why are we just learning about all of this right now? Why didn't you

tell us about it sooner? Second of all, who gave you permission to have him psychoanalyzed by a school psychologist? I don't recall signing a waiver or giving any permission to have this done!

Miss Kirkland: I certainly understand that you are very upset. We put off this communication in order to work with Andrew on his social skills and to give him more time to adjust to the new environment. When we saw that we were not making any progress, we called in the psychologist and notified you right away of her conclusions and recommendations.

Melissa: Well, I don't accept how you went about this at all. You should have involved us from the very beginning. And in no way did you have the right to bring in a psychologist to observe Andrew without our permission. I really believe that this is actionable.

Greg: Honey, please calm down. We're getting off the subject. What is truly important is to determine whether or not Andrew has a behavior problem in the school setting. Let's go home and think this over.

Melissa: You're not getting this, Greg. This is not a small deal. Miss Kirkland is telling us that they are not going to let Andrew come back to school without clearance from a shrink. And that's the least of it. This will all go down on his record. It is certain to hurt his chances of being accepted to a good private school. This is no little deal, and I object strongly to the whole thing. After all we have gone through to get Andrew, I don't believe this is happening to us. I really think that you should talk this over with someone in your law firm tomorrow morning!

On the way home from the meeting with Miss Kirkland, the following discussion took place between Greg and Melissa Kramer:

Greg Kramer: Darling, I know you're upset about Andrew, but I have never seen you lose your cool the way you did with Miss Kirkland. You are a judge and an expert mediator, and you understand that threats and temper outbursts are counterproductive. I thought that Miss Kirkland was only trying to be reasonable and helpful. Now she probably believes that Andrew has learned to be so assertive and inconsiderate by modeling our behavior.

Melissa Kramer: I can't believe I am hearing this from you! You are actually taking a stranger's side against your own wife and son. We are being attacked and you are siding with the enemy.

Greg: Darling, please calm down. I am not your enemy or Andrew's. And I don't think that Miss Kirkland is out to get us or Andrew, either. I believe that we should have Andrew evaluated by a competent child psychologist to see what is what. Perhaps one of the consultants you use in family court.

Melissa: Over my dead body will Andrew be sent to some headshrinker! He's just 3 years old, for Heaven's sake. What is a shrink supposed to tell us at this point? That he has been a victim of abuse by his parents? This could all backfire on us and go down

> permanently on Andrew's record. No way. He is a bright and
> happy child. I'm not going to let this go any further. I will home
> school him myself until he is ready to go to kindergarten. Case
> closed!

Melissa Kramer did exactly what she said she would do. The next
day she had Greg call Andrew's school to say that he would not be coming back. She also instructed her attorney to write a letter to the school
stating explicitly that the Kramer family prohibited the transfer of any
information about Andrew—either written or verbal—without his parents' written permission. She purchased many books and tapes about
the intellectual enrichment of young children and dedicated herself to
educating her son.

Andrew's New Sister, Lana

Melissa had not been feeling well. She was nauseated in the mornings
and felt uncharacteristically listless throughout the day. Initially she attributed her state of health to the stress and anxiety related to Andrew's
experience at pre-kindergarten. Greg insisted that Melissa see her internist, who examined her carefully and took an extensive series of blood
tests. The tests confirmed her doctor's suspicion: Melissa was pregnant,
probably near the end of her first trimester. At first the Kramers
couldn't believe it. They were, in fact, stunned. After being preoccupied
for over a decade with trying conceive a child, and after going through
seemingly countless and almost unbearable procedures in the fertility
clinic, they had given up all hope of Melissa's ever becoming pregnant.
After the adoption of Andrew, they didn't even think about the possibility. Rather, at that point, they were considering adopting a second
child. Their shock quickly changed to unbridled joy. Both Greg and Melissa now understood as well that Melissa's uncharacteristic anger and
moodiness were likely related to the hormonal changes associated with
her pregnancy.

With the birth of their daughter, Lana, 6 months later, Greg made a
conscious effort to spend more of his time with Andrew. Both father and
son loved sports and the outdoors. Greg Kramer was an amateur natu-
ralist with a passion for studying the local ants, spiders, and butterflies,
and he spent many hours sharing his knowledge and love for nature
with his son. Andrew was particularly interested in the habits of spiders and ants, which, as he grew older, he read about and studied
closely in their natural environments. Two incidents occurred when
Andrew was 8 years old that greatly disturbed his parents. The first
event took place one afternoon when Greg Kramer came home early

from work. Greg was told that Andrew was playing by himself in the woods behind their home, so he went outside to join him. He found Andrew crouching by a large fire ant mound, about which had been placed three living frogs. The frogs were struggling to escape being devoured by the ants, but they were unable to get away. Upon closer observation, Greg discovered that the hind legs of each frog had been tied together with white thread, so they could not escape the voracious ants. Greg also noticed that both eyes of two of the frogs had been punctured, making them blind. As Greg had tried to teach his son to respect and not interfere with wildlife, he was horrified by what he observed. He questioned Andrew about what he had done:

> **Greg Kramer:** Andrew, what were you doing with those poor frogs?
> **Andrew Kramer:** An experiment, Daddy. Ants are usually afraid of frogs, because frogs eat insects. I wanted to see if they would attack frogs that couldn't get away from them.
> **Greg:** But, Andrew! Didn't you feel bad about the poor frogs that were being eaten alive by the ants?
> **Andrew:** I don't understand what you mean, Daddy. I don't think the frogs feel sorry for the ants when they eat them.

The second incident, which occurred 7 months later, was even more disturbing to Mr. and Mrs. Kramer. They awakened one evening to piercing screams from their daughter Lana, who at that time was $4\frac{1}{2}$ years old. Her cries were such that both parents ran to her room. They found her thrashing about in her bed, seemingly in excruciating pain. At first the parents were unable to figure out what was the matter with their daughter. Her face was flushed and her skin felt hot. When they removed her pajamas to help cool her off, they immediately noticed that her left upper arm was red and swollen. They quickly observed that her right buttock was also inflamed, and they decided to rush Lana to the emergency room of the children's hospital. Her arm was becoming more swollen by the second, and she seemed delirious from pain. The emergency room pediatrician took her temperature and vital signs and told the terrified parents that her daughter would be admitted immediately to the pediatric intensive care unit. At first none of the doctors would commit themselves to telling the Kramers exactly what was wrong with their daughter. Several hours later, Dr. Weingarten, the director of the intensive care unit, took them into a small, windowless room to speak with them.

> **Melissa Kramer:** Will Lana be all right? Do you know what is wrong with her?

Dr. Weingarten: At this time, we cannot answer with certainty either question, but we are doing our best to save Lana.

Melissa (frantically): Are you saying that Lana might die? I want to see her this very moment. I won't let my daughter die.

Greg Kramer: Please, darling. Try to calm down and let the doctor tell us what they have found out.

Dr. Weingarten: Right now your daughter is in shock. Her heart stopped beating for a few minutes, but we kept her ventilated and got it started again. We are almost certain that she is in toxic shock from an insect bite, probably a spider. We have already given her antitoxins, which, if we are right, should save her life. The extent of damage and the level of her recovery will depend mainly on two things: how her body reacts to the spider bites and whether or not she is allergic to the antitoxins we have given her.

Dr. Weingarten patiently spent an hour answering the parents' questions, but he was not overly reassuring to them. For the next 3 days the Kramers lived a waking nightmare. They never left the intensive care room waiting area. Lana remained in a delirium, and her arm swelled several times the size of her thighs. The arm also turned blue, as did her left forearm and hand. At one point there was concern about whether or not the arm could be saved. Slowly she began to show signs of recovery. After 4 days she recognized and spoke to her parents, and the swelling on her arm and hand began to recede. Lana remained in the intensive care unit for 11 days before being transferred to a private room in the hospital. To the relief of everyone, a slow but full recovery was predicted. At the time of her discharge, Dr. Weingarten spoke to the Kramers:

Dr. Weingarten: Your whole family, especially Lana, has been through a great trauma. We are fairly certain that the bite on her arm was from a brown recluse spider, given the nature and severity of her resulting pathology. This is not that unusual, as they are plentiful around here, and they love to go into homes. We see several children each year who are bitten by these spiders, with severe repercussions. We are uncertain about the type of spider that bit Lana on her buttock; but we know from her reaction to the bite that it was not a brown recluse. The toxicologist is pretty sure that it was a black widow bite, and, as you know, black widows are also abundant in Houston. What is unusual is that Lana had two spider bites from two different types of spiders! None of us has ever seen that before, not even in kids who are on overnights in the woods. It's like being hit by lightning twice in the same day. I guess if you practice long enough you will see everything. I know that you have already had the exterminators in your home several times during the past 2 weeks. I would have them check your home weekly to make sure there aren't some nests under your home or nearby. Now you should have all of Lana's medications, and I will see her next week in clinic.

At the time and through the many years that followed, it never occurred to the doctors or to the Kramers that Lana's spider bites were not the result of unfortunate coincidence. Greg Kramer fleetingly wondered how two spiders were able to crawl into her pajamas, which had elastic around the arms and ankles. He reasoned that they probably entered her pajamas through the collar and was thankful that they didn't bite her on her face. He didn't revisit this puzzle for 15 years.

Elementary School

Andrew was accepted to the most selective private school in the city based on his high entry test scores in math and science; his interpersonal charm during his teacher interviews; his athletic prowess, particularly in sports involving hand-eye coordination such as tennis and baseball; and the prominent professional and personal reputations of his parents. Andrew flourished in elementary school. Not only did he receive good grades, he was also popular and a leader among his peers. He was among the tallest and was considered to be one of the best looking of his classmates. Physical fighting was not permitted in his school, with the penalty of certain expulsion for those who were repeat offenders. Although Andrew never fought in school, many of his best friends got into trouble for skirmishes. A few were expelled. Most of the smaller, less assertive boys in the class felt intimidated by Andrew and his friends and learned to stay out of their way. On the other hand, his teachers in elementary school and the parents of his friends regarded Andrew as a serious and responsible boy. He would look directly into the eyes of the adults with whom he spoke and was unfailingly courteous and respectful to them. Although he could have had starting positions on the school football and baseball teams, Andrew chose to compete on the tennis team. His two favorite extracurricular interests were computers and rocketry. Living in Houston, Texas, he was able to make many trips to the Johnson Space Center and to belong to sophisticated rocket clubs that designed and launched their own missiles. He spent innumerable hours on the Internet, where he learned about rockets and missiles and developed expertise in solid rocket propellants and explosives.

Middle School

Trouble swirled, bubbled, and brewed about Andrew during his middle school years, but he never got burned or seemed to feel the heat. Although his grades stayed strong, some of his school's most experienced teachers distrusted him. The teachers noticed that his best friends were not serious students and did not engage in athletics or participate in the school's outstanding fine arts programs. Most of his friends were on academic probation and were eventually caught violating the school's stringent rules about alcohol and drugs. A few were even prosecuted for felony violations outside of school, an almost unheard-of occurrence for this elite private school. Over the next several years, most of Andrew's friends flunked out or were expelled from school. During the ninth grade, Andrew's history teacher, Mr. West, strongly suspected him of cheating on a final examination. Andrew had received a perfect score on the 2-hour, 150-question, multiple choice and fill-in-the-blank test. Mr. West was suspicious because over his 23 years of giving similar final examinations, no other student had even come close to such an achievement. Not even students whom he knew were outstanding and who had later achieved perfect scores on the history SAT II. Andrew's performance in class and on other tests was average. The trouble was that Mr. West had no proof, and he couldn't figure out how Andrew had managed to pull off the cheating. He called Andrew to his office to question him about the test result.

> **Mr. West:** I am confused and upset about your score on the history final.
> **Andrew Kramer:** Then I'm confused, too, Mr. North. I worked so hard preparing for the test; I thought you would be proud of me for doing so well.
> **Mr. West:** You and I both know there is no way that you could have gotten all those questions right; I even asked one or two questions on subjects that we didn't cover in class.
> **Andrew:** Oh, now I understand what you mean, Mr. West, and you are exactly right. On quite a few of the multiple choice questions, I made what I would call educated guesses. For once I was lucky and got them all right. I really didn't know every answer. But I don't know why you would ask questions on things that we weren't responsible for.
> **Mr. West:** And how do you explain getting all the short answer, fill-in-the-blanks questions correct?
> **Andrew:** Like I told you, Mr. West, I studied very hard for the test— first in order to learn a subject that I am very interested in; and second, to try to pull my final grade up to an A, which I believe I succeeded in doing.
> **Mr. West:** Andrew, I believe that the best way to resolve this is to have you take another final, and, if your grade remains near-perfect, I will have no problem giving you an A in the class.
> **Andrew:** You are accusing me of cheating just because I did well. You have no evidence whatsoever that I cheated. I believe that you have something personal against me. I have always felt that you

disliked me because of my religion; and I have in fact told this to my parents and friends on numerous occasions. Just like you, I can't prove it. One thing you can be sure of: I have no intention of retaking this test or speaking with you about it any further. I can assure you that you will hear from my parents about this sooner than you would like.

After this interchange, Andrew calmly left the office of Mr. West, who was trembling in a state of fury and frustration. The school's principal, Mr. Kelsey, soon called a meeting, which was attended by Mr. West, Mr. and Mrs. Kramer, and himself.

Melissa Kramer: Greg and I are outraged by what we consider a malicious, unsubstantiated charge against our son by Mr. West. We are here to see that this does not go one bit further!

Mr. West: Andrew's perfect score on the final is grossly inconsistent with his classroom performance over the past year as well as his grades on all his other tests in this course. All I did was request that he retake a similar test.

Melissa: I beg to disagree. All you did was accuse him of cheating. He is a student who has been at this school for 9 years without a single blemish on his record. If you give him a much harder test this time, or if Andrew misses a few questions, does that mean—*res ipsa loquitur*—that he is a cheater? I certainly think not.

Principal Kelsey: I am sure we can find some middle ground here that we all can comfortably share.

Melissa: The middle ground is to drop this whole thing right now. As you probably know, Mr. Kelsey, our daughter, Lana, who has just finished the sixth grade here, received perfect scores on three of her finals this term. Does that mean that she has to take the tests over as well? Are you accusing our whole family of being cheaters?

Principal Kelsey: We aren't accusing anyone of cheating. We are just trying to seek clarity and find resolution. Lana Kramer is one of the finest students in the history of the school. I believe that she has come in first in just about every subject in every class since she has been here. All the faculty know and agree that she is an exceptional student, who is beyond reproach in every way. We are not here to talk about Lana.

Melissa: You might not be here to talk about Lana, but I am. If you persist with this unsubstantiated allegation against our son, we will have no choice but to sue you, Mr. West, the board of trustees, and the school for slander and defamation of character based on what we believe is a vendetta against our son over his religion. Under such circumstances, of course, both Lana and Andrew will have to leave this school, adding to the damages. I also believe that the other Jewish students and their parents will not stand for our being treated like this.

Principal Kelsey: I will assume my prerogative as principal to make a decision on this matter by the end of the day. I will first discuss this issue with the chairperson of the board of trustees and the school's legal counsel. I will get back to everyone by late afternoon. I believe that I have sufficient information at this point to make a judicious and fair decision.

That afternoon all parties involved were informed by Principal Kelsey that the score on Andrew's final examination would remain 100% and that he would receive the final grade of A in the history course. Manifestly, Mr. West felt humiliated but remained certain that Andrew had cheated on the final test. He was completely baffled as to how Andrew had managed to pull it off. Two years later Mr. West believed he had figured it out, but that was the least of his problems at the time. Based on an anonymous tip, the Federal Bureau of Investigation (FBI) obtained a court order to confiscate both Mr. West's school and home computers. Mr. West learned that he was being accused of trafficking in illegal child pornography, and he retained an attorney. Because the hard drive on Mr. West's school computer was subpoenaed by the FBI, Principal Kelsey was fully informed of the charges against the history teacher. It turned out that although no pornography was found on his school computer, there was evidence of substantial pornographic material—including illegal child pornography—on Mr. West's home computer. Through his counsel, Mr. West admitted that he occasionally surfed the Web and visited some legal pornographic sites. Some of these sites contained pictures suggesting that the females featured were underage, even though the participants were actually above the age of legal consent. Mr. West's hard drive also contained a substantial amount of illegal child pornography, about which he claimed to have no idea how it got there. After spending his life savings on attorneys and computer experts for his defense, it was ultimately determined that it could not be proved whether or not someone had "hacked" into his computer and inserted the illegal material. The firewall on the Internet carrier of his home computer was far more porous than that of the school.

Although the charges against Mr. West were eventually dropped by the FBI, the private school concluded that they would not renew his contract for the next year. The school maintained that it had to act in the interest of protecting all students, even if Mr. West had not been proved guilty of the charges. Although it was unstated, the school no doubt was unsettled by the embarrassing publicity surrounding the accusations against Mr. West. Mr. West chose not to contest the school's decision; he had neither the resources nor the energy to take on the school's powerful attorneys. During his ordeal, it occurred to Mr. West that

2 years earlier, Andrew must have hacked into his home computer, on which he had written and saved the final test and answer sheet. He also speculated that Andrew might have been the source of the FBI tip and had inserted the child pornography on his computer. When Mr. West advanced this theory to his attorneys, they advised him as follows: "With all due respect, Mr. West, you have enough problems without involving Judge Kramer and Greg Kramer. We can assure you that if you try to involve their son in your problems, you will end up in jail." Mr. West never went to jail, but his career in teaching was over. Of course, Andrew Kramer and his parents felt completely vindicated when they learned of Mr. West's plight.

High School

Long before beginning high school, Andrew had an intense interest in girls, and they in him. His parents thought that their son's main problem with girls was distraction from his studies. His telephone at home was always ringing with their calls, and he was constantly being asked out by them. He seemed to capture the attention of girls who were both considerably older and younger than he, and, truth be told, he also caught the notice of many of their mothers. When Andrew's parents gave him a car at age 16, he gained far more freedom and independence than his parents had anticipated or believed appropriate. He was away from home much of the time, including being out overnight during weekdays and on most weekends. He always had convincing excuses for being away, such as working on school projects with his classmates or going on field trips with his rocketry club. Because the Kramers kept in touch with their son via his cell phone and since Andrew intensely objected when they checked up on him by calling the homes where he was supposed to be ("You are acting as if you don't trust me," he would say), the parents really didn't know where their son was most of the time. Although they were not comfortable with this arrangement, the Kramers rationalized that they would let it go until such time as Andrew got into trouble or his school grades declined.

During Andrew's years in middle school and high school, there were many confusing incidents that his parents chose to overlook. Whenever they questioned the credibility of their son, their queries seemed to backfire. An example occurred when Andrew was in the tenth grade and Melissa Kramer took his new car for its 5,000-mile servicing. While looking for the warranty service book she found, buried deeply in the car's glove compartment, a garage door opener encircled by an envelope and a thick rubber band. Judge Kramer's curiosity got the better of her when she noticed that Andrew's name was written on the front of the envelope in what seemed to be a woman's handwriting. She removed and opened the envelope and discovered inside a page of expensive-appearing stationery engraved with name of Ellen Michael, a person whom she knew fairly well. More an acquaintance than a close friend, Ellen was the divorced mother of two young children, and she lived in an expensive house about 3 miles from the Kramer home. What was handwritten in green ink on the stationery took Melissa Kramer's breath away:

> Dearest Andrew,
> Use this opener, and me,
> At any time and in any way
> You want.
> > Love,
> > Ellen

Judge Kramer's mind raced over the possibilities. Was it possible, as the note clearly implied, that her 16-year-old son was having an affair with a divorced woman? Was Andrew capable of such a thing? Was Ellen Michael the type of woman who could seduce a child? Because Melissa had always made a big point about family members respecting one another's privacy—especially their mail—how could she bring this up with Andrew? She had already made up her mind that she would immediately tell her husband. On the way home from the car dealership, she stopped at Kinko's to make a copy of Ellen's note. Thereafter, she carefully re-attached the note and envelope to the opener, which she returned to the glove compartment. As Melissa was carrying out this task, she was aware of how uncharacteristic this behavior was for her. She could not recall a similar occasion when she had acted so secretively or felt so deceitful. Her heart would not stop racing. That night she told her husband about the garage door opener and showed him the copy of the note:

> **Melissa Kramer:** Why do I feel so upset, Greg? I have been shaking all day.
> **Greg Kramer:** Because you are so used to being in control. You always know the right thing to do; but there is no "right thing" to do in this case. We both expect that Andrew will be angry and confused if he finds out that we read one of his personal letters.
> **Melissa:** Do you really think this is about ethics, Greg? If so, whose ethics—Andrew's or ours?
> **Greg:** What really matters is our responsibility to protect our son, so we must speak to him about this.

Melissa: I am not so sure about that. I think we are taking a very big chance. He will know that I violated his trust by reading his personal mail, and this could be very confusing to him.

Greg: Let's not miss the big picture, here. Andrew is still a minor, and there is a strong possibility that he has gotten himself into something that is way over his head. Our overriding responsibility is to protect him. Let's speak with him this evening.

Melissa: I will go with you on this one, Greg. But I am very nervous about it.

That evening the parents told Andrew that they had found the garage opener in the glove compartment of his car and had read the note that was addressed to him. The discussion that ensued was as follows:

Andrew Kramer: You both look so intense and serious. You're acting as if I have committed some sort of crime. You are really confusing me.

Greg Kramer: We understand your confusion. At the same time, we want an explanation from you about what was found in your car.

Andrew: This is so embarrassing. The note and opener are a joke we are playing on my friend, Conner. Conner's sister babysits for Mrs. Michael's two little children. Conner drives her there and picks her up when she's through. This is hard to say to your parents, but Conner thinks that Mrs. Michael is "hot." It's a stupid, harmless crush, but he's always talking about her, to the point that it's been bugging all of us, especially his sister. We got his sister to take some of Mrs. Michael's stationery and write that dumb note that you read. We tied the note to my friend Larry's garage door opener and were going to give it to Conner as a joke. I was going to pretend that Mrs. Michael had a crush on me to make him jealous. This is all so stupid and so embarrassing. Conner would have never believed the note was real, anyway. I can't believe that you fell for it.

Melissa and Greg Kramer were both relieved and upset. They apologized profusely to Andrew for the misunderstanding and for doubting him. They also were deeply concerned about damaging the relationship with their son. And Andrew didn't make it any easier for them.

Andrew: This is so upsetting to me. I never want to hear another word about this non-event again. I'm pretty sure that our relationship won't be the same again, either. How do you expect me to trust you? Don't you know that I truly believed all of those things you preach to me about not going through each other's private stuff? You even have me leave the room when you're talking to your stupid clients over the phone. As if I were interested, anyway. I really and truly don't know what to believe anymore. Both of you are just going to have to give me a whole lot more space. No more calling me on my cell phone every minute to check up on me. I'll call you when I think you need to know where I am.

Greg thought about calling Mrs. Michael and Conner to check out the story, but Melissa protested vehemently.

Melissa: Have you lost your mind? What would you say to them that wouldn't make you sound sick and paranoid? And that would be the end of our relationship with Andrew. I shouldn't have let you talk me into telling him about this in the first place. Greg, I really must question your judgment about your son. We are just going to have to trust him, and that's it.

Needless to say, Melissa and Greg did not pursue this matter any further. In addition, at age 16, Andrew had used this episode to maneuver himself into being almost completely free from parental oversight.

Senior Year of High School

In October of his senior year of high school, Andrew's best friend, Larry, was responsible for a serious automobile accident in which he was determined by blood analysis to have been driving while under the influence of alcohol, marijuana, and the prescription sedative alprazolam (Xanax). One of the passengers in the car that he sideswiped sustained a brain injury that left her with a permanent disability. In the ensuing police investigation, Larry implicated Andrew as being the source of the marijuana and alprazolam. A search warrant was issued for the Kramer home, where they found in Andrew's room several kilograms of marijuana, large quantities of cocaine, and hundreds of pills. In addition, a cache of several thousand dollars in cash was also discovered hidden in Andrew's bedroom. It was clear to the police that Andrew was a drug dealer, and once again his parents were incredulous. At first Andrew feigned surprise and protested that he had no idea how the drugs and cash came to be in his room. To his parents he suggested that the police had planted the illegal substances as a possible vendetta against his mother for her rulings against several police officers during their divorce hearings. To the police he disclosed that the husband of the Kramers' housekeeper of many years had a record of incarceration for car theft, and that he had access to Andrew's room when the family was away on holidays. But this time, for the first time in his life, Andrew could not talk his way out of trouble. However, although he may have been down, Andrew was by no means out. Because he was legally a minor, because he had never before been in any legal trouble, and because the assistant district attorney prosecuting the case and the presiding judge had great respect for his parents, Andrew was placed on probation with the condition that he undergo a minimum of 1 year of professional counseling. Melissa Kramer chose one of her close friends, Dr. Henrietta Roth, a psychoanalyst who specialized in family treatment, to evaluate and treat Andrew. Greg Kramer disagreed with this selection, because he believed that a more impartial professional with expertise in problems related to substance abuse would be more appropriate. As usual, Melissa Kramer prevailed.

The Kramers were at a loss as to why Andrew would need to make money by dealing drugs. Neither parent could recall his ever requesting anything that they did not buy for him. Dr. Roth rapidly arrived at a psychological formulation endorsed by Andrew. She posited that Andrew felt that he was unwanted by his biological parents, who had given him up for adoption, and that he endured a second rejection and abandonment by his adopted parents when his sister, Lana, was born. Andrew also felt that his parents favored Lana because she was their biological child and because she was such an exceptional student. Treatment consisted of the therapist's exploring with Andrew his deepseated sense of not belonging, its implications, and of family work that encouraged the parents to find better ways to communicate to Andrew how much they cared for him. Both parents were led to believe that they had let Andrew down and that they were responsible for his bad behavior. Needless to say, the Kramers felt considerable guilt for unwittingly harming their son. No clinical attention whatsoever was paid to the possibility that Andrew might have specific psychiatric diagnoses, including a problem with chemical dependency. Andrew was not tested for the presence of cocaine or marijuana in his hair, nor was he monitored during his treatment through random urine and blood tests for the ongoing presence of illegal substances. The following interchange occurred during one of the Kramers' family sessions with Dr. Roth:

> **Greg Kramer:** We have spent a lot of time discussing Andrew's problems with us, but I believe that we should also focus on his drug abuse.
> **Dr. Roth:** I happen not to agree with you, Greg. I am convinced that Andrew's substance use was the symptom and not the true problem. The real problem is his sense of being disenfranchised by both sets of parents: his biological parents because he was adopted, and the two of you after the birth of Lana. Any time we spend talking about drug use deflects our attention from the real issues.

Greg: You used the term *symptom,* which implies to me that Andrew has a specific diagnosis. I, for one, would like to know what that diagnosis is.

Dr. Roth: I was using the term generically. I do not believe that it would be in Andrew's best interest to label him at this point. In fact, I believe that such labeling does more harm than good. Apart from all the negative connotations and stereotyping associated with diagnoses, it tends to give the parents of adolescents a false sense of certainty that a simple problem can respond to a simplistic remedy, such as a medication. No, Greg, I think you are way off base here; probably because you are threatened by my and Andrew's delving into his parents' prominent role in the causation of his problems.

This dialogue between a psychiatrist and the parents of her patient exemplifies much that goes very wrong when an incompetent clinician is out of step with the modern practice of behavioral medicine. Unfortunately, such malfeasance is not uncommon. Presented in Table 7–1 is a summary of the errors in Dr. Roth's treatment of Andrew Kramer and his parents.

As a consequence of Dr. Roth's incompetence (which in my opinion constitutes malpractice), Andrew's psychiatric disorders went undiagnosed and untreated. Not only were the Kramers' time and resources wasted, but Andrew missed a critical opportunity to grow and to change. Because Andrew's encounter with the police did not occur at school and because he was not convicted of a crime, his school record remained unblemished. Although his many assets, including high intelligence and charm, enabled him to graduate from high school with high grades and good recommendations, his misuse of these assets to manipulate people and to avoid responsibility for misbehavior would work against him in the long run.

In adolescents, the primary treatment of the two psychiatric disorders for which Andrew met diagnostic criteria—conduct disorder and polysubstance dependence—is behavioral, with emphasis on establishing clear limits and following through on delineated consequences when these limits are violated. Psychodynamically informed psychotherapy can be a useful complement to the behavioral treatment, but the diffuse, divisive, and formulaic type practiced with such confidence and condescension by Dr. Roth certainly cannot. The DSM-IV-TR criteria for conduct disorder (American Psychiatric Association 2000) are summarized in Table 7–2.

TABLE 7–1. Dr. Roth's errors in the assessment and treatment of Andrew Kramer

1. By accepting the referral of a patient who was the child of a close friend, Dr. Roth failed to heed psychiatry's prerequisite for impartiality and clear therapeutic boundaries. She continued to see Melissa Kramer socially while caring for her son.

2. Dr. Roth did not conduct or oversee a systematic medical/psychiatric workup on Andrew that should have included, at minimum, a detailed history taken from parents and teachers, physical examination (including nasal assessment for cocaine abuse and dermal assessment for intravenous substance abuse), and laboratory testing (including hair analysis for past substance abuse and urine and serum analysis for current substance abuse).

3. Dr. Roth initiated treatment without a specific or even a tentative diagnosis.

4. Dr. Roth's entire approach to understanding and treating Andrew was guided by a single theoretical framework, psychodynamic psychiatry. She thereby discounted biological features and factors such as the possibility that Andrew had inherited a genetic predisposition to chemical dependencies from his biological parents or that his thinking and mood were influenced and impaired by substance abuse.

5. By ascribing the causation of his behavioral problems to his parents, Dr. Roth tacitly absolved Andrew from assuming the primary responsibility for their remediation.

6. By attributing the source of and responsibility for Andrew's psychological and behavioral problems to his parents, Dr. Roth burdened Mr. and Mrs. Kramer with the guilt of having harmed their son.

7. When queried by Greg Kramer about his son's diagnosis, Dr. Roth became defensive and confrontational, rather than thinking about and directly answering his question.

8. Dr. Roth failed to consider, diagnose, or treat *two* serious mental illnesses for which Andrew fully met DSM-IV-TR (American Psychiatric Association 2000) criteria: 1) conduct disorder; and 2) polysubstance dependence.

Andrew Kramer and the Diagnosis of Conduct Disorder

About Conduct Disorder

The diagnosis of conduct disorder is restricted to children and adolescents who habitually break the rules of society and disrespect the rights

TABLE 7–2. Diagnostic criteria for conduct disorder
(slightly modified from DSM-IV-TR)

A. A repetitive and persistent pattern of behavior in which the basic rights of others or major age-appropriate societal norms or rules are violated, as manifested by the presence of three (or more) of the following criteria in the past 12 months, with at least one criterion present in the past 6 months:

Aggression to people and animals

1. Often bullies, threatens, or intimidates others

2. Often initiates physical fights

3. Has used a weapon that can cause serious physical harm to others (e.g., a bat, brick, broken bottle, knife, gun)

4. Has been physically cruel to people

5. Has been physically cruel to animals

6. Has stolen while confronting a victim (e.g., mugging, purse snatching, extortion, armed robbery)

7. Has forced someone into sexual activity

Destruction of property

8. Has deliberately engaged in fire setting with the intention of causing serious damage

9. Has deliberately destroyed others' property (other than by fire setting)

Deceitfulness or theft

10. Has broken into someone else's house, building, or car

11. Lies frequently to obtain goods or favors or to avoid obligations (i.e., "cons" others)

12. Has stolen items of nontrivial value without confronting a victim (e.g., shoplifting, but without breaking and entering; forgery)

Serious violations of rules

13. Stays out frequently at night despite parental prohibitions, beginning before age 13 years

14. Has run away from home overnight at least twice while living in parental or parental surrogate home (or once without returning for a lengthy period)

15. Is often truant from school, beginning before age 13 years

B. The disturbance in behavior causes clinically significant impairment in social, academic, or occupational functioning.

C. If the individual is age 18 years or older, criteria are not met for antisocial personality disorder.

Source.   Adapted from American Psychiatric Association: *Diagnostic and Statistical Manual of Mental Disorders,* 4th Edition, Text Revision. Washington, DC, American Psychiatric Association, 2000, pp. 98–99. Used with permission.

of others. In a British population study, approximately 5% of 10- and 11-year-old children were diagnosed with this condition, and it was found to be 10 times more prevalent in boys than in girls (Rutter et al. 1970). Using DSM criteria, an American study of both male and female teenagers in Missouri reported a prevalence of 8.7% (Kashani et al. 1987). Most important, conduct disorders of childhood and adolescence foreshadow a greatly increased incidence of adult antisocial behaviors, as documented in a series of excellent studies by Robins and co-workers (Robins 1991; Robins and Price 1991). Other investigators have determined that children and adolescents with the most severe disorders of conduct have increased chances of becoming adults who exhibit the most extreme and persistent antisocial behaviors (Moffitt 1993). Somewhat more hopefully, 25%–40% of children with conduct disorder will meet criteria for antisocial personality disorder as adults (Robins 1987).

Although I believe that there is strong evidence of genetic and neurobiological underpinnings for both conduct disorder and antisocial personality disorder (reviewed later in this chapter; see "Diagnostic Features of Antisocial Personality Disorder"), experiential and social factors also influence the development of these conditions in many individuals. Children and adolescents are notoriously suggestible and highly subject to peer pressure. The misbehavior of some adolescents may occur principally in the context of dysfunctional group behavior. In such instances, the youth might go along with substance abuse, thefts, and assaults to be included with the group, but he or she does not instigate or pursue such behaviors on his or her own. Adolescent death rates among those who are serious delinquents are 50 times greater than for their nondelinquent peers, and the causes of death are usually traumatic or violent: accidents, overdoses, suicides, and homicides (Yeager and Lewis 1990). As a result of these data, I believe that all children and adolescents who meet criteria for conduct disorder deserve constructive professional involvement and guidance from teachers and coaches, from community leaders (such as in police programs and local volunteer clubs), and from knowledgeable and skilled mental health professionals (in contrast to the treatment offered to Andrew by Dr. Roth). With such help, not only will many of these children be spared from wasting their lives in the throes of addiction and imprisonment, but also countless innocent people will not become their victims.

Andrew Kramer and Conduct Disorder

Although Andrew Kramer fully met DSM diagnostic criteria for conduct disorder, his diagnosis was more difficult to determine than that of most other children and adolescents with this condition. He used his superior intelligence to cover up his transgressions, most often by getting others to do his "dirty work." For example, rather than personally engaging in a physical altercation with a high school rival, Andrew would induce one of his friends to take on his adversary. In addition, he manipulated his devoted, successful parents into using their resources and political connections to help him elude responsibility and consequences on the few occasions when he was found out. Nonetheless, throughout middle school and high school Andrew tortured animals, bullied his schoolmates, abused and sold illegal substances, used deceit to miss school, spent many nights away from home, and engaged in sexual activities with numerous females, including some who were much younger and much older than he. He showed no empathy or remorse for those whom he deceived, used, and abused. In summary, because of his intelligence, attractiveness, and cunning, Andrew was difficult to detect and catch, making him among the most dangerous of human predators.

The Case of Andrew Kramer: College and Launching a Life of Crime

College

Andrew attended a prestigious institute of technology in the Northeast. In this competitive environment he was, at best, an average student in mathematics and computer sciences, the subjects in which he had excelled in high school. During the first semester of his freshman year, Andrew became involved with Alexandra Bishop, a gifted graduate student in mathematics and the leader of one of the breakout study sections in his calculus course. He moved into her apartment, and soon Alexandra was completing almost all of his homework assignments as well as tutoring him for his examinations. Andrew rarely attended classes. Rather, he slept much of the day, after spending all night, almost every night, playing high-stakes poker with upperclassmen and graduate students. At the games Andrew would drink about a fifth of bourbon nightly, and he often smoked marijuana on the way back to Alexandra's apartment. With the help of Alexandra, he was able to pass his first-semester courses, but he was becoming more and more involved in gambling. He began to place daily wagers on college basketball and professional football and basketball games. By spring of his freshman year, Andrew owed tens of thousands of dollars in gambling debts, much of it to underworld bookies in Boston and Las Vegas. When he returned to Houston for spring break, Andrew convinced his parents that he needed to take his car back to college to perform a community service project in the inner city. During the same visit Andrew also stole his father's credit card and a valuable antique diamond brooch from his mother's hidden jewelry box. To pay off his gambling debts (and to keep from getting beaten up by criminal enforcers), Andrew sold his car and his mother's brooch for cash and sent his father's credit card to one of the bookies in Las Vegas. His parents could not figure out how these items had been stolen, but they blamed the construction workers who at the time were remodeling Mrs. Kramer's bathroom.

After Andrew managed to cover most of his gambling losses, he became determined to "get in on the other side" of the gambling business. That summer Andrew told his parents that he wanted to stay in the East to take extra courses and to work on his community service project that involved teaching computer skills to disadvantaged children in the inner city. However, with several of his college friends, he set up an illegal business in which wagers from college students around the country were solicited through e-mail and Web sites and then processed through gambling connections in Las Vegas. By that fall, Andrew was raking in large sums of money, with rapidly growing profits. He took many trips to Las Vegas and Atlantic City to develop "business connections" at those sites. With his gambling profits he bought himself a new red Ferrari. Even though he was involved with many other women, Andrew managed to stay with Alexandra, who continued to prepare all of his homework, write his term papers, and tutor him for tests. Nonetheless, because Andrew rarely attended classes and was always behind in his courses, he had to drop many subjects because of low test grades. He was placed on probation at the end of his sophomore year, a fact that he carefully hid from his parents. He failed to make up required courses in summer school or during the first semester of his junior year. In fact, that semester he had withdrawn from most of the courses in which he had enrolled and thereby had violated the conditions of his probation. Although Andrew made up many excuses about having health problems, he could not talk his way out of this situation. He was asked to leave the university. By that time his illegal gambling business was thriving, so he had plenty of money. He dealt with the problem of explaining to his parents about being expelled from college as follows:

Andrew Kramer: I have decided to leave college for now, because I need to work full time on my computer sports business.

Melissa Kramer: What are you saying? Why would you drop out now, with only a little more than a year to go? We don't have any financial problems. You can always go into business after you graduate.

Andrew: In the computer business, 18 months is a lifetime. The window of opportunity would surely close on my ideas. I am not the first person to do this. I am sure you know that Bill Gates dropped out of Harvard during his freshman year there. I think he did all right without a college degree.

Greg Kramer: Son, are you sure you are telling us everything? You haven't let us see your grades since you were a freshman.

Andrew: I expected as much from you, Dad. You have never trusted me, much less ever encouraged anything I have tried to do independently. Lana can do no wrong, but everything I do is wrong in your eyes. Dr. Roth was right—the only way I could ever please you would be if I were your "real" son. Don't worry, Dad, I won't ask you for any help. You can give everything to Lana.

Andrew was no more forthcoming with Alexandra:

Andrew Kramer: I think it would be best for us to date other people for a while.

Alexandra Bishop: Are you telling me that you're leaving me?

Andrew: You can look at it any way you want. All I'm saying is that I'm moving out today and am getting my own apartment.

Alexandra: Do you know what I think, Andrew? I think you have used me all this time. Now that you have been asked to leave college, you don't need me any more to help you with your studies and are dropping me.

Andrew: If you were such a great help to me in school, why did I flunk out? If you want to know the truth, Alexandra, I think you have been holding me back since the day I met you. You're such a nerd and so boring. I think we would both be better off if you went back to your equations and just left me alone.

Alexandra: Since you're going to leave me now, when do you plan to pay me back the $10,000 I lent you from my trust?

Andrew: I don't have a clue what you're talking about. You never lent me any money. I don't owe you a penny.

Alexandra: Andrew, I have the cancelled check. When I had to get my father's permission to take money from my trust, he made me have you sign a notarized document that I still have.

Andrew: Listen to me carefully, Alexandra. You have broken every university rule and honor code that there is—writing papers for me, telling me what was going to be asked on the calculus tests. I think you even changed some of my test grades. You also took advantage of a freshman. You used your power and position as a teacher to seduce me. I believe that you fucked me up psychologically, and that is why I flunked out of school. I wouldn't threaten me over that so-called loan, if I were you. Not only will you never get a job in a university, but my parents would sue you and the university for compromising my morals and ruining my college career. Let's just call it quits and leave each other alone.

New Business

Getting Started

During the next several years, Andrew lived in Boston and traveled to the many colleges and universities throughout New England to advance his gambling business. On the various campuses, he would find undergraduate and graduate students who were already involved in gambling, and he would enlist one or two on each campus to be his site representatives. They, in turn, would recruit other students to place bets with him over the Internet (and, with trusted customers on special occasions, over his cell phone), which he in turn would place with underworld bookies in Las Vegas and Boston. His college-student agents would both collect the bets and distribute the payoffs. Compared with most in this illegal business, Andrew was highly sophisticated in computers and software. He was aware that his college student agents would be vulnerable to discovery if they used their university-based Internet networks, as do almost all college and graduate students. Universities own these networks and are free to access student communications—even private e-mail exchanges—when they deem it to be in the best interest of the student or the university. He therefore provided his agents with sophisticated computers and well-protected Internet software systems and carriers. One weak link in his system was that almost all of his customers communicated their bets to agents or his central site in Boston over their university-based Internet connections. Andrew had discovered a very profitable business, and he also proved to be an excellent administrator. The nature of college campus life is that there is a continuous turnover of students—both a problem and an advantage for Andrew's business. The problem was that he needed a continuous succession of new customers because the old ones would graduate and would often move far away from his "distribution region," where bets were collected and winnings paid off. On the positive side, Andrew had the opportunity to try to recruit the most trusted and talented graduating agents to become key middle managers in his system. As his business involved modest personnel and human resource investments and paid no taxes, it was incredibly profitable. Andrew made hundreds of thousands of dollars each year and spent at least that much on a lavish lifestyle. He lived in an expensive Boston condominium and leased jet planes to attend parties and participate in high-stakes gambling adventures throughout the world. His covers were several legitimate Internet businesses, such as fantasy football Web sites that were supposed to make money through advertising to the clients, who could use the sites for free. To his parents and other people in the legitimate world, Andrew's all-too-obvious success came from these sports-related "dotcom" businesses.

Andrew's business was not all fun and glamour, however. His financial success in the niche college gambling business caught the attention of several types of competitors. First, established gambling enterprises comprising seasoned criminals tried, to use their parlance, to "shake him down for a piece of his action" or to "muscle in on his territory." Andrew was constantly being threatened, so it was necessary for him to hire bodyguards and thugs to protect himself and his territory and to reciprocate in kind if required. In addition, enterprising college students on various campuses would start competitive businesses that on occasion became rapidly profitable. Andrew dealt particularly harshly with the upstarts, whom he sometimes would have beaten up and their computers and phone systems destroyed. There was a rumor that one fledgling collegiate entrepreneur turned Andrew in to campus security. According to the widely circulated rumor, the campus police were receiving bribes from Andrew, and they did not respond to the student's allegations. Furthermore, shortly thereafter the college entrepreneur was involved in a suspicious hit-and-run car accident in which he was seriously injured. Nothing could be proved against Andrew or his associates, and no charges were filed.

Unfriendly Competition

As Andrew's college gambling business grew, he began to branch out into subsidiary products, some quasi-legal and most illegal, such as producing and selling counterfeit ID cards for underage students to use to get into bars and nightclubs. One of his quasi-legal enterprises was an Internet-based student travel service. This company featured deeply discounted charter trips and tours abroad for college students and graduate students. Problems would frequently occur whereby the planes and participating hostels were oversold and the customers would be unable to get their money back. On several occasions, some students were stranded in distant foreign countries and had to wire their families to send money so that they could return to the United States on other air carriers. Andrew was no stranger to lawsuits, and he supported several Boston attorneys who worked nearly full time for him to protect his interests. Because Andrew himself was far removed from most of the operations and because most students did not have the resources to pursue their grievances in court, he was never convicted of a crime.

One of Andrew's most profitable businesses was dealing drugs on college campuses. He mostly sold addictive prescription drugs such as amphetamines, barbiturates, benzodiazepines such as alprazolam (Xanax) and diazepam (Valium), narcotic analgesics such as hydrocodone bitartrate (Vicodin) and oxycodone (OxyContin), and so-called designer drugs such as Ecstasy. Andrew's operation would also sell marijuana and cocaine. It was the latter two illicit drugs that required his involvement with international drug distributors who were hardened criminals involved in large organized crime syndicates. Shortly after having a heated dispute with one of these drug distributors over payment for a large shipment of marijuana, Andrew was discovered at 4:00 A.M. on the street in front of his condominium, beaten up and unconscious. In the emergency room of the general hospital he was diagnosed as having multiple fractures of his skull and facial bones as well as a dislocated right shoulder, broken right arm, shattered pelvis, and fractured left femur. X-rays of his skull revealed significant bleeding between his skull and the membrane surrounding his brain, called a subdural hematoma. Comatose and in shock, he was rushed to surgery, where teams of neurosurgeons, plastic and reconstructive surgeons, and orthopedists painstakingly worked to save his life and put him back together. He was in surgery for more than 15 hours and did not regain consciousness for 2 days. One of Andrew's business associates called Andrew's parents, who rushed to Boston. By the time they saw their son, he was unable to communicate with them. He had sustained multiple fractures to both sides of his mandible, which required the insertion of surgical pins and screws. His jaw required immobilization for at least 6 weeks, which meant that his jaws were wired shut. Andrew could not write with his right hand, because of a large cast and the immobilization of his shoulder joint. A waist-to-toe cast of his left pelvis and leg left him nonambulatory. The Kramers' discussion with Andrew's physician, Dr. Janicak, went as follows:

> **Greg Kramer:** What can you tell us about our son's condition?
> **Dr. Janicak:** When he first arrived in the emergency room, we were not sure that we could save him. At this point we are fairly certain that he will survive but are uncertain about what deficits he will be left with.
> **Melissa Kramer:** What do you think happened to him?
> **Dr. Janicak:** We know from the nature of his injuries that he was assaulted. The emergency room surgeon believed him to have been beaten severely with a large, blunt instrument, like an aluminum baseball bat. Whoever did this wanted more than his wallet. They tried to kill your son and almost succeeded.

Greg: You mentioned that you were concerned that he might be left with some defects, could you tell us more about that?

Dr. Janicak: I believe that I said "deficits." I don't like to speculate, as my predictions might turn out to be inaccurate or misleading. I will say that, while there certainly can be many complications and problems associated with his multiple fractures and soft tissue injuries, I am most concerned about the long-term implications of his traumatic brain injury. Only time can tell whether or not he suffered permanent damage to his memory and intellectual functions. Brain trauma can also lead to difficulties in the regulation of mood and emotions. It will take some time to see where we are with these.

Rehabilitation in Houston

Andrew spent 6 weeks in the general hospital in Boston, and his parents were at his bedside for most of this time. Because his jaw was wired shut and he was unable to write, communication with him was minimal. The medical team indicated to the Kramer family that Andrew would require extensive physical rehabilitation to regain motor function of his arm and lower limbs. They also believed that the assessment of Andrew's intellectual and cognitive functioning should be delayed until after his jaw healed and he could resume speaking. They all agreed that this portion of his rehabilitation was best accomplished in Houston, where there are excellent medical facilities and personnel and where he was also able to have the support of his family. On discharge from the general hospital in Boston, Andrew was flown by private air ambulance to a rehabilitation hospital in Houston. Six weeks later, Andrew was evaluated by Dr. Gerhardt George, a neuropsychologist, to determine the cognitive and psychological effects of the traumatic brain injury that he had sustained. After extensive testing and interviews, Dr. George found him not to have lasting cognitive deficits from his traumatic brain injury. However, he diagnosed a psychiatric condition that he was confident antedated, by many years, Andrew's brain injuries: antisocial personality disorder.

Diagnostic Features of Antisocial Personality Disorder

Diagnosis

DSM-IV-TR diagnostic criteria for antisocial personality disorder (American Psychiatric Association 2000) are presented in Table 7–3, and key principles regarding this condition as exemplified by the case of Andrew Kramer are summarized in Table 7–4.

TABLE 7–3. Diagnostic criteria for antisocial personality disorder (adapted from DSM-IV-TR)

A. A pervasive pattern of disregard for and violation of the rights of others, occurring since age 15 years, as indicated by three (or more) of the following:

  1. Failure to conform to social norms with respect to lawful behaviors as indicated by repeatedly performing acts that are grounds for arrest

  2. Deceitfulness, as indicated by repeated lying, use of aliases, or conning others for personal profit or pleasure

  3. Impulsivity or failure to plan ahead

  4. Irritability and aggressiveness, as indicated by repeated physical fights or assaults

  5. Reckless disregard for safety of self or others

  6. Consistent irresponsibility, as indicated by repeated failure to sustain consistent work behavior or honor financial obligations

  7. Lack of remorse, as indicated by being indifferent to or rationalizing having hurt, mistreated, or stolen from another

B. The individual is at least age 18 years.

C. There is evidence of conduct disorder [see Table 7–2] with onset before age 15 years.

D. The occurrence of antisocial behavior is not exclusively during the course of schizophrenia or a manic episode.

Source.   Adapted from American Psychiatric Association: *Diagnostic and Statistical Manual of Mental Disorders*, 4th Edition, Text Revision. Washington, DC, American Psychiatric Association, 2000. Used with permission.

Lack of Conscience

Theoretical Considerations

The hallmark of the psychopathology of people with antisocial personality disorder is their lack of feelings of guilt or remorse over harming others. This absence of conscience or a moral sense is also termed by psychoanalysts a *superego deficit*. According to psychoanalytic theory, the superego oversees the drives and behavior of the individual and keeps them in check by a set of values and ideals that have been derived from the parents. According to classic Freudian theory, a male child develops this capacity before age 5 as the result of his conflict between his sexual desires for his mother and his fear of the retaliation of his father. The male child resolves this conflict by repressing his libidinous feel-

TABLE 7–4. Key principles of antisocial personality disorder exemplified by the case of Andrew Kramer

Historical fact	Key principle	Interpretation
Andrew was adopted.	When adopted children develop antisocial personality disorder as adults, fundamental questions about the causality of this condition are raised (the role of "nature vs. nurture").	It is not possible to separate the contributions of 1) the psychosocial stresses associated with being adopted and 2) the role of genetics in the causation of Andrew's personality disorder.
Andrew was nurtured, prioritized, and protected by both of his adoptive parents.	Antisocial personality disorder can develop in people who have no history of parental neglect or abuse.	Although Andrew might have perceived that he was unwanted by his adoptive parents, the role of his genetic predisposition to antisocial personality disorder is strongly implicated in his case.
When Andrew was 3 years old, he could not be taught to share toys or play amicably with the other children in his pre-kindergarten class.	Most children who later develop antisocial personality disorder as adults bully their childhood peers.	Even as a very young child, Andrew was aggressive with his peers and did not understand that they also had rights and feelings.
Melissa Kramer blamed the pre-kindergarten teacher for saying that Andrew had a behavioral problem.	Often a parent or spouse will unknowingly enable the destructive behaviors of a person with antisocial personality disorder.	Melissa Kramer's vulnerability to the manipulations of Andrew had deep roots.
As a child, Andrew tortured animals.	Extreme cruelty to animals by children is often diagnostic (in part) of conduct disorder and predictive of antisocial personality disorder in adulthood.	Throughout his life, Andrew showed no more compassion for human beings than he exhibited for the frogs that he tortured as a child.

TABLE 7–4. Key principles of antisocial personality disorder exemplified by the case of Andrew Kramer *(continued)*

Historical fact	Key principle	Interpretation
As an infant, Lana Kramer was bitten by two venomous spiders while in her crib.	Children with conduct disorders and adults with antisocial personality disorder commit far more crimes than they are caught committing.	At the time of Lana's spider bites, no one considered that Andrew might be the culprit. With the benefit of hindsight and logic, one can conclude that his responsibility is likely.
Andrew has many assets, including high intelligence, good looks, leadership qualities, and excellent verbal skills.	The more personal assets possessed by a person with antisocial personality disorder, the more dangerous he or she is.	Andrew used his assets in the commission of crimes and in the avoidance of blame and punishment.
When Andrew's teacher accused him of cheating, the teacher got in trouble.	Even when you have evidence, it is dangerous to accuse people with antisocial personality disorder of misdeeds. They will stop at nothing to protect themselves.	From a young age, Andrew was conniving and vindictive.
Andrew sexually abused his sister from the time that she was a little girl.	Adults with antisocial personality disorder have histories of being ruthless and dangerous when they were children and adolescents.	Andrew regarded his sister, Lana, both as a rival and as an object for his aggressive and sexual drives.
As a teenager, Andrew was sexually active with younger girls and older women.	People with antisocial personality disorder discover, at a very young age, how to gratify their sexual drives.	Andrew understood how to use his good looks and powers of persuasion to exploit vulnerable girls and women.

TABLE 7–4. Key principles of antisocial personality disorder exemplified by the case of Andrew Kramer *(continued)*

Historical fact	Key principle	Interpretation
During high school, Andrew both abused and sold drugs.	Children and adolescents with conduct disorder and adults with antisocial personality disorder characteristically abuse alcohol and other addictive substances.	Andrew chronically abused alcohol and illicit drugs from the time he was a young teenager through his adult life. Dealing in drugs became a lifelong occupation for Andrew.
Dr. Henrietta Roth did not diagnose or treat Andrew's alcohol abuse or substance use disorders.	Many mental health professionals are not competent to diagnose and treat children with conduct disorders and adults with antisocial personality disorder.	Neither systematic nor data-based in her assessment of Andrew, Dr. Roth failed to diagnose his conduct disorder or substance use disorders.
Andrew co-opted Dr. Roth in blaming his parents for his misdeeds.	Well-intentioned but incompetent mental health professionals are putty in the hands of intelligent people with antisocial personality disorder.	Dr. Roth's incompetence resulted in a missed opportunity to help Andrew change his behavior or, at a minimum, to protect his sister from his abuse.
In college, Andrew used Alexandra Bishop to help him pass his courses.	People with antisocial personality disorder prey on trusting, kind, and capable people.	To Andrew, Alexandra was like a vending machine: an object that he would use to fulfill his needs and advance his ambitions.
Andrew was angered that Alexandra asked him to repay his $10,000 loan from her.	People with antisocial personality disorder are predators who feel neither gratitude nor compassion for their prey.	Andrew's relationship with Alexandra was based solely on the fulfillment of his needs. When his needs changed, she was threatened and discarded.

TABLE 7–4. Key principles of antisocial personality disorder exemplified by the case of Andrew Kramer *(continued)*

Historical fact	Key principle	Interpretation
Illegal gambling operations and drug dealing became Andrew's occupation.	Many criminals have antisocial personality disorder, making them doubly dangerous.	Although Andrew had the requisite family support, intelligence, and interpersonal skills to achieve professional success, he chose a life of crime.
Andrew's criminal activities eventually resulted in his being seriously injured.	People with antisocial personality disorder are at high risk of serious injuries and premature death from violence.	Although Andrew got away with almost all of his crimes, other criminals finally got to him.
Andrew's parents and sister were severely traumatized by his misbehavior.	People with antisocial personality disorder harm those with whom they have close relationships, as well as people with whom they have no relationship.	Family members, friends, and strangers became victims of Andrew's abuse.
Andrew felt no guilt or remorse over harming his parents, his sister, or Alexandra.	The absence of a conscience or a sense of morality is the defining feature of people with antisocial personality disorder.	Andrew felt completely justified for his manipulative, harmful, and exploitive behavior of his family and Alexandra.

ings for his mother and aggressive feelings toward his father by identifying with and internalizing the strength and values of the father. The result of this unconscious process is the development of the superego and the establishment of a strong masculine identity. Freud would conceptualize this as a healthy resolution of the child's *Oedipal complex.* According to Freud and other psychoanalysts, the correlate of this developmental process in women would be the *Electra complex,* with the positive resolution being her identification with her mother, accepting a female identity as an adult, and the internalization of the mother's moral standards. However, if there are problems with the process, such as an absent, inattentive, or overly punitive parent, the child might grow up to have deficits in the development or application of his or her conscience or moral sense.

Although most experienced clinicians have uncovered these dynamics in the family histories of *some* patients with antisocial personality disorder, there are also many family situations—such as that of Andrew Kramer—where these psychodynamics do not seem to apply for people with this condition. There are multifarious alternative explanations for the development of a conscience or moral sense, and these range from modeling and learned-behavior theories to conceptualizations that involve genetics and brain biology. For the reader who wishes a critical assessment of Freudian theories of the development of conscience as well as an excellent review of the work of cognitive psychologists such as Jean Piaget and Lawrence Kohlberg on moral development, I recommend Chapter 14 of David R. Shaffer's textbook, *Developmental Psychology: Childhood and Adolescence* (Shaffer 1999). Although there is merit and value in many diverse theoretical avenues to conceptualizing and understanding moral development, I believe that recent research results render the genetic and neurobiological theories especially compelling.

Multiple Killers

The most dangerous and notorious people with antisocial personality disorder are the small minority who commit multiple murders over extended periods of time. A form of multiple killers are serial killers, who have histories of being physically abused by their fathers as children, exhibit the features of conduct disorder during their adolescence, and meet criteria for antisocial personality disorder by the time that they are adults. Sadomasochistic sexual involvements and pleasure from tormenting animals and torturing human beings are common concomitants to the homicides of serial killers. Several biographies and videotaped interviews of serial killers portray the chilling details of their cunning ruthlessness, lack of empathy for their victims, and absence of guilt or remorse over the broad repercussions of their crimes. One book recounts the life and exploits of the multiple killer (because he was a professional hit man, he may not qualify as a serial killer) Richard Kuklinski, known as the Iceman, who is estimated to have killed approximately 100 people (Bruno 1993). An interview with Mr. Kuklinski conducted by psychiatrist Park Elliott Dietz was presented on cable television as part of the HBO *America Undercover* documentary series ("The Iceman Confesses" 2001). These portrayals graphically demonstrate the consequences of the failed development of moral conscience in a person who fully meets DSM criteria for antisocial personality disorder. The confluence of antisocial personality disorder, a predilection for murder, and great political power—such as can occur in the leader of a totalitarian government—can result in genocide.

Biological Aspects of Antisocial Personality Disorder

Epidemiology

In Chapter 17 of his textbook *Psychodynamic Psychiatry in Clinical Practice,* Glen Gabbard, M.D., reviews the evolution of the diagnosis of antisocial personality disorder and reveals that at the present time there is scientific disagreement about the specific criteria for the diagnosis of this condition (Gabbard 2000). This absence of diagnostic uniformity necessarily leads to confusion and uncertainty in the epidemiological and genetic studies of the disorder. Nonetheless, there are useful conclusions that can be drawn about the epidemiology of antisocial personality disorder. First of all, antisocial personality disorder is not a rare condition: the lifetime prevalence for the disorder among men ranges from 2% to 4% of American populations (Cadoret 1986; Robins 1987/1992). This rate may be an underestimation of the prevalence of the disorder, because the survey did not include samples of the approximately 2 million people in the United States who are incarcerated, many of whom would certainly meet DSM criteria for this condition. Other statistics, stemming from the National Comorbidity Survey, indicate an overall rate for antisocial personality disorder of 3.5% of the population, an estimate that includes both men and women (Kessler et al. 1994).

A second area of agreement regarding the epidemiology of antisocial personality disorder is that the condition is much more common in men than in women. Various studies indicate that men are two to seven times more likely to have the condition (Cadoret 1986; Robins 1987).

Third, comorbidity of antisocial personality disorder with alcoholism and substance use disorders is very high (Smith and Newman 1990). Up to 70% of people with antisocial personality disorder are also diagnosed with alcoholism or a substance use disorder at some point in their lifetime (Black 2001).

Genetics

Twin Studies

Although there is excellent research in this realm, to date no published study or area of research either proves or disproves that antisocial personality disorder has genetic origins. That being said, however, there is strong circumstantial evidence of a prominent genetic component to the condition. A problem regarding research on twins with antisocial personality disorder is that many studies derive inferences based on research conducted on criminal populations. Almost all of these studies indicate that there is a heritable component to criminality. For example, one study found that among monozygotic twins, if one twin has a criminal background, there is a 66% chance that the other identical twin will also have a history of criminality. By contrast, among dizygotic (fraternal) twins the concordance is 31% (Brennen and Mednick 1993). The results of these twin studies and the studies of other investigators strongly implicate a genetic predisposition among people with certain types of criminal records, particularly those who have committed violent crimes. However, do these findings about the genetics of criminality also apply to people with antisocial personality disorder? The answer is that at this point we cannot be certain. Depending on the study and the diagnostic criteria used, there are wide divergences in the percentage of imprisoned people who have antisocial personality disorder, with rates ranging from 25% to 80% (Hare 1983; Hare et al. 1991).

One recent study of antisocial personality disorder evaluated 5,150 twin pairs who served on active military duty during the Vietnam War (Fu et al. 2002). Of this group, 3,360 pairs (1,868 monozygotic and 1,492 dizygotic) completed extensive diagnostic interviews and were assessed for the lifetime heritability of several psychiatric conditions, including antisocial personality disorder, major depression, alcohol dependence, and marijuana dependence. Importantly, antisocial personality disorder evidenced the highest degree of heritability among these conditions. For the total twin sample (including both monozygotic and dizygotic twins), if one twin had antisocial personality disorder, there was a 69% likelihood that the other twin would also have this condition over his or her lifetime. For the other conditions the results were as follows: major depression, 40%; alcohol dependence, 56%; and marijuana dependence, 50%. A similar study conducted earlier on this population had found that environmental factors had significantly more influence on juveniles than on adults with antisocial traits but that genetic factors were more influential on the development of antisocial personality disorder in adults (Lyons et al. 1995). Finally, researchers Rhee and Waldman (2002) carefully reviewed all published twin and adoption studies to estimate the magnitude of genetic and environmental influences on the development of antisocial personality disorder. Their findings indicated a stronger role for genetic influences than for environmental and experiential factors.

Laboratory Genetics

Scientist Dean Hamer (2002) has provided an overview of the past, present, and future of the genetic research of behavioral disorders. Describing the progress of the last 100 years, he wrote:

> The basic approaches…were to compare identical and fraternal twins, other family members, and adoptees that had been raised together or apart. The results were striking, albeit slow to be accepted. Genes were shown to influence virtually every aspect of human personality, temperament, cognitive style, and psychiatric disorder. The effects of heredity were substantial, typically representing 30 to 70% of total variation, and highly replicable across societies and cultures. The long reach of genes extended from a friendly disposition to xenophobia, from bipolar disease to bedwetting, from getting married to keeping a job. (Hamer 2002, p. 7)

Dean Hamer's overview of the current and future approach of behavior genetics is a bit more difficult for the layperson to follow:

> The current aim is to identify the specific genes that contribute to individual differences and determine what they do in the brain. The approach is to search for DNA sequence variations that correlate with behavioral and personality traits, either by tracking anonymous markers close to the genes of interest in family members (linkage analysis) or by directly comparing the coding and regulatory sequences of candidate genes (association analysis). (Hamer 2002, p. 71)

The hope and promise of the new era of medicine is that more will be understood about the origins and fundamental pathology of illnesses at the molecular and genetic levels. With this discovery and knowledge will come more precise ways of diagnosing, treating, and preventing devastating psychiatric illnesses. As applied to antisocial personality disorder, this basic understanding would have profound social implications, given the association of this condition with violence, criminality, alcoholism, and substance use disorders. A strategy of genetic research in this area is to isolate a fundamental element of antisocial personality disorder—such as impulsivity, aggressiveness, or lack of empathy—and then try to discover an abnormal gene associated with that trait. An example of this genre of research is that of Avshalom Caspi and co-workers (2002), who studied the genetics of the neurotransmitter metabolizing enzyme monoamine oxidase A (MAO-A), which is thought to moderate the effects of childhood abuse. These scientists investigated a large sample of males from birth to adulthood to try to pinpoint the genetic factors that explain why some children who are maltreated develop antisocial personality disorder as adults whereas others do not. The researchers reported that abused children with genes that give rise to high levels of MAO-A are less likely to develop antisocial problems; the authors concluded that their findings help to explain why not all victims of maltreatment grow up to victimize others. However, another study was not able to confirm this finding in Chinese males with antisocial personality disorder (Lu et al. 2003). I chose these two, among many recent papers on behavioral genetics, to demonstrate the process, promise, and problems associated with modern genetic research in behavioral disorders. Could the differing findings in these two studies be a result of cultural influences—because one study was conducted in an American population and the other in a group of males from China? Throughout this book I have emphasized the inseparability of biological, psychological, social, and spiritual influences on human emotions and behavior. This principle certainly applies to scientific progress in isolating genes responsible for human psychiatric disorders, as Dean Hamer cogently articulated:

> The results [of finding specific genes that are responsible for specific behavioral disorders] have been disappointing and inconsistent....What's the problem? It's not the basic premise of linkage and candidate gene analysis; these approaches have identified dozens of genes involved in inherited diseases. Nor is it the lack of DNA sequence information; virtually the entire code of the human genome is now known. The real culprit is the assumption that the rich complexity of human thought and emotion can be reduced to a simple, linear relation between individual genes and behaviors. This oversimplified model, which underlies most current research in behavior genetics, ignores the critical importance of the brain, the environment, and gene expression networks. (Hamer 2002, p. 71)

To the reader who is interested in understanding more fully how this science is conceptualized and conducted, I recommend Hamer and Copeland's (1998) book *Living With Our Genes*.

What can be concluded about the role of genes and inheritance in antisocial personality disorder? Although no single gene has yet been linked conclusively to a specific trait of people with this condition, there remains good evidence that there are critical genetic components to antisocial personality disorder. I and other academicians interested in this area also believe that, as with other psychiatric conditions, experiential, environmental (social), and biological factors intermix with genetics to give rise to this condition (Cadoret et al. 1985, 1995; Gabbard 2000; Jacobson et al. 2002; Reiss et al. 1995). Thus, as with most psychiatric conditions, nature *and* nurture are essentially and indelibly intertwined in the genesis of antisocial personality disorder. Later in this chapter (see "The Interplay of Nature and Nurture in Antisocial Personality Disorder: Murky Waters"), I speculate about how this works.

Biology

Reduced Autonomic Response

Several compelling lines of evidence suggest that people with antisocial personality disorder are biologically different from those without the condition. One such difference involves reduced responses in their brains and peripheral nervous and endocrine systems to certain types of stressors, particularly to danger or the threat of personal harm. Our *autonomic nervous system* helps to regulate somatic reactions during times of danger by coordinating what are often referred to as fight-or-flight reactions. The autonomic nervous system comprises sensory and motor nerve cells (neurons) that integrate the brain with key systems in the rest of the body. It accomplishes this through two subnetworks, the *sympathetic nervous system* and the *parasympathetic nervous system*. It is the sympathetic nervous system that is most involved with fight-or-flight responses. Presented in Table 7–5 is a summary of how the sympathetic nervous system works in the case of a dangerous fire in one's home.

Each of the sympathetic nervous system–mediated responses in the body listed in Table 7–5 is designed to facilitate escape or attack responses, and each can be measured in the laboratory.

Raine and co-workers (1990a, 1990b) demonstrated that *reduced physiological and autonomic arousal* (comprising lower resting heart rate, lower rate of skin conductance responses during rest, and higher

---

TABLE 7–5. The response of the sympathetic nervous system to a dangerous fire

---

1. **Sensory input** from the eyes (seeing flames), nose (smelling smoke), nerve endings in the skin (feeling heat), and ears (hearing children screaming) is conducted through peripheral nerves to the brain.

2. The brain's **cerebral cortex** processes the sensory input, concludes that there is danger, and determines what needs to be done to escape the danger.

3. The cerebral cortex sends messages (flight responses) to deeper regions of the brain—including the **amygdala, hypothalamus,** and **brainstem**—that coordinate the neurological and endocrine responses to the danger (Smith and DeVito 1984).

4. Stimulation of the **adrenal gland (adrenal medulla)** causes the release of the hormone and neurotransmitter **noradrenaline** (also called norepinephrine).

5. Noradrenaline stimulates glycogen in the liver to convert to glucose, which fuels the muscles.

6. Noradrenaline stimulates the muscles in the iris of the eye to cause the pupil to dilate.

7. Noradrenaline stimulates the muscle in the heart to cause increased heart rate and stronger contractions.

8. Noradrenaline stimulates the muscles in arteries to cause increased blood pressure.

9. Noradrenaline stimulates the muscles in the walls of the trachea and in the air passages of the lungs so that they will dilate and permit more oxygen and carbon dioxide flow.

10. Noradrenaline stimulates salivary glands to *reduce* saliva production.

11. Sympathetic stimulation results in the release of acetylcholine that acts on sweat glands in the skin to *increase* perspiration.

---

slow-wave [theta] electroencephalographic responses) in 15-year-olds is predictive of increased criminal behavior in this group when they are 24 years old. Several years later, the same group of researchers reported that *increased* physiological and autonomic arousal among 15-year-olds is associated with reduced rates of criminal behavior by age 29 (Raine et al. 1995). These findings correlate with personal reports of criminals with antisocial personality disorder, as well as the observations of the clinicians who have evaluated them. When asked how they feel and react somatically while torturing and killing their victims, serial killers will respond that they feel "calm" or "normal." In their recounting of the specifics of their crimes to interviewers, these criminals show no evidence of increased autonomic responses such as elevated heart rate and blood pressure, heightened perspiration, or dry mouth. Their somatic responses differ widely from those who do not have antisocial personality disorder as they report on witnessing murders, accidents, or disasters. Perhaps the term "cold-blooded killer" has its basis in the reduced autonomic responses of people with antisocial personality disorder.

Brain Differences

Functional brain imaging is a term applied to a variety of new technologies that have been developed to image discrete regions of the living brain as the subject works on specific tasks. Given the strong suggestion from epidemiological studies and twin research of a heritable component to antisocial personality disorder, behavioral scientists have used functional brain imaging to search for evidence of brain differences in people with this condition. Although several investigators have reported that criminals and people with antisocial personality disorder have abnormalities in limbic (Kiehl et al. 2001) and hippocampal (Laakso et al. 2001) areas of the brain, mounting research evidence has been documenting reduced brain activity in frontal and temporal cortical brain regions (Raine et al. 1998, 2000; Soderstrom et al. 2002). Frontal and temporal areas of the cortex regulate judgment, abstraction, social skills, and what are termed *executive brain functions*, which include impulse control, planning, and developing strategies for problem solving. Criminality and antisocial behaviors are characterized by failure to accept societal rules and norms, reduced emotional responses to stressors, and impaired capacity to anticipate consequences for misbehavior; frontal and temporal regions of the brain regulate these functions (Damasio 1996; Veit et al. 2002). The absence of empathy for victims is often a component of criminality and is a distinguishing feature of antisocial personality disorder. Functional brain imaging studies have localized the regulation of empathic feelings and behaviors to the frontal cortex, specifically the left lateral inferior frontal gyrus of that lobe of the brain (Farrow et al. 2001). Thus, if neuroscientists and neuropsychiatrists were asked to localize brain regions, circuits, and systems that were responsible for the moral sense and social conscience of humans, most would look first to the frontal and temporal cortex and would explore for links to the limbic system, a region that regulates emotion. Not surprisingly, when there are lesions—such as tumors—in these areas of the brain, behavioral changes similar to those seen in antisocial personality disorder can occur. Two neurologists reported the case of a 40-year-old schoolteacher with the recent onset of sexual obsessions and inappropriate sexual behavior, including pedophilia (Burns and Swerdlow 2003). The teacher collected pornographic material involving children, frequented child-oriented Web sites on the Internet, and for the first time in his life solicited prostitutes. He made sexual advances toward his prepubescent stepdaughter, who informed on him. He was found guilty of child molestation, was removed from the home by court order, and was sentenced either to enter an inpatient rehabilitation program or to go to jail. He chose the former, but this did not alter his sexual compulsions or inappropriate solicitations of sex. Finally he was evaluated by neurologists, who documented a 2-year history of headaches and several localizing neurological signs. Magnetic resonance imaging revealed an egg-sized tumor in the right orbitofrontal region of his brain, an area associated with "poor judgment, reduced impulse control, and sociopathy" (Burns and Swerdlow 2003, p. 437). With the surgical removal of the tumor, his sexual obsessions and impulsive behavior stopped.

Biochemical Abnormalities

Abnormal levels of several body hormones and brain transmitters are associated with prominent features of conduct disorder and antisocial personality disorder. Elevated levels of the male hormone dehydroepiandrosterone sulfate were found to be specific to the diagnosis of oppositional defiant disorder in children, which implicates dysfunction in adrenal androgens in this condition (van Goozen et al. 1998, 2000). Reduced plasma levels of the brain serotonin metabolite 5-hydroxyindoleacetic acid and the brain dopamine metabolite homovanillic acid were found in boys with oppositional defiant disorder, along with a correlation between the degree of serotonin reduction and the severity of their aggressive and delinquent behaviors (van Goozen et al. 1999). Reduced brain levels of serotonin in children who show excessive aggression is not surprising, because serotonin (also called 5-hydroxytryptamine; 5-HT) has a modulating and calming effect on the behavioral responses of human beings and other primates. For example, in rhesus macaque monkeys it has been documented that low levels of a brain serotonin metabolite in the cerebrospinal fluid are associated with severe aggression and other socially disruptive behaviors (Higley et al. 1996). Finally, and remarkably, concentrations of brain serotonin metabolites have been demonstrated to be significantly lower in infants with family histories of antisocial personality disorder (Constantino et al. 1997).

The Interplay of Nature and Nurture in Antisocial Personality Disorder: Murky Waters

Parental Perspectives

The research data presented in the preceding sections suggest that heredity, biological factors, and life experience combine to result in the features and behavioral patterns of antisocial personality disorder. Many questions remain about *how* these factors intermix to produce this dangerous and destructive personality disorder. Why, for example, might one child more be more vulnerable to develop this condition than his or her sibling of the same gender, born and raised by the same biological parents in the same environment? To try to answer this question, let us begin by reviewing what we know: 1) adults with antisocial personality disorder are impulsive, irritable, and aggressive, and they most often show these traits from childhood; 2) irritability, impulsivity, and aggressiveness can be inherited predispositions; and 3) like other hereditary traits and conditions (e.g., body size and shape, eye color and hair color, juvenile-onset diabetes), inherited traits of temperament and personality are not necessarily shared by all siblings. Wouldn't it be likely, therefore, that a child who is genetically predisposed to be irritable, impulsive, oppositional, and aggressive would evoke different responses (from his parents, siblings, and peers) than would his or her sibling who is calm, affectionate, and obedient? Understandably, most mothers would become angry and frustrated with a child who does not reciprocate her love and nurturance and who resists her efforts to set limits on his or her behavior. This mother would most likely have an entirely different experience and relationship with the sibling who is calm, affectionate, and compliant. For purposes of explanation, I label the genetic predisposition of a child to be aggressive, irritable, and oppositional as the **phenomenon** and the dysfunctional cognitive, behavioral, and emotional responses of the "difficult child" to the differential treatment of significant others as **epiphenomena.** Both the phenomenon and epiphenomena encompass signs and symptoms of dysfunction that comprise the diagnostic criteria of antisocial personality disorder. In the next sections I will explore how the genetically predisposed phenomenon and experientially derived epiphenomena are perceived by different members of the family.

The Patient's Perspective

During my career in psychiatry I have interviewed many adults with antisocial personality disorder and have asked them three related questions. First I ask why they feel they have the right to harm and take advantage of others. The essence of their response is *"I take because nobody gives."* Where does this particular sense of entitlement come from? The irritable, aggressive, and impulsive child with a genetic predisposition to antisocial personality disorder will be confused and frustrated by the mother who does not seem to meet his or her needs and who seems perennially impatient and upset. This child is certain to notice that the sibling has an entirely different, more positive relationship with parents, teachers, and other figures of authority. The difficult child will begin to distrust, resent, and resist all authority figures *and* what they represent: *rules.* Perceiving that he or she is being treated unfairly, the difficult child will feel entitled to violate the rules (e.g., by lying, cheating, and exploiting others) to get a fair shake and a fair share.

A second question that I have asked people with antisocial personality disorder is "Do you ever feel sorry for your victims?" The essence of their responses is *"I won't give what I never got."* By not feeling understood, loved, or prioritized by parents and other important caregivers, those who grow up as difficult children are less able to experience compassion or empathy for others. Furthermore, they envy and resent what other people have, and they feel no responsibility to share anything, especially their positive feelings.

Third, when I have asked people with antisocial personality disorder if they ever feel guilty about the suffering of their victims, they respond, *"If it doesn't hurt me, it doesn't hurt."* In essence they are saying that feeling guilty over causing pain to someone else does not make any sense to them. They don't get anything back from feeling guilty, so what's the point? My medical students and psychiatry residents who have watched me interview patients to whom I have posed these questions have dubbed the responses "Dr. Yudofsky's Three Laws of Sociopathy."

The Sibling's Perspective

The sibling, or the "easy child," is most often both fearful and resentful of the antisocial sibling. Experience has taught him or her that the other sibling does not play by the rules and is dangerous. The easy child is resentful because the sibling gets away with breaking the rules and because of the disproportionate share of parental attention required to control the difficult child. This sibling will say, "I do everything right and get nothing for it, while he/she does everything wrong but gets everything." Such children especially resent their parents for letting their siblings get away with breaking all the rules. To use the terms introduced above under "Parental Perspectives," the phenomenon is that a child was genetically predisposed from birth, irritable, aggressive, and oppositional. The epiphenomena are *both* the responses of the difficult child's parents, teachers, and siblings to his or her behavior (e.g., anger and frustration) *and* the difficult child's response to *their* responses (e.g., distrust of authority, breaking rules, and lack of empathy).

Parent-Child Interactions

The phenomenon of a child who does not have the brain-based capacity to *perceive* love and affection will lead to many epiphenomena that are characteristic features of antisocial personality disorder. The child almost certainly feels frustration, anger, and resentment toward the parent who does not appear able to connect with him or her emotionally or gratify his or her needs. This creates a vicious cycle in which the negative responses of the child lead to frustration in and even retaliation by the parent. In innumerable cases this cycle devolves to child abuse. The child might mistakenly believe that he or she is not worthy of the affection or prioritization of the parent or is a bad child who is being punished through this perceived deprivation. A self-image of being a bad person may unfetter the child from the need to follow the rules that are meant for the good people. The bad child would feel free and entitled to take from others his or her rightful due (i.e., "I take because nobody gives"). In addition, a person who did not have the experience of feeling loved would understandably have difficulty expressing loving, empathic feelings for others, including compassion for those whom they harm ("I won't give what I didn't get"). This person most likely would not feel pangs of conscience or remorse over hurting or exploiting others.

The Complex Interaction of Genetics, Life Experience, and Environment in the Development of Antisocial Personality Disorder

A research study by Reiss and colleagues (1995) explored differences in parenting styles in the development (and nonexpression) of depressive symptoms and antisocial behavior in adolescence. To accomplish their goal, the scientists evaluated same-sex adolescent children in 708 families, including 93 sets of monozygotic twins, 99 sets of dizygotic twins, 95 sets of siblings from the same biological parents who were living with their biological parents, 181 sets of siblings born from the same biological parents but who were living with stepparents, 110 pairs of half-siblings who were living with stepparents, and 130 pairs of genetically unrelated siblings living with stepparents. This study found the following: "Almost 60% of the variance in adolescent antisocial behavior and 37% of the variance in depressive symptoms could be accounted for by conflictual and negative parental behavior directed specifically at the adolescent" (Reiss et al. 1995, p. 925). Thus, experiential and environmental factors were found to be highly important in the development of behaviors that comprise the criteria for antisocial personality disorder. However, a second finding in the siblings of children with antisocial behaviors was the following: "In contrast, when a parent directed harsh, explosive, and inconsistent parenting toward the sibling, we found *less* psychopathologic outcome in the adolescent" (Reiss et al. 1995, p. 925). What this indicates is that *both* genetic *and* experiential/ environmental factors are implicated in the development of adolescent antisocial behavior: the child who developed such behavior likely had a genetic predisposition to this condition that was aggravated or triggered by harsh parenting, whereas his or her sibling, who also suffered parental mistreatment, either lacked a genetic predisposition to antisocial behavior or had genes that were protective against the development of this condition.

To date there has been only one solid study that shows a direct genetic link between emotional stress and a psychiatric disorder. A group of scientists from England, the United States, and New Zealand discovered that there are two forms of a gene regulating a serotonin transporter called 5-HTT (for 5-hydroxytryptamine transporter) that moderates the influence of stressful events on depression (Caspi et al. 2003). The serotonin transporter is critical to the reuptake of serotonin at the brain synapses, where selective serotonin reuptake inhibitor (SSRI) antidepressants are known to act. There are two common variants located in the promoter region of the gene that regulates 5-HTT: long-allele and short-allele forms. The investigators discovered that individuals with one or two copies of the short allele in the promoter region of the 5-HTT gene were more vulnerable to depression in response to stressful events than were those with longer variants of this gene. In fact, if the subjects in the study had a documented history of childhood abuse, those with two short-allele variants ran a 63% risk of having a major depressive episode, compared with a 30% risk for subjects carrying the long allele (Caspi et al. 2003, p. 388).

Treatment of Patients With Antisocial Personality Disorder and Their Families

As is emphasized throughout this book, a serious and motivated patient is essential to achieving a meaningful therapeutic outcome in psychiatry. Like the majority of patients with antisocial personality disorder, Andrew Kramer did not regard himself as having a psychological problem and therefore did not seek—nor would he accept—psychiatric treatment of any kind. Expressed another way, there was nothing that Andrew believed that he could "get" from a mental health professional. Examples of what an antisocial patient might want from a psychiatrist would include 1) drugs, 2) help with obtaining a plea bargain for treatment in lieu of incarceration, 3) testimony to a parole board to support his or her release from prison, and 4) help in persuading a family member to provide money to support his or her recovery. People with antisocial personality disorder try to con and manipulate their therapists in the same ways that they do all other people. It is therefore not surprising that J. Reid Meloy, an expert in the treatment of people with this condition, wrote the following: "There is as yet no body of controlled empirical research concerning the treatment of antisocial personality disorder or severe psychopathy. Also, no demonstrably effective treatment is available, although this finding does not prove the null hypothesis that no treatment will ever exist for these troublesome conditions" (Meloy 2001, p. 2253).

I believe that there are certain circumstances in which treatment can be helpful, and these include the following:

- Intensive treatment of children with conduct disorders. Such treatment *might* (there is little confirmatory research) help prevent *some* of these children from developing antisocial personality disorder as adults.
- Treatment of comorbid disorders of people with antisocial personality disorder. Such treatment would include psychopharmacology for mood and anxiety disorders and intensive inpatient treatment for alcoholism and substance use disorders.
- Treatment of the family members and victims of people with antisocial personality disorder. Such people often seek the help of and are benefited by mental health professionals.

To begin our therapeutic consideration on a somewhat positive note, let us first consider the treatment of the family of Andrew Kramer.

Treatment of the Kramer Family

Getting Andrew's Story Straight

Two months after Andrew was transferred from Boston to Houston, Mr. and Mrs. Kramer scheduled a consultative appointment with me. Before their meeting with me they forwarded to my office Andrew's extensive medical record. The interchange at our first meeting began as follows:

> **Greg Kramer:** Thank you for agreeing to see us. We know how busy you are, but we believe that we need your help.
>
> **Dr. Y.:** I have read your son's medical record. How can I be of help to you and your son?
>
> **Greg:** Andrew's doctors in Boston gave us your name and suggested that he see you. They said you specialize in neuropsychiatry, especially neuropsychiatric aspects of traumatic brain injury. Unfortunately, at this point, our son refuses to see any psychiatrist. He says, "I've been there and done that, and it was a waste of my time." Since he won't see you, we decided to come ourselves to ask you some questions.
>
> **Dr. Y.:** Of course I will do my best to help you and Andrew. However, please understand that I am at a great disadvantage in advising you since I do not have the opportunity to meet with Andrew in person and evaluate him directly.
>
> **Greg:** At least he has given consent for you to see his medical records, including his diagnostic tests. This should help somewhat. What we want is your advice about whether or not we should support his request to return to Boston. Is he able to live there independently?
>
> **Dr. Y.:** I certainly cannot answer that question definitively without evaluating Andrew in person, but I can tell you what I have learned from his medical records and can ask you some questions that might help you make a decision about whether or not to support his going back to Boston. First of all, from the skull films, EEGs and fMRIs of his brain that were done in Boston, Andrew suffered serious brain injury, especially to the temporal and parietal regions of his brain. These brain regions comprise the side portion of his brain and are involved, among many things, in memory, mood regulation, and certain types of thinking. Fortunately, according to his neuropsychological testing reports and the medical notes from his doctors and nurses, these functions seem to have recovered fully. Is that your impression?
>
> **Melissa Kramer:** We believe that his memory, intellect, and personality have fully recovered. Most of the people in Houston who know him well agree with us about this.
>
> **Dr. Y.:** Then what seems to be the problem with Andrew returning to his life in Boston?

Greg: Doctor, my wife doesn't agree, but I believe that Andrew had serious psychological problems before his injuries. In fact, I strongly suspect that his problems may have had a role in why he was injured in the first place.

For the next hour and a half, Greg Kramer detailed a rough outline of Andrew's history that has been presented thus far in this chapter. Clearly, Greg had mistrusted his son for a long time. On the other hand, Melissa Kramer had a different point of view:

Melissa Kramer: I think that it is Greg who has the problem with Andrew. Our son is brilliant and independent. Since he was a little boy, he has never taken the path most traveled on; and I for one believe that that has been his greatest strength. Not one bit of what Greg has alleged about Andrew would stand up in court. It is all hearsay and circumstantial evidence. The facts are that Andrew has been a superachiever all his life, and he has never been convicted of a single crime. I have a big problem with criminalizing a person just because he is an independent thinker and does not lead a conventional life. Who do you think is right, Doctor?

Dr. Y.: I believe that we need more information before coming to any sort of determination. I suggest we start by inviting his sister, Lana, to join us at our next meeting. I also would appreciate it if you could get hold of Andrew's official transcript from college. Also, if Andrew would give you or me permission to speak with his college dean and dormitory advisor, that would be illuminating.

Lana Kramer Drops a Bombshell

The Kramers agreed to have Lana join us for the next session. Lana was at home for the summer after having completed her first year of college.

Dr. Y.: We are here to try to help your parents determine how best they can help your brother, Andrew. Of course, ideally, it would be best if Andrew would be willing to join us, but he has declined. I thought that you might have some special insights about your brother that would shed some light on our understanding of how best to help him.

Lana Kramer: Doctor, I don't completely agree with you. I think that it is much better that Andrew isn't here. Much of what I am going to say, I would be afraid to say in his presence. I have been waiting for my entire life to say many of these things. I still don't feel safe doing so. For as long as I can remember, I have been terrified of Andrew. I think…no, I know that my own brother is a monster! As far back as I can remember, he would do the most terrible things to me and would say that he would kill me if I ever told our parents. I believed him then, and I believe him now. That's why I am shaking.…

Lana spoke, uninterruptedly, for more than an hour. She spoke of being physically, sexually, and emotionally abused by her brother since her early childhood. Her examples were legion and chilling. She never felt safe while he was in the house, even when her parents were also home. Lana recounted how Andrew felt that he owned her body; that from the time that she was a little girl, he would examine her "private parts." When she began to go through puberty, he would examine her, "like a gynecologist" almost every day and would take pictures. Lana was certain by the ways Andrew's friends looked at her and laughed at her in school, that he had shown his friends the pictures of her being exposed. At about the same time, when Lana was 12, Andrew began to have sex with her whenever he had the chance. Lana said that she tried to stay away from home as much as possible after that time. She spent hours away from home participating in extracurricular activities and studying in the library of a local college. She did whatever she could to stay out of Andrew's reach. Lana also disclosed that throughout childhood and adolescence, until Andrew left for college, she would not invite girlfriends to the house. Andrew would spy on them and, when they grew older, try to seduce them. By the time she was 14, Andrew stopped having sex with his sister. Lana reasoned that he was having sex with so many other people, including several girls in her own grade, that he didn't need her any more. However, until he left for college, Lana said that he would from time to time make her undress so that he could "inspect" her. In tears throughout her account, Lana said, "I have only told you the tip of the iceberg when it comes to this monster— I could go on for days."

> **Melissa Kramer:** Then just answer me this, Lana. Why didn't you tell us any of this until now?
>
> **Lana Kramer:** For two reasons. One, I was terrified of Andrew. I thought if I told on him that he would kill me. He threatened to kill me many, many times. I hate to say this, but I still think that he will kill me someday to get my part of your estate. Second, even worse than him killing me was that I thought that you, Mom, would never believe me. Andrew has you wrapped around his little finger. Every time he got into trouble, he would use you to turn things around so that his victim would become your victim. It was enough being tortured by my own brother, but I didn't want you piling on me as well. Every kid at school and most of their parents knew that Andrew is a pervert. Everyone but his own parents! My own parents! That part is worse even than what Andrew did to me.
>
> **Dr. Y.:** I believe that it is essential to maintain Lana's confidentiality in this matter. Let me be very specific: Not one word of what Lana

has said can be communicated to Andrew. I have no reason to doubt Lana's judgment that she would be in great danger—over time—if Andrew finds out what she has said. In fact, I see no reason to disclose to Andrew that Lana has attended this meeting at all. Secondly, I would like for the three of us to meet together at least three more times to craft a plan about how best to deal with the issues that have been raised this morning. Although these disclosures and revelations are disturbing, I believe strongly that what we fail to discuss and deal with is far more distressing and destructive.

Mr. and Mrs. Kramer Confront the Reality of Andrew

As a result of these consultative sessions, Greg Kramer indicated that he had for a long time suspected Andrew of being "untrustworthy." He went on to reveal that the combination of Andrew's ability to "talk his way out of trouble" and Melissa Kramer's "unwavering support of Andrew on every front" resulted in his never having directly confronted his son. As I had requested, Greg retrieved information from the university in Boston that his son had attended and learned that Andrew had been lying for years to his parents about his grades, his school status, and why he left school. On his own initiative, Mr. Kramer also called Alexandra, whom he had met previously, and reported, "Her story confirmed, totally and in painful detail, what Lana had revealed and what I had long suspected: our son is a pathological liar, a predator, and most likely a dangerous criminal." Through Alexandra, Greg also learned that it was Andrew who had stolen his credit card, Mrs. Kramer's antique brooch, and many other valuable family items. Melissa expended great effort to learn how Andrew's biological parents had fared in the 24 years since his adoption. She found out that Andrew's mother was doing well. The mother of three teenagers, she had married a man who was a career officer in the United States Navy. However, his biological father was a different story. He was imprisoned for armed robbery at age 19. On being paroled 6 years later, he was soon rearrested for possession of illegal substances and for violating his parole by carrying a concealed, unregistered semiautomatic pistol. While in prison he was involved in a riot in which he murdered another prisoner and seriously injured a prison guard. Andrew's biological father is currently serving a life sentence. Finally, with Andrew's consent, I secured the test results from the comprehensive neuropsychological battery of tests taken at the rehabilitation hospital in Houston and spoke with Dr. Gerhard George, his neuropsychologist. Dr. George advanced his diagnostic impression of Andrew, based on his evaluations and the results from the Minnesota Multiphasic Personality Inventory (MMPI) component of the testing: antisocial personality disorder. Based on this information, I recommended a treatment plan for the Kramer family as summarized in Tables 7–6 and 7–7.

TABLE 7–6. Treatment plan for the Kramer family

1. Dr. George's diagnosis of Andrew as having antisocial personality disorder was reviewed and accepted by the family. This diagnosis was entirely consistent with Lana's and her parents' experience with Andrew, as well as with the information that Greg Kramer had obtained from many other sources.

2. Mr. and Mrs. Kramer agreed that Andrew had the potential to endanger his sister, Lana Kramer. Many steps were taken to protect her confidentiality, to restrict Andrew's access to her, and to protect her personal and inherited assets from him.

3. Greg Kramer successfully petitioned the court to issue a restraining order forbidding Andrew to have any contact or communication whatsoever with his sister Lana. Mr. Kramer assured Andrew that if this order were violated in any way, he would use all of his influence and resources to see that Andrew was put directly in prison.

4. Lana Kramer was referred to Dr. Lynn Marie Martin, a psychiatrist in the city where Lana attended college, for ongoing treatment of the psychological consequences of the abuse by her brother.

5. Greg Kramer informed Andrew that he had found out about his thefts from the family. He therefore denied Andrew access to the family residence and summer home until a psychiatric consultant of their choosing indicated that Andrew was trustworthy.

6. Authority for Andrew's access to family assets and trusts was placed in the hands of a tough, experienced, and informed (about Andrew) estate attorney in a large local law firm.

7. The Kramers notified Andrew that they would no longer discuss, or provide him with, monetary support for any purpose other than for him to see a psychiatrist of their choosing.

8. Mr. and Mrs. Kramer would remain in couple treatment with me, the objectives of which are summarized in Table 7–7.

Andrew's Adult Life

When he had sustained sufficient physical recovery, Andrew returned to Boston and to his life of crime. On several occasions he sought out the help of his parents, primarily for loans of large sums of money for various projects. When he learned that they would not accede to his re-

TABLE 7–7. Objectives of the couple treatment of Melissa and Greg Kramer

1. **Work on repairing their relationship with each other.** The stress and confusion associated with their dealing with Andrew resulted in bitterness and poor communication between them.

2. **Work on protecting and repairing their relationship with their daughter, Lana.** Because her parents had not protected her from Andrew and because of the disproportionate amount of attention and family resources that Melissa and Greg Kramer had bestowed on her brother, Lana was bitter toward her parents.

3. **Work on understanding and dealing with their guilt.** The parents blamed themselves for causing Andrew's bad behavior and failures. They felt even greater guilt for not protecting Lana from her brother.

4. **Work on maintaining firm boundaries with their son.** Andrew used his considerable skills of manipulation and persuasion to refute what his parents had discovered about him and to get back into the good graces of the family.

5. **Prepare them emotionally to expect a tragic outcome for their son.** Andrew had refused all psychiatric treatment, and many people with antisocial personality disorder who do not accept help end up in jail, murdered, or dead from an accident or drug overdose.

6. **Help them grieve for the loss of the "idealized image" of their son.** Melissa Kramer had the most difficulty understanding and accepting that their son is a dangerous, inveterate predator—as opposed to an intelligent, hardworking, and successful computer entrepreneur. For her, this realization was emotionally akin to the death of her son.

quests, he gradually stopped calling them. From various sources the Kramers learned that Andrew had opened up several nightclubs that were, for a while, quite successful. However, he was convicted of arson and insurance fraud after one of these clubs burned down, a crime for which he spent several years in jail. On another occasion Andrew told his parents that he was married and had two young children. He claimed that he desperately needed money from them to pay for medical and educational expenses for their grandchildren. He told them, "Just because you and my 'real' parents abandoned me, it doesn't mean you have to write off your poor, innocent grandchildren." Greg Kramer hired a private detective, who discovered that Andrew had in fact married, and then divorced, an employee in one of his nightclubs. She was a stripper who had two young children from a former relationship. There was no evidence that Andrew had tried to adopt these children or had shown any interest in their support. Each encounter battered the emotions of Mr. and Mrs. Kramer, and they used their couple treatment with me to try to come to terms with their painful and conflicted feelings regarding their son. Presented in Table 7–8 is a summary of certain principles in treating people with antisocial personality disorder and their families, as exemplified by the case of Andrew Kramer.

In the remainder of this chapter I review the pros and cons of various types of treatment for people with antisocial personality disorder.

Psychotherapy of Antisocial Personality Disorder

Psychoanalyst Glen Gabbard, M.D., a leading authority on both personality disorders and insight-informed psychotherapy, wrote the following:

> Outpatient individual psychotherapy of the severely antisocial patient is doomed to failure. Affects will be discharged through action, because there is no contained environment in which to control such channeling. In addition, the patient's lies and deceptions are so pervasive that the therapist will have no idea what is really going on in the patient's life. (Gabbard 2000, p. 508)

In my view there is considerable danger when psychotherapy is attempted for people with antisocial personality disorder by 1) therapists who are inexperienced in the treatment of people with this condition, 2) incompetent clinicians such as Dr. Roth, 3) and so-called professionals who themselves have problems establishing therapeutic boundaries and setting limits with patients. In these circumstances, the patient will subvert the treatment and manipulate the clinician to get things that he or she wants. For example, Andrew Kramer convinced Dr. Roth that he had been mistreated by his parents because he was adopted. In turn, Dr. Roth colluded with Andrew to exact special privileges from his parents. Another all-too-common example is when a well-intentioned therapist who works in a prison system is deceived, seduced, and manipulated by an antisocial inmate to advocate to the parole board for his early release. The prisoner's sole therapeutic goal is not to learn about himself and change but to convince the therapist that he has changed and is no longer a danger to society. I therefore strongly advise limiting the use of psychotherapy for people with antisocial personality disorder to the rare patient with this condition who wants nothing more from the clinician than treatment, and to therapists with extensive experience and expertise in this area. On a more positive note, there are preliminary indications that a highly structured and targeted form of treatment,

TABLE 7–8. Key principles in the treatment of patients with antisocial personality disorder as exemplified by the case of Andrew Kramer

Historical fact	Key principle	Interpretation
Andrew's childhood alcohol abuse, substance use disorders, and conduct disorder were neither diagnosed nor treated effectively by Dr. Henrietta Roth.	Many mental health professionals are not competent to diagnose and treat children with conduct disorders or adults with antisocial personality disorder.	Dr. Roth was neither systematic nor data based in her assessment of Andrew. Her treatment approach—psychodynamically informed psychotherapy—is not effective for most children with conduct disorder.
Andrew co-opted Dr. Roth in blaming his parents for his misdeeds.	Well-intentioned but incompetent mental health professionals are easily manipulated by intelligent people with antisocial personality disorder.	Dr. Roth's incompetence resulted in a missed opportunity to help Andrew change his behavior or, at a minimum, to protect his sister from his abuse.
In family treatment, Lana Kramer finally disclosed Andrew's abuse of her to her parents.	People with antisocial personality disorder are expert at concealing their cruel and abusive behaviors.	The structure, confidentiality, and impartiality of the therapeutic setting helped Lana feel sufficiently safe to reveal the truth about her brother.
Lana Kramer required treatment to recover from the physical and sexual abuse of her brother.	Psychiatric care is usually more helpful to the victims and families of people with antisocial personality disorder than it is to the people with the condition.	Even though Lana was a successful student and was socially adept, she nonetheless required psychotherapy to deal with her emotional responses to Andrew's abuse.

TABLE 7–8. Key principles in the treatment of patients with antisocial personality disorder as exemplified by the case of Andrew Kramer (*continued*)

Historical fact	Key principle	Interpretation
Mr. and Mrs. Kramer could not agree about how best to deal with Andrew.	People with antisocial personality disorder often cause splits among their family members along the lines of those whom they can deceive and those whom they do not.	Couple treatment helped Melissa Kramer to accept the truth about her son and repair her relationship with her husband.
As an adult, Andrew Kramer refused to accept psychiatric evaluation or treatment.	People with antisocial personality disorder usually will not accept that they have psychological problems.	Andrew never evidenced any interest in changing his cruel, manipulative, and exploitive behaviors.

cognitive-behavioral therapy, has been used with some success in cor-
rectional treatment programs to treat juvenile and adult offenders with
conduct disorder and antisocial behavior (Gacono et al. 2000). Although
psychotherapy with some people with less severe forms of antisocial
personality disorder might be attempted in highly structured environments such as in hospitals or prisons, there are many pitfalls to such
treatment, as summarized in Table 7–9.

TABLE 7–9.   Pitfalls of psychotherapy for people with antisocial
personality disorder

1. The patient does not believe that there is anything wrong with him or her
   and therefore is not motivated to change his or her behavior.
2. The patient will lie to the therapist.
3. The patient will try to manipulate the therapist to get something, such as
   drugs, a recommendation for early parole from prison, or a premature
   discharge from the hospital.
4. The patient will threaten and try to intimidate the therapist.
5. The patient might not have the capacity for establishing a therapeutic
   relationship with the clinician or the cognitive ability to gain insight into
   his or her behavior.
6. The patient might be motivated to "defeat" the therapist and to undermine
   the therapeutic goal of changing and improving the patient's behavior.
7. The therapist might be fearful of the patient.
8. The therapist might be repulsed by the patient's revelation of his or her
   cruel and sadistic thoughts and behavior.
9. The therapist might be vulnerable to the patient's manipulations and
   attempts to violate therapeutic boundaries.
10. The therapist might set unrealistic treatment goals and become frustrated
    by and resentful of the patient's slow progress.

Psychopharmacology of Antisocial Personality Disorder

Several of the characteristic signs and symptoms of antisocial personality disorder—such as impulsivity, irritability, and aggressiveness—may
respond to psychiatric medications. In addition, comorbid disorders
(including alcoholism, substance use disorders, and, in less severe
cases, depression) may also benefit from the use of medications.

However, other classic features of this condition—such as deceitfulness, manipulation, irresponsibility, and lack of remorse—are not amenable to psychopharmacology.

Irritability and Aggression

Impulsive and disinhibited aggression have long been known to be associated with damage to the cerebral cortex, which can be the result of many factors ranging from brain trauma to Alzheimer's disease (Silver and Yudofsky 1987; Yudofsky et al. 1989). Many people with antisocial personality disorder have histories of brain injuries from accidents, abuse, or fights, and their impulsive aggression that results from these lesions will often respond to treatment with medication. This form of anger, irritability, and aggression can be responsive to a broad range of medications, including antihypertensive (e.g., propranolol), anticonvulsant (e.g., carbamazepine), antimanic (e.g., lithium), and antidepressant (e.g., SSRIs) drugs (Yudofsky et al. 1998).

People with antisocial personality disorder are notorious for using violence to coerce, exploit, and torment others to gratify their own needs and desires. Eichelman (1992) and other investigators term this type of aggression *predatory aggression.* Predatory aggression, which is most often premeditated, is not responsive to medications. The most dangerous criminals usually demonstrate both impulsive and predatory aggression. A study of 15 death-row inmates who had committed murder found that *each* criminal had a history of severe head injury and evidence of significant neurological impairment (Lewis et al. 1986). The subjects were selected for this study because of the imminence of their executions, as opposed to evidence of neurological dysfunction. I advocate using medications to treat the impulsive aggression of people with both antisocial personality disorder and demonstrable neurological impairment. Although this approach will not likely affect premeditated predatory aggression, injuries will be prevented and lives will be spared by reducing the impulsive, disinhibited violence in this population.

Comorbid Conditions

People with antisocial personality disorder frequently abuse alcohol and illegal drugs. Such substances intensify their core behavioral pathology so that they become even more reckless, impulsive, irritable, and aggressive when they are "high" on or withdrawing from drugs and alcohol. The use of medications like disulfiram (Antabuse) to treat alcohol dependency or methadone to treat heroin addiction may be a helpful adjutant to the rehabilitation of antisocial patients and inmates.

Laboratory research has shown that criminals with antisocial personality disorder do not feel the high levels of anxiety experienced by criminals without the disorder, nor do they worry as much (Ogloff and Wong 1990), and hospitalized patients with severe forms of the condition do not usually evidence major depression (Gabbard and Coyne 1987). Therefore the use of nonaddictive antianxiety medications and antidepressants has limited use in this population. I discourage the use of any addictive drugs—including benzodiazepine types of antianxiety agents, stimulants, and narcotic types of pain killers or sleep medications—for people with antisocial personality disorder.

How to Protect Yourself From People With Antisocial Personality Disorder

The principles and guidelines presented in the paragraphs that follow will help you protect yourself from people with antisocial personality disorder.

Prevention

Be Aware of Your Vulnerability

Ted Bundy, a serial killer with classic and severe antisocial personality disorder, had little difficulty gaining the trust of and trapping young women. First of all, he was quite aware of the attractiveness of his clean-cut good looks, which he used as bait. He would groom and dress himself in ways that made him appear successful and safe. Second, he understood his prey. He knew that college-age women tend to be trusting, helpful, and adventurous. Many of these women believe that they are worldly and self-sufficient and can handle themselves in all situations. As you will see, they were in way over their heads when it came to Ted Bundy, however. Third, Bundy was cunning. He would park his rigged van in locations at the fringes of college campuses that he knew young women would frequent and where they would feel safe. Next, he would position a sofa on the ground outside the rear door of his van. Donning a false cast over his left arm, he would wait for his preferred prey (he had a predilection for young women with long, dark hair) to walk by the trap. He would approach the targeted woman, apologize profusely for interrupting her day, and explain that, because of his broken arm, he had been struggling unsuccessfully to load the sofa into his van. Bundy would explain to the woman that she would be most helpful if she would guide the sofa from the inside of the vehicle, a task that "takes two good hands." At the instant that the sofa was fully in the van, with the victim was at the farthest point in its interior, Bundy would slam the rear door shut and lock it from the outside. He would then drive to a remote location where, at his leisure, he would sexually abuse, torture, and ultimately kill the trusting young woman.

There are very few people with sufficient vigilance to escape the predations of a Ted Bundy, once he has them in his sights. And with serial killers, there are rarely second chances for escape. Fortunately, only a small fraction of the people with antisocial personality disorder are serial killers, and of this group, very few are as intelligent and clever as was Ted Bundy. Nonetheless, people with antisocial personality disorder are always exploitive and sometimes dangerous in their important relationships. In most cases, however, their victims will usually have opportunities to protect themselves—if they acknowledge, understand, and try do something about their problem. Prevention is the best medicine.

Be Vigilant in _All_ New Involvements

As reviewed above under "Epidemiology," conservative epidemiological data indicate that 2%–4% of the population meet criteria for antisocial personality disorder. Given how dangerous and destructive people with this disorder can be, it is prudent to be vigilant and mildly suspicious about any new involvement. I fully understand that spontaneity and free-spiritedness are romantic ideals, but it is still wise to look both ways before running across a busy street. Metaphorically speaking, I believe that such vigilance especially applies to the most exciting and glamorous streets like Rodeo Drive, Fifth Avenue, and 42nd Street. Individuals with antisocial personality disorder are expert at spotting and exploiting people when they are most distracted and vulnerable. Examples include people with nonsuspicious, kindly, and generous dispositions; those who are going through difficult transitions in their lives, such as divorce, illness, or loss of employment; and those who have something that others especially want, like money, social position, or access to power. I recommend that you ask yourself the following question about all important new involvements, especially those that might involve sexual intimacy or a large monetary investment on your part: _"How do I know that this 'new' person is honest and safe?"_ If the honest answer is, _"I really don't know whether he or she is being honest and is safe,"_ your index of suspicion should be elevated. Your next question to yourself should be the following: _"What else do I need to find out about this person to be confident that the person is portraying him- or herself honestly and is safe?"_

Monitor the Relationship

Pay Attention to Your Feelings

When questioning many of my patients about their *initial feelings* on meeting someone whom they later discovered had antisocial personality disorder, I have listened for common threads in their seemingly varied responses. My patients will frequently tell me that their initial feelings were "unusually strong," often passionately positive. Admittedly my sample is skewed, because if the relationships turned out to be "marriages made in Heaven," these people probably would not have sought treatment in the first place. Probably as the result of my experience in helping to repair lives that have been ravaged by relationships with people with personality disorders (and with apologies to my wonderful, ingenuous readers who are incurable romantics), I have come to be suspicious of "instant passion." Far too often one party is overselling himself or herself, and the other party—usually my patient—is not being sufficiently cautious, critical, or self-protective. Certainly, "chemistry" has great importance in a relationship, but so does accurate information and common sense. My recommendation is that on feeling extremes of passion very early in a relationship, a red flag should go up before your pants come down. Tell yourself to slow things down until you have more facts about the background and past of that particular person.

A second common response that I receive from my patients about their initial feelings in a relationship with someone who turns out to have antisocial personality disorder is the following: *"At first I felt uncomfortable, but I couldn't quite figure out why."* Not wanting to be judgmental or willing to rain on their own parades, my future patients chose to ignore this feeling—with uniformly disastrous consequences. My strongest recommendation is that you pay close attention to *any* feelings of discomfort that you experience early in a relationship, and then do your best to determine why it is that you feel uncomfortable— before getting too close. You had better determine whether or not the exciting new feline is a tiger before tickling it.

Ask Yourself These Questions

Summarized in Table 7–10 are questions to ask yourself to assess whether or not you are likely to be in a relationship with a person who has antisocial personality disorder. Many of these questions are derived from the Fatal Flaw Scale (see Chapter 2, "Does This Person Have a Fatal Flaw?").

TABLE 7–10. Questions to help you assess whether or not a person with whom you are in a relationship has antisocial personality disorder

---

1. Do I distrust this person?
2. Do I believe that this person is dishonest?
3. Does this person have an inconsistent record of employment?
4. Has this person failed to repay the loans that I have made to him or her?
5. Has this person failed to return expensive items that he or she has borrowed from me?
6. Does this person come through on promises and personal commitments?
7. Is he or she unfaithful to me?
8. Does this person disrespect rules and disobey laws?
9. Am I uncomfortable in the presence of this person?
10. Do I always feel physically safe with this person?
11. Has this person ever stolen anything from me, from members of my family, or from my friends?
12. Has this person ever been violent with me, members of my family, or my friends?
13. Has this person harassed me, members of my family, or my friends?
14. Does this person have a prison record for theft, drug offenses, sexual abuse, or assault?
15. Is this person dependent on alcohol, prescribed narcotics, or illegal substances?
16. Do my most trusted friends and family members think that he or she is dangerous?
17. Do my most trusted friends and family members think that he or she is "bad for me"?
18. Do my most trusted friends and family members encourage me to break off with him or her?

If you answer "Yes" to even a few of the questions listed in Table 7–10, you should seek immediate consultation with an experienced mental health professional to help you determine whether or not this person is dangerous to you and likely has antisocial personality disorder or some other personality disorder. Combinations of personality disorders, such as narcissistic personality disorder along with paranoid personality disorder, can also result in unacceptable and dangerous behaviors that are identified by your responses to these questions. The bottom line is that you need professional help with assessing the full implications of your relationship, especially the dangers that it might pose.

Take Definitive Action

Prioritize Your Personal Safety

If you or a loved one is in imminent danger, you must immediately contact the local police. In this communication, you must be clear and factual about why you believe that the person with antisocial personality disorder has endangered you or your loved one. Listen carefully to the instructions of the police and follow their advice. On occasion, particularly after notifying the police in a large urban precinct, a person who feels that he or she is at risk of being harmed will conclude that the police are responding with insufficient alacrity or protectiveness. At that point I would advise the person to engage the counsel of an attorney who will help secure the appropriate police response.

Seek the Help of an _Experienced_ and _Knowledgeable_ Mental Health Professional

I do not advise you to attempt to extricate yourself from a relationship with a person with antisocial personality disorder without competent professional help. If you are correct about the diagnosis, you will be playing by one set of rules and the other party will be presuming that no holds are barred. No possible outcome will be fair or to your advantage. Take care in choosing a professional; this is no job for an amateur—whether a friend or a mental health "professional." Mistaken advice or inaction can literally be lethal. No matter how worldly or well-intended friends and family members may be, they will be over their heads in providing you with safe and effective help in dealing with a person with this personality disorder. Unfortunately, many mental health professionals are untrained and inexperienced in this clinical area, and as such are dangerous. Also, this is not the time to expend precious therapeutic hours with the clinician taking a history of your early life experiences, toilet training, relationships with siblings, and the like. Rather, the professional must know how to assess rapidly the implications of your relationship with this person and what course of action you should take that will be both safe and definitive. For example, in some instances your going to court to obtain a restraining order against the other person will be life-saving; in other circumstances it will provoke and incense the other party and increase the danger to you.

TABLE 7–11. Questions to ask when selecting a mental health professional to help you deal with a person with antisocial personality disorder

1. Do you have experience in treating patients who are in relationships with people who have antisocial personality disorder?

2. Are you comfortable in advising me about how to deal with someone who might be dangerous?

3. Will you give me direct advice about how I should best protect myself from this person?

4. If necessary, will you consult with my attorney and the police to help ensure my safety or resolve problems associated with the relationship?

5. If it is safe and indicated, will you include this person in some of my treatment sessions to help me resolve the problems associated with terminating the relationship?

6. After I have safely extricated myself from this relationship, how will you go about helping me understand why I became involved in the first place?

7. After I have safely extricated myself from this relationship, how will you go about helping me to avoid making the same mistake in future relationships?

In general, people with antisocial personality disorder require the establishment of clear boundaries and firm consequences for their violation. However, if the individual is impulsive by virtue of substance abuse or has paranoid and other psychotic tendencies, other strategies may be required. You need a mental health professional with skills and experience who will know how to work with you to assess—immediately—your risk of being harmed and to devise a specific action plan reduce this risk. I know of cases in which too much time was taken by the professional in the assessment phase, with fatal consequences for the patient. Once you are safe, this professional can work with you to further extricate yourself from the relationship, deal with its consequences, and move forward with your life. Outlined in Table 7–11 are questions to pose when selecting such a professional.

Some mental health professionals will be unaccustomed to and uncomfortable with being asked questions about their therapeutic approach. Some might even *resent* your queries. If so, move on to your next option. You have a responsibility to yourself to make your best effort at selecting a clinician who is capable of and predisposed to helping you to make judicious, far-reaching decisions in your relationships and fundamental changes in yourself. The reason you are seeking help in the first place is that you have experienced the painful and destructive repercussions of unhealthful involvements, and you do not want to repeat this mistake by choosing an incompetent therapist. In general, people are far more thorough about interviewing architects and checking the references of homebuilders than they are in selecting their medical and mental health practitioners. A new home can be wonderful, but you must be safe and healthy and have peace of mind to enjoy it. Again, you owe it to yourself to do the requisite to engage a clinician who is expert and experienced in helping you deal with the consequences of a relationship with a person who has antisocial personality disorder.

Afterword

The remorseless exploitation of others to gratify their own often perverted drives and needs characterizes people with antisocial personality disorder. As was evident in the case of Andrew Kramer, the genes that he inherited from his biological parents (whom he never met) were clearly more responsible for his ruthless behavior than were his treatment by his parents or the environmental influences of his childhood. Throughout this chapter, I have elaborated on the discussion of these research findings because I believe that the results and conclusions of the research are likely applicable to the other personality disorders reviewed in this book. Although I believe that genetic predispositions will ultimately be proved to be the key variable in the causation of most personality disorders, I also believe that genetics, environment, and experience are critical, indelible, and ineluctable "co-conspirators." My conclusion is hopeful in at least two ways: 1) symptomatic expression of genetic-based predispositions to personality disorders can potentially be mitigated by early detection of the condition and interventions involving the reduction of stress by the modification of harmful relationships and damaging environments; and 2) the revolution in genetic medicine should open new avenues for early detection, rapid and precise diagnosis, effective treatment, and even prevention of the severe and disabling disorders of personality and character that have harmed individuals and plagued societies throughout the history of mankind.

References and Suggested Readings

American Psychiatric Association: Diagnostic and Statistical Manual of Mental Disorders, 4th Edition, Text Revision. Washington, DC, American Psychiatric Association, 2000

Black DW: Antisocial personality disorder: the forgotten patients of psychiatry. Primary Psychiatry 8:30–81, 2001

Black DW, Baumgard CH, Bell SE: A 16- to 45-year follow-up of 71 men with antisocial personality disorder. Compr Psychiatry 36:130–140, 1995

Brennen PA, Mednick SA: Genetic perspectives on crime. Acta Psychiatr Scand Suppl 370:19–26, 1993

Bruno A: The Iceman: The True Story of a Cold Blooded Killer. New York, Delacorte, 1993

Burns JM, Swerdlow RH: Right orbitofrontal tumor with pedophilia symptom and constructional apraxia sign. Arch Neurol 60:437–440, 2003

Cadoret RJ: Epidemiology of antisocial personality, in Unmasking the Psychopath: Antisocial Personality and Related Syndromes. Edited by Reid WH, Dorr D, Walker JI, et al. New York, WW Norton, 1986, pp 28–44

Cadoret RJ, O'Gorman T, Troughton E, et al: Alcoholism and antisocial personality: interrelationships, genetic and environmental factors. Arch Gen Psychiatry 42:161–167, 1985

Cadoret RJ, Yates WR, Troughton E, et al: Genetic-environmental interaction in the genesis of aggressivity and conduct disorders. Arch Gen Psychiatry 52:916–924, 1995

Caspi A, McClay J, Moffitt TE, et al: Role of genotype in the cycle of violence in maltreated children. Science 297:851–854, 2002

Caspi A, Sugden K, Moffitt TE, et al: Influence of life stress on depression: moderation by a polymorphism in the 5-HTT gene. Science 301:386–389, 2003

Constantino JN, Morris JA, Murphy DL: CSF 5-HIAA and family history of antisocial personality in newborns. Am J Psychiatry 154:1771–1773, 1997

Damasio AR: The somatic marker hypothesis and the possible functions of the prefrontal cortex. Philos Trans R Soc Lond 351:1413–1420, 1996

Eichelman B: Aggressive behavior: from laboratory to clinic. Quo vadit? Arch Gen Psychiatry 49:488–492, 1992

Farrow TFD, Zheng Y, Wilkinson ID, et al: Investigating the functional anatomy of empathy and forgiveness. Neuroreport 12:2433–2438, 2001

Fu Q, Heath AC, Bucholz KK, et al: Shared genetic risk of major depression, alcohol dependence, and marijuana dependence: contribution of antisocial personality disorder in men. Arch Gen Psychiatry 59:1125–1132, 2002

Gabbard GO: Cluster B personality disorders: antisocial, in Psychodynamic Psychiatry in Clinical Practice, 3rd Edition. Washington, DC, American Psychiatric Press, 2000, pp 491–516

Gabbard GO, Coyne L: Predictors of response of antisocial patients to hospital treatment. Hosp Community Psychiatry 38:1181–1185, 1987

Gacono C, Nieberding R, Owen A, et al: Treating juvenile and adult offenders with conduct disorder, antisocial, and psychopathic personalities, in Treating Adult and Juvenile Offenders with Special Needs. Edited by Ashford JB, Sales BD, Reid WH. Washington, DC, American Psychological Association, 2000, pp 99–120

Hamer DH: Genetics: rethinking behavior genetics. Science 298:71–72, 2002

Hamer DH, Copeland P: Living With Our Genes: Why They Matter More Than You Think. New York, Doubleday, 1998

Hare RD: Diagnosis of antisocial personality disorder in two prison populations. Am J Psychiatry 140:887–890, 1983

Hare RD, Hart SD, Harpur TJ: Psychopathy and the DSM-IV criteria for antisocial personality disorder. J Abnorm Psychol 100:391–398, 1991

The Iceman Confesses: Secrets of a Mafia Hitman. Directed by Ginzberg A. HBO Home Video, 2001

Higley JD, King ST JR, Hasert MF, et al: Stability of interindividual differences in serotonin function and its relationship to severe aggression and competent social behavior in rhesus macaque females. Neuropsychopharmacology 14:67–76, 1996

Jacobson KC, Prescott CA, Kendler KS: Sex differences in the genetic and environmental influences on the development of antisocial behavior. Dev Psychopathol 14:395–416, 2002

Kashani JH, Beck NC, Hoeper EW, et al: Psychiatric disorders in a community sample of adolescents. Am J Psychiatry 144:584–589, 1987

Kessler RC, McGonagle KA, Zhao S, et al: Lifetime and 12-month prevalence of DSM-III-R psychiatric disorders in the United States: results from the National Comorbidity Survey. Arch Gen Psychiatry 51:8–19, 1994

Kiehl KA, Smit AM, Hare RD, et al: Limbic abnormalities in affective processing by criminal psychopaths as revealed by functional magnetic resonance imaging. Biol Psychiatry 50:677–684, 2001

Laakso MP, Vaurio O, Koivisto E, et al: Psychopathy and the posterior hippocampus. Behav Brain Res 118:187–193, 2001

Lewis DO, Pincus JH, Feldman M, et al: Psychiatric, neurological, and psychoeducational characteristics of 15 death row inmates in the United States. Am J Psychiatry 143:838–845, 1986

Lu RB, Lin WW, Lee JF, et al: Neither antisocial personality disorder nor antisocial alcoholism is associated with the MAO-A gene in Han Chinese males. Alcohol Clin Exp Res 27:889–893, 2003

Lyons MJ, True WR, Eisen SA et al: Differential heritability of adult and juvenile antisocial traits. Arch Gen Psychiatry 52:906–915, 1995

Meloy JR: Antisocial personality disorder, in Treatments of Psychiatric Disorders, 3rd Edition. edited by Gabbard GO. Washington, DC, American Psychiatric Publishing, 2001, pp 2251–2272

Moffitt TE: Adolescence-limited and life-course-persistent antisocial behavior: a developmental taxonomy. Psychol Rev 100:674–701, 1993

Ogloff J, Wong S: Electrodermal and cardiovascular evidence of a coping response in psychopaths. Crim Justice Behav 17:231–245, 1990

Raine A, Venables PH, Williams M: Autonomic orienting responses in 15-year-old male subjects and criminal behavior at age 24. Am J Psychiatry 147:933–937, 1990a

Raine A, Venables PH, Williams M: Relationships between central and autonomic measures of arousal at age 15 years and criminality at age 24 years. Arch Gen Psychiatry 47:1003–1007, 1990b

Raine A, Venables PH, Williams M: High autonomic arousal and electrodermal orienting at age 15 years as protective factors against criminal behavior at age 29 years. Am J Psychiatry 152:1595–1600, 1995

Raine A, Meloy JR, Bihrle S, et al: Reduced prefrontal and increased subcortical brain functioning assessed using positron emission tomography in predatory and affective murderers. Behav Sci Law 16:319–332, 1998

Raine A, Lencz T, Bihrle S, et al: Reduced prefrontal gray matter volume and reduced autonomic activity in antisocial personality disorder. Arch Gen Psychiatry 57:119–127, 2000

Reiss D, Hetherington EM, Plomin R, et al: Genetic questions for environmental studies: differential parenting and psychopathology in adolescence. Arch Gen Psychiatry 52:925–936, 1995

Rhee SH, Waldman ID: Genetic and environmental influences on antisocial behavior: a meta-analysis of twin and adoption studies. Psychol Bull 128:490–529, 2002

Robins LN: The epidemiology of antisocial personality disorder [1992], in Psychiatry. Edited by Michels RO, Cavenar JO, Brodie HKH, et al. Philadelphia, PA, JB Lippincott, 1987, pp 1–14

Robins LN: Conduct disorder. J Child Psychol Psychiatry 32:193–212, 1991

Robins LN, Price RK: Adult disorders predicted by childhood conduct problems: results from the NIMH Epidemiologic Catchment Area project. Psychiatry 54:116–132, 1991

Rutter M, Tizard J, Whitmore K: Education, Health and Behaviour. London, Longmans, 1970

Shaffer DR: Aggression, altruism and moral development, in Developmental Psychology: Childhood and Adolescence, 5th Edition. Pacific Grove, CA, Brooks/Cole, 1999, pp 509–556

Silver JM, Yudofsky SC: Aggressive behavior in patients with neuropsychiatric disorders: the scope of the problem. Psychiatr Ann 17:367–370, 1987

Smith OA, DeVito JL: Central neural integration for control of the autonomic responses associated with emotion. Annu Rev Neurosci 7:43–65, 1984

Smith SS, Newman JP: Alcohol and drug abuse-dependence disorders in psychopathic and nonpsychopathic criminal offenders. J Abnorm Psychol 99:430–439, 1990

Soderstrom H, Hultin L, Tullberg M, et al: Reduced frontotemporal perfusion in psychopathic personality. Psychiatry Res 114:81–94, 2002

van Goozen SH, Matthys W, Cohen-Kettenis PT, et al: Adrenal androgens and aggression in conduct disorder prepubertal boys and normal controls. Biol Psychiatry 43:156–158, 1998

van Goozen SH, Matthys W, Cohen-Kettenis PT, et al: Plasma monoamine metabolites and aggression: two studies of normal and oppositional defiant disorder children. Eur Neuropsychopharmacol 9:141–147, 1999 van Goozen SH, van den Ban E, Matthys W, et al: Increased adrenal androgen functioning in children with oppositional defiant disorder: a comparison with psychiatric and normal controls. J Am Acad Child Adolesc Psychiatry 39:1446–1451, 2000

Veit R, Flor H, Erb M, et al: Brain circuits involved in emotional learning in antisocial behavior and social phobia in humans. Neurosci Lett 328:233–236, 2002

Yeager CA, Lewis DO: Mortality in a group of formerly incarcerated juvenile delinquents. Am J Psychiatry 147:612–614, 1990

Yudofsky SC, Silver J, Yudofsky B: Organic personality explosive type, in Treatments of Psychiatric Disorders: A Task Force Report of the American Psychiatric Association. Washington, DC, American Psychiatric Association, 1989, pp 839–852

Yudofsky SC, Silver JM, Hales RE: Treatment of agitation and aggression, in Textbook of Psychopharmacology, 2nd Edition. Edited by Schatzberg AF, Nemeroff CB. Washington, DC, American Psychiatric Press, 1998, pp 881–900

OBSESSIVE-COMPULSIVE PERSONALITY DISORDER

Time for you and time for me,
And time yet for a hundred indecisions,
And for a hundred visions and revisions
Before the taking of a toast and tea....

I have measured out my life with coffee spoons

—T.S. Eliot, "The Love Song
of J. Alfred Prufrock"

Essence

Have you ever had an important relationship with an "emotional alchemist?" Through his alchemy, can this person transform your joy, pleasure, and fun into misery, worry, and drudgery? Are the hard times embraced, and the happy times distrusted? Do good times get put off for the future, but the future never seems to arrive? Does he reproach you for resting and resent your recreation? Does he transform the slightest disagreement between you into a fight to the death? Can he inject the amphetamine of urgency and intensity into the veins of your most leisurely and complacent pursuits? Do data, details, and deadlines obscure the tasks at hand, the big picture being buried under mounds of planning and minutiae? Like molten lava oozing across a level field, do his constant checking, monitoring, and rechecking stifle your initiative and suffocate your creativity? Does his preoccupation with your productivity blind him to your purpose?

Does his fear of catastrophes paralyze your planning for happy events? Will he reduce everything—even feelings—to some measurement: how much, how long, how far, how big? Is he so blinded by the inessential that your essence is always eluding his grasp? Does his imposition of rules, formalities, and obligations squeeze the oxygen from the flames of your passion? Does everything have a price for him, and is it always too much? Do you fear you are starting to think like him, becoming too much like him? Are you losing your "sense of self?" With that in mind, is this relationship becoming too expensive? Is it costing you much more than it's worth?

The Case of Karl Adler

The Outskirts

For Karl Adler, life, and the *meaning* of life, were enviably simple: "winning" is life's purpose, and competition is its essence. When he had become famous and admired, he liked to say that the key to his success was "my being so ordinary that I had to fight hard to become extraordinary." The middle child of a hardworking father who owned a successful electrical engineering firm, Karl was born at the hem of Indianapolis's finest neighborhood. Among his earliest memories were of his mother driving him deep into the oak-treed fabric of the elegant neighborhoods nearby to peer through the iron gates and fences that protected the homes of Indiana's most established families. Karl instinctively understood two things: that the blackened wrought iron that was forged in the steaming mills of Gary served not as protection from criminals but as barriers to the encroaching middle class. He also knew that, more than anything else in life, he wanted to be on the other side, to look out rather than to look in. On returning from these Sunday afternoon outings, Karl would be struck with how small and modest his family's modern, ranch-style home seemed by comparison. On those occasions, Karl would feel small. Indeed, he was of diminutive stature compared with his father, his two brothers, and almost all of his Hoosier friends. They all seemed to have elongated their limbs as they stretched to lift basketballs over the omnipresent rims and nets that floated like orange and white jellyfish above the driveways in their neighborhood.

Overcoming "Average"

An enriched environment that the offspring of parents with established Midwestern wealth skittishly shared with the children of striving professionals, the private academy that Karl and his brothers attended was considered to be the best in the region. Several of the Lilly children attended this school, as did the progeny of the scientists and financial and marketing executives employed in the Lilly family's pharmaceutical company. The intellectual apples clung close to the parental trees, yielding bountiful harvests of soaring aptitudes in both the sciences and the humanities. In most classes, Karl had to work hard to achieve average grades, and often he was below the median. It seemed to Karl that many of his peers had taken similar Sunday drives and were being beckoned by the imposing estates beyond the wrought-iron gates and fences.

Karl calculated that sports could be his way over the barriers, and hard work and strict schedules his catapult. Although he was too frail for football and not particularly fleet or coordinated, Karl had dreams of being a dominating point guard in basketball. Starting in the third grade, Karl worked tirelessly and systematically to mold himself into an accomplished player. He tried to attend as many high school and college games as possible, and he would watch countless college and professional basketball games on television. He would focus on the smaller players to learn how these Lilliputians managed to survive amid the giants who ruled the confining, varnished rectangles. He studied how the premier point guards positioned themselves, how they moved, and— most importantly—how they anticipated the flow of the game. How they knew where the sphere was going before it was even passed. Far in advance of his friends, who effortlessly and mindlessly stretched hands and wrists beyond the rims above their asphalt driveways, Karl understood the principles and poetry of the game: posting up, setting screens, picks and rolls, and passing lanes. Every day before class in middle school, he would run 6 miles in under 40 minutes, work out with weights for 45 minutes, and complete a strict routine of shooting free throws and field goals in the gym of his church. His shooting routine would go as follows: first he would take 100 shots from the foul line, which he would make himself repeat if he made fewer than 85. He would then take 20 shots from each of 10 spots on the court's floor that he had previously marked with magic marker. He would make himself repeat this entire cycle if he missed more than 3 shots from any of the locations. From age 10, Karl played in several winter and summer basketball leagues and attended basketball camps. He also read extensively about the sport. He knew something about every player in the National Basketball Association (NBA) and a great deal about all of the more successful players and their individual teams. His friends would delight in asking Karl esoteric questions about the statistics of the sport, such as "What was the final score of the third game of the 1956 NBA championship series?" They would marvel in disbelief when Karl would not only tell them the score of the game but also many other details, such as the names and scoring totals of the high scorers on each of the teams.

By the time he was a freshman in high school, Karl was the best player on his private school team and one of the better players in the prep school league. Watching him from the stands, a knowledgeable fan would first note the high level of intensity with which he played the game. Although he was in constant motion, there was purpose to each move and action. Excelling as a passer and shooter, he was also attentive to the less obvious aspects of the game. Before every game, Karl would do his best to find out what he could about his opponents—especially the player whom he would be guarding. He would spend hours preparing for the game, trying to understand the opposing team's strengths and to think though effective defensive strategies. Often defending an opponent who was 6 inches taller than he, Karl nonetheless was usually able to keep the ball away from him and disrupt his accustomed scoring patterns. For his 3 years of high school, Karl led his team in scoring, assists, and steals. Remarkably, for a player who was about 5 feet 9 inches tall, he was also his team's second best rebounder, after the center, who was 6 feet 10 inches tall.

Overshooting the Mark

Aiming High

In high school, Karl set for himself two ambitious goals that he used to motivate himself to maintain his grueling training regimen. First, he had a burning ambition be recruited by either Indiana University or the University of Kentucky, two perennial powerhouses in the sport. He was confident that he would be a valuable asset to either team and that he would continue to develop athletically under their outstanding coaching. Their high visibility would help him attain his second goal—to be drafted by an NBA team. Like a general preparing for a military campaign, Karl planned out each detail of his strategy to make one of the two towering college basketball teams. He attended summer basketball camps organized by the coaching staffs of each program and worked tirelessly during these camps to prove his abilities to the coaches. Directly after each practice in summer basketball camp, while the other players would be resting or recreating, Karl, in painstaking detail, would record the lessons of the day. He would bring to the camp the other notebooks that he had laboriously prepared over the years and would make references and links to related material in these tomes.

Occasionally his peers would look over his shoulder and tease him about the complex and detailed diagrams that Karl crafted and studied:

> **Teammate:** Wow. What is that stuff? It looks like the electrical wiring of a Boeing 747 jet.
>
> **Karl Adler:** It's the new defense formations that Coach Nelson was teaching us today. I'm trying to get it down in writing so I can understand it better.
>
> **Teammate:** You take all of this stuff too seriously. It's just a game, man. You'd play a lot better if you chilled out and had some fun on the court.
>
> **Karl:** It's much more than a game to me.

Losing His Temper

At the end of each day, Karl would study his notes and prepare questions that he would ask his basketball coaches the next day. He worried that if he hadn't mastered every aspect of their teaching, the deficiency "would come home to roost at a critical point in a critical game." Karl strove for perfection on the basketball court and chastised himself mercilessly when he made mistakes. Most of the time, Karl's temper was directed toward himself for making a mistake on the court. However, as he gained recognition and confidence from his ball-playing skills, he would occasionally lash out at others. When it came to basketball, Karl had difficulties understanding and accepting others who were not so motivated as he in the pursuit of excellence. He would silently seethe when players on his team would goof off in practice, and he would yell at them—sometimes during the games—when they made careless errors that led to turnovers or missed scoring opportunities. He showed no tolerance for players who got by on their innate athletic talents but who were not serious about fulfilling their potential in basketball. He did not believe that these individuals had the right to be on the team, and he felt that their attitude had corrosive effects on morale.

When he became captain of his high school team in his junior year, Karl's temper outbursts worsened. Several younger players quit the team as a result of his merciless criticism of them. One tearful, departing freshman told Karl something that would become a recurring theme throughout his personal and professional life: "You jump all over me when I make a mistake, but you never say anything when I do something right." Mistaken calls by referees were another common source of pique for Karl. Although he understood fully that it was counterproductive to argue with officials, Karl occasionally lost control. During a closely contested championship game in his senior year, a referee called three questionable fouls on Karl for setting "moving picks"; although he was furious, Karl didn't say a word. With several seconds left to go in the game and the team behind by two points, Karl made a shot from behind the three-point line. However, the same referee who had called the three fouls on Karl signaled that the shot should be counted as a regular two-point field goal, and indicated that Karl's foot was touching the line. It was obvious to many in the stands with good views of the play, and especially to Karl, who had endlessly practiced this very shot in his preparatory routine, that the referee was mistaken. He knew exactly and had checked where his foot was positioned, and it was behind the line. The dam restraining the fathomless reservoir of feelings fueled by years of self-discipline and self-deprivation burst. Karl grabbed the referee by the shirt, pulled him within an inch of his face and screamed, "You blind, stupid, incompetent asshole! You lost the game for us. You ruined our whole season!" It took a while for his coach and several players to pry the stunned referee from Karl's unrelenting grip, and even more players were required to restrain him and drag him, writhing in fury, from the court. Of course, Karl was thrown out of the game, which was lost when the opposing team made the technical foul resulting from his outburst. After the game, rather than feeling humiliated for losing control, losing the game, and making a public spectacle of himself, Karl was entirely focused on finding a videotape of the fateful three-point shot. He unshakably believed that if the tape proved that both of his feet were in fact behind the line, his actions would be vindicated. Through persistence, he procured several still shot photographs and a tape from a parent of a player he knew on the opposing team that indicated clearly that the referee was wrong: both feet were several inches behind the line, both before and after he made the shot. Even though he was reprimanded by the coach and the school principal and received a month of after-school and weekend detention for his unsportsmanlike conduct, Karl never admitted or accepted that he was in the wrong. He reasoned, "Why have rules of the game if they don't mean anything? Why work for excellence if incompetents have the last word?" Karl concluded that he had long ago outgrown the mediocrity of high school basketball and would mark time until he could play for a major college team.

The Best Athlete

Karl averaged almost 30 points and more than 10 assists per game in his junior year of high school. Unprecedentedly for a basketball player in his private school league, he was scouted by many college teams, including Indiana University and the University of Kentucky. Over the summer he hoped to hear from both schools. When he didn't hear from the coaching staff of either school, he asked his high school coach, Mr. West, to try to find out the reason. The following conversation ensued:

> **Coach West:** I was finally able to talk to the head coaches at both schools. I know how hard you have worked toward the dream of playing for either Indiana or the University of Kentucky, but they did not indicate any interest in recruiting you.
>
> **Karl Adler (visibly upset):** Did they indicate why?
>
> **Coach West:** I pushed them on just that question. They complimented you on your attitude and work ethic, but told me that their experience had taught them to go with the best athletes. They do not feel that you have the height, speed, quickness, or jumping ability to play at their level. They suggested your looking into an Ivy League school or a strong junior college.
>
> **Karl:** What bullshit. I don't have the grades to play for the Ivies; and you know that they don't give athletic scholarships anyway.
>
> **Coach West:** You don't need a scholarship. Your family will pay your tuition.
>
> **Karl:** I have worked far too hard to be a "walk on." I'm too good to be a walk on. They are so wrong. I know that I can play and contribute to any school. There is no way in the world that I will drop off the earth playing for some junior college team in the boonies, either. Thanks for all the help.

Although Karl was bitterly disappointed, he would not accept defeat. Reasoning that he would have to sell himself to be able to play for a premiere college basketball team, he assembled a videotape that highlighted his best performances. Karl also carefully compiled his statistics, featuring head-to-head comparisons with other well-regarded point guards against whom he had competed within leagues and at the summer basketball camps. He narrowed down his college wish list to about 10 programs, based on the quality of their coaching. National Collegiate Athletic Association (NCAA) rules permitted him to visit several of these colleges in his senior year, and he showed up on their campuses uninvited and unannounced. So unconventional was this approach that several college coaches refused to even speak with him. A few, however, looked at his tape and read his statistical material, and even watched him work out and play in informal scrimmages. In one workout Karl made 26 out of 30 unguarded shots from behind the three-point line, a feat rarely accomplished even by professional athletes. Ultimately, two top-tier basketball schools showed some interest, but neither would offer him a scholarship. Karl's high school coach and father tried to persuade him to attend a smaller school with a less prominent basketball program. They argued that the academic opportunities would be better and that he would have a greater chance of making the starting squad at a smaller college. But with Karl there was no such thing as compromise. He never wavered from his goal of playing for an elite college basketball team, which he believed was essential to attain his second goal of being drafted by an NBA team.

College

Betting on a Long Shot

Through perseverance, Karl hammered out an arrangement with a large Midwestern university with a first-rate basketball program. He would only be guaranteed a spot on the team during his freshman year, however, and he would not receive a scholarship. If, in his first year, he showed some promise of making a contribution to the team, there would be the possibility of a scholarship in his sophomore year. Coach West and Karl's father were not impressed:

> **Coach West:** I have to be frank with you. I am convinced that you are making a big mistake. It's a mediocre school academically, and they're not even giving you a 4-year commitment to be on the team. You will be a little fish in a big basketball pond.
>
> **Karl Adler:** I am getting exactly what I want: the chance to prove myself on a great team with excellent coaches.
>
> **Coach West:** Have you thought at all about the alternatives? First of all, you are passing up other real offers from outstanding smaller schools like Lehigh, Rice, Army, and Vanderbilt, where you are certain to make the team for 4 years and get playing time. Even though you don't like to think about it, there will be life for you after basketball. At any of these schools you are certain to get a fine education.
>
> **Karl:** I don't see it that way at all. Where I'm going I will have stiffer competition, better coaching, more national visibility, and a much greater chance of making the NBA.
>
> **Coach West:** Let's be realistic for a moment. The chances of any college player making the NBA are remote, less than one in a thousand. And how many athletes who are less than 6 feet tall get drafted? Because this university hasn't invested in you by giving you a scholarship, they are unlikely to give you much playing time. Not to mention the possibility of injuries. You're betting your entire future on a long shot.
>
> **Karl:** I hear you; but I'm sticking to my plan. I know what I'm doing.

Matching Up

Karl attended his university's basketball training camp during the summer before his freshman year of college. Although the upperclassmen on the team complained bitterly about the practices and the new recruits were unprepared mentally and physically, Karl was totally in his element. For the first time in his long experience with basketball, the level of the workouts matched his own intensity and seriousness. Although he impressed the coaching staff with his basketball skills and incomparable work ethic, Karl found himself surprised by the quick reactions, speed, and athleticism of the other members of the team. By a large margin, Harris "Happy" Jefferson was the cream of the freshman crop. Loose and limber as a rag doll, Happy moved his 7-foot frame and 300-pound torso with fluidity and grace. Through sheer athletic ability he could compensate during practices for what he had not learned or did not understand about the complex offensive strategies and defensive formations. He did not pay the slightest bit of attention during the classroom strategy and teaching sessions. The coaches understood that excelling in practices is one thing, but playing against equally gifted athletes in NCAA division 1 competition is something entirely different. He would have to learn the intricacies of the game to fulfill his enormous potential. Concerned that Jefferson might have attention-deficit disorder, the director of athletics had Happy tested by the team's sports psychologist. The final report read as follows:

> I was unable to arrive at definitive diagnostic conclusion, because the client kept falling asleep during the course of my evaluation. I am certain, however, that Type A personality and obsessive-compulsive personality can be ruled out at this time.

At the conclusion of the summer practice session, Head Coach Larry Everett asked Karl to see him in his office. Certain that the coach wanted to compliment him on his overall performance and hopeful that he would disclose his playing role when the season started in late fall, Karl was ebullient.

Coach Everett: I want to let you know that you will be rooming with Happy this coming year. We hope you will be a good influence on him. We want you to keep a close eye on him to be sure he doesn't get in any trouble and help him with his homework when he gets stuck. Your fancy private school education and high board scores are going to pay off for us.

Karl Adler: Of course, I'll do my best to help out the team.

Coach Everett: You help out Happy, and you help the team. We expect that he will get a lot of playing time this year, even though he is just a freshman.

Karl: Do you see any playing role for me this year?

Coach Everett: Not really. We have two experienced point guards coming back. Bide your time.

Having worked diligently during summer practice and thinking that he held his own with his teammates, he was shocked and demoralized by the coach's request. Not being someone who was particularly drawn to the irony of being paired with a person who was his dispositional opposite, Karl came to the following conclusion: "This is what it comes down to: they want me to be a babysitter for this lazy moron."

Walking into their dormitory room, even the casual observer would by struck by the dichotomy. One side could have been in a surgical suite. Beneath the textbooks that were lined up according to size and perpendicular to the base of the bookshelf, the bedspread was tucked in neatly and was trampoline tight. A rectangular green blotter was precisely centered on the shining surface of Karl's metal student desk, and it looked like the lawn for his house-like stack of spiral-bound notebooks. Happy's side of the room lacked only gliding seagulls above and poisoned birds below to become the combination of a landfill and toxic waste dump. About a dozen grease-darkened, empty pizza boxes competed for space on the floor with scattered crushed Coke cans, countless empty cellophane cookie and potato chip bags, fountain-like magazines that sprayed their colorful pages in all directions, 14 weight-lifting discs, and one iron bar. His desk was buried under assorted socks, jock straps, undershorts, tent-like sweatshirts, and silo-sized sweat pants. Lying on its side like a beached whale on the sheetless mattress, a gigantic boom box blasted forth rap music. Not surprisingly, Karl had never been more miserable in his life. Not only did he find it impossible to concentrate or study in the room, but he was unable to establish any sort of sleeping schedule. Despite having a 10:00 P.M. curfew on weekdays, Happy would stay up until early hours of the morning talking on the telephone with his many friends and listening to the blaring music. Rarely awakening before noon, Happy missed many classes and was often late for practice. Karl thought that it would only be a matter of time until Happy flunked out of school or was kicked off the team. If he were only patient, some order, peace, and predictability would be restored to his life.

"Nothing but Net"

Growing up, Karl had never had a best friend, nor was he particularly close to either of his two brothers. Although he idolized his older brother, Norman seemed to have resented him from birth. Even more painful to Karl was the fact that Norman formed a close and lasting relationship with the youngest brother, an alliance from which Karl was excluded. Because his mother worked closely with his father in the family business, much of Karl's childhood was spent in the care of house-keepers. Almost all of his early memories were of playing by himself, unwelcome to join his two brothers, who were having fun together. He felt as if he were on the outside looking in. He also recalled being the brunt of his brothers' frequent pranks and constant, mean-spirited remarks. In the Adler family, intelligence, especially in math and science, was held in the highest regard. Both of his brothers were intellectually gifted in computational sciences such as physics, computer sciences, and physical chemistry, and Norman took special delight in pointing out how much more advanced the younger brother was than Karl in these subjects. On the other hand, Karl was stronger and more coordinated than his brothers, and he surpassed them in all sports.

Although Indiana's "state passion" is basketball, Karl's parents and brothers were among the minority of Hoosiers who have no interest whatsoever in the game. Karl recalled being disappointed that they rarely attended his games, even the important championship ones, nor did they show interest in the coverage of his exceptional performances in the local newspapers or on television news. Karl himself did not derive much pleasure from his own fine games and was uncomfortable with the congratulations and admiration of others. However, after team losses or poor personal performances, he would criticize himself mercilessly, ruminate about his mistakes, and take the constructive critiques of coaches as mean-spirited reproaches. The overall result was that Karl was lonely and unhappy.

"Happy" Days

Karl did not like to be surprised. He approached his life very much like a military campaign: clear objectives, realistic assessments of his strengths and weaknesses, great emphasis on preparation and flawless execution, objective measures of success, and ongoing assessments of and adjustments to failure. Feelings—which Karl regarded as nonmeasurable, distracting "noise" in his system—were deliberately excluded from his grand design. Notwithstanding his extraordinary emphasis on predictability and control, Karl was completely unprepared to like Happy, much less to become his best friend. Even before they became roommates, Karl was perennially frustrated by Happy's laissez-faire approach to everything. As freshman members of the ball team, they trained together daily. During scrimmages, Karl was always screaming instructions to Happy, who was usually out of position on both offense and defense. On the innumerable occasions that Happy would not move in the right direction after a pick, would not be expecting a pass that would lead to an easy score, or would miss a defensive assignment that led to points for the opposing team, Karl would take him aside to chastise him for his indolence and ignorance and try to explain what had happened. Any other player would have bridled at being so harshly reprimanded and being given remedial instructions by a peer, but Happy took Karl completely in stride. In fact, to the other players' astonishment, Happy, who was universally popular with his team-mates and nationally regarded as a basketball player, seemed to look up to Karl. He respected Karl and was proud to be his roommate. Not only did he not mind Karl's constant harpings, but Happy seemed to pay more attention to Karl than to the team coaches. Happy never failed to invite Karl to join him at the countless parties and school events he at-tended, and he tried to include him in the fun and horsing around when his many friends visited their room.

Gradually, Happy's good nature and respect thawed Karl's defenses against intimacy—protective barriers frost-hardened by the rejections of his family and of class-conscious Indianapolis, into which he had never found a fit. Not because of Coach Everett's mandate but because he cared about Happy, Karl worked with his friend to salvage his first-semester grades. It was mid-semester when Karl went with Happy to all of his professors and found that he was failing every course. He se-cured all of the course requirements and the exact grades on tests and papers that would result in Happy's remaining eligible to play basket-ball. Karl developed and daily updated precise records to track both Happy's academic and sports performances. At any given time, Karl could produce Happy's grade-point average in any course or his cur-rent statistics for scoring, rebounding, assists, and turnovers. Karl also discovered something about Happy that had been missed during the 18 years of his life: in addition to being an outstanding athlete with a win-ning temperament and personality, Happy was highly intelligent. What Happy lacked and Karl provided were organizational and time man-agement skills. For the first time in his life, Happy prepared for his classes, paid attention to his teachers, and learned the material. His grades soared.

Hitting Bottom

By the time the basketball season began in late October, it was evident that Happy had earned a starting position as center. His performance against his experienced counterparts on the many highly ranked teams on their schedule was disappointing, however. He was consistently out-maneuvered on defense and outscored on offense.

As the season progressed, the team was losing many of its games against its most competitive opponents. Karl, who saw no playing time whatsoever, was beside himself. He believed that the formations and style of play of his team were outmoded and did not make optimal use of the players' abilities. While watching from the bench his team's futile struggles, he would buffer his pain by devising novel configurations and plays.

At night, after the games, he would diagram and record in his notebooks what he had devised. At the practice the day after a particularly devastating defeat, he asked to meet with Coach Everett, with whom he shared his ideas. The coach responded defensively, saying, "Son, get this straight, you are here to play, and I'm here to coach. As far as I can tell, you are just taking up valuable space on the bench." This interaction marked a low point for Karl. He began to doubt himself. Because he was a nonscholarship player, no one seemed to notice him, and he couldn't work any harder. He began to think that he had made the wrong choice of schools. As such a small fish in a big pond, Karl again had the hated feeling of an outsider looking in.

Getting His Shot

It turned out that Coach Everett was wrong about one thing: completing that year with a disappointing record of 13 wins and 12 losses and with no postseason tournament bids, he was fired after 22 years of coaching the team. A new coach, who had achieved some success as head coach of the basketball team of one of the military academies, was hired. Although he was very young, Coach Brodie brought in an entirely new coaching staff. To Karl's amazement, after their initial workout in the fall of Karl's sophomore year, Coach Brodie said to the team, "I want to meet with each of you personally to learn about your basketball goals and your life goals. I also welcome any ideas that any of you have for making practices more interesting and effective—or helping the team be more competitive." After considerable trepidation, Karl decided to approach Coach Brodie with his ideas. He reasoned that at this point, he did not have very much to lose.

> **Karl Adler:** Thank you for making some time to see me. I have some ideas that I think might help the team, both on defense and offense. To save you time, I've brought some notebooks in which I have outlined my suggestions.
>
> **Coach Brodie:** Four notebooks! It seems you've done a lot of thinking about this, Karl. I'll have a look at them and get them back to you when I'm done. Thanks a lot.

A week passed without Karl hearing a word from his coach. In truth, Karl did not hold out much hope that the coach would even read the notebooks. When Coach Brodie approached him and asked to see him briefly after practice, Karl's first thought was that he was going to tell him that he was going to be cut from the team.

> **Coach Brodie:** Thank you for letting me take a look at your notebooks. While I don't agree with everything that you have proposed, Karl, most of it is very interesting to me. It's very different from anything I've tried before. I want to spend more time going over it, and I'd like your permission to Xerox your books for the other coaches. After they study them, I am going to hold a meeting to go over your ideas with them. You're welcome to join us for the session.
>
> **Karl Adler:** It's fine with me, except that I hadn't planned on anyone else reading this stuff. I would have done a more careful job if I had known anyone would be looking at it.
>
> **Coach Brodie:** The only way you could have put more care into your notes, Karl, would have been to have written them in iambic pentameter. Let's get together on this in about a week.

Saturday practice ended at noon, and Coach Brodie asked Karl to remain to discuss his ideas with the other coaches. The session lasted though the evening, with the coaches being astonished by Karl's knowledge of the abilities and limitations not only of his fellow teammates, but also of the opposing teams they would play that season and most of their key players. Karl recommended a radical change in the team's traditional offensive style, departing from Coach Everett's more free-wheeling, fast-breaking, undisciplined approach to adopt a more deliberate, slower-paced half-court offense with many intricate set-plays:

> **Karl Adler:** The offense should center around Happy, who should receive the ball on nearly every series of plays in the high post position. The one and two guards would cut around him and either cut toward the basket or move laterally to the three-point line. Happy can pass off to one of the guards or use the pick to drive toward the basket.
>
> **Coach Brodie:** What keeps the defense from collapsing on Happy, double-teaming or even triple-teaming him?
>
> **Karl:** You have two guards who are outstanding three-point shooters. Happy has "soft hands" and is a great passer—with good vision, judgment, and timing. He can hit the open man, or take a pass underneath if they drop off of him to cover the outside. Also, I have been working this past year with Happy on his spot-up jump shot from about 22 feet out. He's not there yet, but by the end of this

season we could have another dangerous option from this basic set. Of course, there will also be fast breaks and opportunistic variations, but not so many that we go back to playing out of control.

The team opened that season with two victories against weak opponents. They were underdogs in their third game, which was against a team that was ranked number three in the nation and had beaten them by a large margin the previous year. By the end of the first quarter they were behind by 11 points. Coach Brodie called over to Karl, who was sitting at the very end of the bench.

Coach Brodie: We're getting blown out. Go in as point guard, tell Happy to move out to the high post and work your newfangled offense.

It was Karl's first appearance in a college game, and a moment for which he had been preparing since the third grade. The first two times that Happy hit him with crisp passes as he broke behind the three-point line, no player from the opposing team even bothered to guard Karl. He hit both shots. When, on the third offensive series, two players rushed to block his shot, Karl hit Happy breaking under the basket with a spectacular lofting pass that Happy jammed home. That game, Karl sank 9 of 11 three-point attempts, had 12 assists (8 of which went to Happy), and hit all 7 of his foul shots. They won the game by 19 points, and Karl started in every game for the remainder of his college career. In their sophomore year, Happy and Karl led their team to a record 22 wins and 4 losses, with an overtime loss in the "round of 16" of the NCAA tournament. In the succeeding year they lost in the final game of the NCAA tournament, and the following year the team won the tournament and was voted a first-place national ranking by both the college coaches' and *New York Times* polls. Happy was voted to the first-team All-American squad after his sophomore year and was joined by Karl for their junior and senior years of play.

Happy was picked in the first round of the NBA draft, but because of concern about his lack of size, speed, and quickness, Karl was drafted late in the third round by a team that was on the opposite coast from Happy's.

Life on the Road

Everything Is Relative

By age 22, Karl had achieved his life's goal: playing in the NBA. Having to switch from the zone defense played in college to the mandatory "man-to-man" defense of the professional league took a severe toll on Karl's game. He commonly had to defend against (and was guarded by) players who were nearly a foot taller than he and who were able to jump much higher. As a result, he had difficulties guarding players in his position and had trouble getting his shots off. He fought valiantly to compensate through Herculean physical conditioning and meticulous mental preparation. At this level, however, hard work was insufficient. Although some of his statistics appeared to be excellent (near the top of the league in three-point, field-goal, and free-throw percentages; leading his team in assists per amount of time played), most of the starting players in his position around the team had higher scoring averages. A great college player, Karl was an average professional. In his role as backup guard, his playing time per game averaged about 15 minutes, or about one quarter of the game. Other players in similar circumstances adjusted to their roles. They rationalized that they were receiving huge salaries to play the game they loved and that by playing less time in each game, their bodies would be spared the brutal wear and tear that limited careers. Unable to accept such rationalizations, Karl drove himself relentlessly in a frenetic effort to overcome being average. Never in his life happy or content, Karl, as an NBA player, was miserable.

Ellen

First impressions.   Shy, distrusting of intimacy, and fearful of dependence, Karl did not have a steady girlfriend in high school and rarely dated in college. In fact, he viewed sexual drives and needs for closeness with women as personal weaknesses to be overcome. He met Ellen Brophy during his senior year of college, when she was a junior. He was fulfilling a community service requirement for graduation by teaching basketball skills to developmentally challenged young adults, most of whom had Down syndrome. Ellen, who was working with the same group as a part of her special education major, first noticed Karl's earnestness. Whereas the other college students just showed up and were friendly at the scheduled supervisory sessions, Karl came prepared with individualized programs and training materials. To help his "clients" find and remember their positions on the court, he gave them colored wristbands that matched pieces of colored tape he placed on the floor. He would find a special ability in each person and would work with him or her tirelessly to develop it further. He would prepare homework drills that he would patiently explain to their parents. He drew up simple graphs that illustrated each person's accomplishments and progress from week to week. In other words, Karl treated his charges with no less respect, intensity, or seriousness than he did himself. Ellen observed all of this and was moved. She also noticed that although the other college students would spend much of their time talking and kidding around with one another, Karl didn't waste a moment. She projected her compassion and generous nature onto his actions and thereby saw a great deal in Karl that was fine. After quietly watching him for several weeks, she built up her courage to introduce herself to him. She was working with several of the same young people whom Karl was teaching, and she asked his insights and ideas about the nature of their disabilities and how best to help them. Over the next several months, they would speak with one another about their clients, but Karl would never ask Ellen anything of a personal nature or speak about himself. She had no idea that he was a celebrated athlete who, at that very time, was helping to bring a national basketball championship to their university.

On one bleak, icy Midwestern midwinter evening, the parent of a client had a minor car accident and was delayed by several hours in picking up her child. Ellen and Karl remained with the young man until the parent arrived, and it was after dark. To Ellen's surprise and delight, Karl asked her if she would like to join him for dinner in the varsity athletic facility. Thereafter, neither of them dated another person, and they married a year later.

Married life.   Ellen adored and idealized Karl, whom she saw as being mature, serious, honest, reliable, and ambitious. She also loved and felt close to his brothers and to his parents, whom she called "Mom" and "Dad." Karl, however, was uncomfortable and standoffish with Ellen's large, close-knit, emotionally expressive, Irish-American working-class family. Although Ellen's younger brothers were thrilled to have a professional basketball player in the family and closely followed all of his games, Karl paid little attention to them. During the 6 months of the basketball season, when he was mostly away from home, Karl did not call Ellen's brothers or ask how they were doing. Ellen's parents suspected that Karl felt superior to them, but Ellen reassured them that the all-consuming demands and pressures of playing in the NBA were the sole source of his distance and seeming disinterest.

On graduating from college, Ellen accepted a position as a special education teacher in the public school system in the city of the professional team that had drafted Karl. Although he earned an annual salary of more than $300,000, Karl thought it wise to put that money away in case he became injured and they should lose their main means of support. In stark contrast to the lavish lifestyles of his NBA teammates, Karl and Ellen lived mostly on her $26,000 annual salary. Residing in a modest one-bedroom rental apartment did not bother Ellen at all. However, Karl always seemed unhappy, and Ellen took this to heart. She felt it was her responsibility to make her husband happy, and she made this her principal mission in life. Because Karl seemed so beleaguered during the basketball season, Ellen tried to protect him from all competing responsibilities and distractions. Thus she assumed all of the household responsibilities—from shopping to cooking his meals; from computing the taxes to paying the bills. During the first year of their marriage, Ellen had hoped for some respite during the off-season months, but Karl seemed to have little time to help out and to be under great stress during that period as well.

At first Ellen did not seem to notice that her husband did not express his appreciation for her considerable efforts to make his life easy, pleasant, and comfortable. Rather, she was aware of how critical he was of her when things did not go perfectly. One example occurred when a check that Karl wrote bounced because there were insufficient funds in the checking account:

> **Karl Adler:** That check was written to our landlord. Don't you realize that they keep records on those things? Not only will our credit be damaged because we were late on our rent payment, but also the bank knows that we are unreliable with our accounts. We might want to get a mortgage from them someday.
>
> **Ellen Adler:** I'm so sorry, Karl. I was trying to do what you told me about not keeping too much money in our checking account, because of the low interest rates.
>
> **Karl:** Haven't you ever heard of keeping accurate records? If you are careful—and what I mean by that is, if you care just a little bit about what you do—these crises can be avoided.
>
> **Ellen:** I'm so sorry that I upset you. I know you are under so much pressure from the team. I'll try harder, I promise.
>
> **Karl:** Apologies and promises just don't cut it, Ellen. As far as I'm concerned, effort and results are the only things that count.

Ellen went on personal campaign after personal campaign to "better herself." No matter how hard she tried, she never seemed to accomplish her two main goals in life: pleasing her husband and making him happy. A pattern developed whereby she would have to "walk on eggshells" during the 6 months of the basketball season (including training), because of Karl's unrelenting intensity and tenseness. She was always looking for the right time to communicate with him, to bring up important issues for discussion. However, the right time never seemed to arrive. Karl always seemed to be brooding about something related to his job—not having sufficient playing time; missing a free throw or field goal attempt; turnovers; losing a game; not being able to contain

the offensive production of a player he was guarding. On those occasions he would barely speak with Ellen, other than to criticize her for
not doing on time or perfectly some task that he had assigned. No matter what issue Ellen brought up for discussion, Karl would respond angrily, "Why are you doing this to me? Can't you see that I am under
immense pressure and must concentrate? I don't think you have a clue
about what I do for a living and how much is expected from me each
day." In truth, most of Ellen's thoughts were about Karl and how to
make life easier and more uplifting for him. During the off months, Karl
would ruminate about his chances of being traded to another team or
being cut altogether. He worried that each new guard whom his team
recruited would beat him out for the backup point guard position, and
that possibility would drive him to train and prepare for the pending
season like a madman. Ellen and Karl seemed to communicate only
about accomplishing tasks and solving problems. When Ellen would
try to bring up lighter subjects such as going out to dinner, taking weekend trips, or making plans for summer vacations, Karl would dismiss
the conversation as being trivial or defer it as being of a lesser priority
than some goal-related project.

Family planning.   There was one issue that Ellen would not let drop:
planning a family. She first brought up having a baby after their third
year of marriage, during Karl's off-season:

> **Ellen Adler:** I know that you are busy, honey, but there is an important
> issue that I would like to discuss with you.
>
> **Karl Adler:** You are so right. I am unusually busy right now trying to
> do my homework on the new drafts to the league. One of them
> will most likely take away my position, and take food off our table
> and out of our mouths. What is it you would like to talk about?
>
> **Ellen:** I think it is a good time for us to try to have a baby.
>
> **Karl:** I can't imagine a worse time to do such a thing. How do you pro-
> pose that we would support a child? You work for practically
> nothing, and I have a job that could end at any given moment.
>
> **Ellen:** I read in the newspaper that you have just been signed to an-
> other year at a salary of almost a half million dollars. We have
> saved almost every penny from all of your previous paychecks.
> Many of the teachers where I work have families, and they are
> paid the same salary that I get.
>
> **Karl:** First of all, we pay huge taxes on my salary. I take home only a
> small fraction of the total. Secondly, we have no idea of the other
> sources of income of the teachers where you work. They might
> have inheritances from their families. As you know, we can't
> count on our parents for a red cent.
>
> **Ellen:** Having a family isn't just about money.

Karl: Oh, isn't it? The first thing we would have to do is buy a house—probably an expensive one in a neighborhood where the public schools are good. With taxes, utilities, and insurance, it will probably turn out to be a terrible investment. Second, you will either have to drop your job or hire an expensive housekeeper. With her benefits, the housekeeper will probably cost us considerably more than you are making. Then we could have unexpected medical expenses. Everyone always believes that their babies will turn out normal and healthy; however, the children's hospitals always seem full and busy, don't they?

Ellen: Are you saying that we will never be able to afford children?

Karl: I don't think we are accomplishing anything with this conversation. I think that you should work up a long-range business plan that takes into consideration the real costs of having children. When you've done that, I'll go over it with you in light of our true income and our future prospects, such that they are. At that point we might have some idea when, if ever, we can afford to start a family.

Ellen dutifully did what her husband requested. When she had completed the task, Karl contested every fact and projection in Ellen's "business plan" and ultimately concluded, "It would be irresponsible to bring a baby into the world at this time, given our financial circumstances. Let's put this on hold for a year or two and reconsider it at a time when our finances are much stronger." Ellen felt stymied on several accounts. First, she could not understand why Karl believed that they could not afford to start a family, even though they had no debts whatsoever and savings of over a million dollars. Second, she was frustrated that the entire discussion about children revolved around money. She could never find the opportunity to talk with Karl about what she considered to be the real point: the pleasures and wonders of having babies and raising a family.

Ellen, who loved babies and children, experienced great anguish whenever she would encounter mothers with their infants and young children. So she did not give up. Every year in late spring, when the NBA season had concluded, Ellen would submit to Karl her updated and revised "long-range business plan" for having children, and every year he would reject her proposal based on what he described as "insufficient attention to unexpected contingencies," which would include such things as catastrophic illnesses of the parents and child or the loss of his job as the result of injury or poor performance.

Gaining a Son and Losing a Step

Karl played for 9 consecutive years on the same team—an unusual accomplishment for a player in the NBA who was not of star caliber. Although he averaged fewer than 12 points per game, he earned the reputation of being a dependable player who never hurt the team and who could be counted on in the clutch. Although he rarely started games, he was often playing at the end of games, especially those that were very close. He almost never made turnovers or committed foolish fouls, and he was consistently among the best in the league at setting up plays and feeding the ball to the open man. When he was able to get open, he was among the NBA's top three-point shooters. In addition, when he was fouled, he could be depended on to make the free throws. Over his years of play, Karl was the hero of several important games that enabled his team to get into or advance in the postseason playoffs. During his seventh and eighth seasons, his team reached the championship round. In his eighth season, Karl's last-second three-point shots brought home victory in two of the games in the championship series. These performances earned Karl national attention and admiration, and that year he was given an award as the league's "Best Sixth Man."

That summer his agent negotiated a 3-year renewal of his contract with a generous salary increase. Ellen, who was then 29 years old, pleaded with Karl to start their family at that time. Given their substantial wealth and the security of a 3-year contract, Karl reluctantly acquiesced. Within 3 months Ellen was pregnant, and at the beginning of Karl's tenth NBA season, she gave birth to their son, Mitchell.

As he had done throughout his career in athletics, Karl compensated for his relative deficiencies in physical prowess through intensive preparation and unparalleled knowledge of the game. He had long understood and accepted that the only way he could outplay his opponents was by outthinking them. However, by his tenth year of play in the NBA, Karl had lost another increment of speed and quickness. This fact was not lost on the league's younger point guards, who were blessed with incredible speed, quickness, and hand-eye coordination. Watching tapes of their play, Karl would often think to himself that the younger players had better reflexes than cats. More and more frequently, Karl would have the ball taken away from him while he was dribbling or would have a pass stolen. On the floor of play, Karl knew exactly what to do, but he could no longer depend on his body to get it done. In the parlance of athletics, Karl had "lost a step." The result was that the very element of his game that made him so valuable to his team—his reliability not to make mistakes and hurt the team—was being compromised by the natural course of aging and the years of wear and tear on his body. An inveterate fighter, Karl drove himself mercilessly to counter and overcome the inevitable, and in the process he was driving himself and Ellen nearly crazy. Brooding obsessively about each turnover and missed opportunity, he was chronically angry, and he turned his anger both outward and inward. He was pervasively irritable and contentious with fellow players, and he felt himself to be embattled on every front. In his mind his struggles had assumed epic proportions, but to others he appeared depressed and self-involved. On the home front, Ellen felt that she was abandoned and was raising their son entirely by herself. She could not help noticing in her neighborhood, at church, or even in the pediatrician's office how other couples would jointly participate in the care and nurturance of their infants, whereas Karl was entirely detached from his child. When Karl would come home from a day's practice, he would not ask Ellen how her day had been or what Mitchell had done that day. Not only did he not hold or pick up his son, but most of the time he did not even look at him when they were in the same room. Rather, he would come home and immediately complain to Ellen about his injuries or about the impending catastrophe of his career, would then stretch for an hour, ice down his aching joints, study scouting tapes, and go to bed early. Despite Ellen's heroic efforts to try to involve him in the joy and miracle of their new baby, Karl remained largely uninterested and wholly self-involved. Although for years she had been willing to make a greater investment in their relationship for an unequal partnership, she would not accept this bargain for her child. The result was that for the first time, Ellen began to question her marriage.

Out and Down

While diving for a loose ball in an NBA conference game, Karl collided with the opposing team's center, a massive man twice his weight. Like a gigantic pestle, the center rolled across Karl's extended right leg with the full force of his accelerating bulk, and Karl's kneecap was pulverized against the playing floor. It was later discovered that several of the ligaments critical to stabilizing the knee joint were also torn. An open surgical procedure was required to repair the damage to bone and tissue, and an intensive rehabilitation plan was prescribed to restore joint function. The team's orthopedic surgeon told Karl that although it was certain that he would not be able to return to play that season, it was uncertain—in fact unlikely—that he would ever again be able to play basketball at a professional level. So accustomed to being told what he could not accomplish, Karl paid little attention to his doctor's pessimistic prognosis. He became fully committed to and absorbed in his rehabilitation process that focused on restoring mobility to his knee and strength to his leg. His plan was to work fiercely through the spring and summer on his medical recovery in order to be back on his team's active squad in time for practice in early fall. The restoration of his muscular strength and coordination was indeed considered remarkable by his medical team, but the team coaching staff was less impressed. His coaches quickly noted that Karl could not plant his right foot with authority, an action that is essential for cutting rapidly to the left or making crisp passes to the left. After 2 weeks of practice, the head coach called him to his office to tell him he was going to be cut from the active squad of the team. By NBA rules he was at that point eligible to be picked up by another team in the league. Karl was shocked and felt humiliated when no team showed interest in recruiting him. His agent pulled strings to arrange tryouts with several organizations, each of which clearly communicated to Karl that the residual effects of his injury precluded any value that he would have to their team. Eventually what was obvious to others became apparent to Karl: he had sustained a career-ending injury.

For the first time since he was a child, Karl did not have a life goal or a guiding plan. He was bitter that his team had not given him the benefit of the doubt, or at least one chance to prove his worth under game conditions. He was also furious with Ellen:

Karl Adler: Since Mitchell was born, you have abandoned me. You didn't lift a finger to help me with my rehabilitation, and I don't think you have an inkling about what I have been going through emotionally.

Ellen Adler: That's unfair. I know how much you are suffering, and I know that you are devastated that you can't play basketball anymore.

Karl: Your pity doesn't help me. Don't you have anything positive to suggest?

Ellen: As a matter of fact, I do have a suggestion. Perhaps your injury could be a blessing in disguise. Finally, you have time to be with your family without being harried and hassled by your job. Mitchell is almost 2 years old, and I don't think you have ever spent one uninterrupted hour with him. On most days, for most of his life you haven't been with your son at all.

Karl: Is this supposed to make me feel better? You've made your point, Ellen. Not only am I a failure as a professional athlete, but I am also a failure as a father. I know you believe I have failed you as a husband.

Over the next several months, Karl became more and more withdrawn and isolated. Formerly, his practice was to awaken at daybreak and to rush to the gym to begin his strength conditioning and mental preparation for the work of the day. After being cut from his team, he gradually developed a pattern where he would stay up most of the night watching sports on satellite television and would sleep and stay in bed during the day. He rarely came out of his bedroom suite, which included his office. (Since the birth of Mitchell, Karl had asked to sleep in a separate bedroom so that Ellen would not disrupt his sleep when the baby cried at night.) He seemed to lose interest in almost everything. Ellen would bring his food to the bedroom, and he stopped reading or returning his mail or accepting phone calls. Ellen was certain that Karl had become depressed, but she was not successful in convincing her husband to see a psychologist or psychiatrist. Ellen herself was beginning to feel more disillusioned than ever before, and she was fearful that she also would become depressed. Since the first year of her marriage, she had harbored the hope that when Karl's demanding career as a professional athlete would end he would have much more time and peace of mind to participate in and enjoy their relationship. She now knew that she had been deluding herself—if anything, Karl was more self-absorbed, distracted, and emotionally unavailable since he had stopped working.

In desperation, Ellen called Karl's friend and teammate from college, Happy Jefferson, and asked him for help with her husband. At that time, Happy was still an active player in the NBA and was considered one of the league's premier centers. Through the general manager of Happy's ball team in a city on the opposite coast from where Ellen and Karl lived, I was identified as the clinician to evaluate Karl, and an appointment was arranged.

> **Ellen Adler:** Happy, there is no way that I will be able to get him to go to the doctor's office. He is offended and gets angry with me every time I ask him to accept some professional help. These days, I can't even get him to leave his bedroom.
> **Happy Jefferson:** Then don't tell him about the appointment or your call to me. I'll make arrangements to fly into town the day of his appointment and will pick him up and take him to the doc.

On the designated day, Happy appeared at Karl's house and told him that he was going to take him to see a doctor.

> **Karl Adler:** It's great to see you, old buddy, but I'm just don't feel up to talking to some doctor today. I'll have Ellen cancel and reschedule for a different day.
> **Happy Jefferson:** Remember what you taught me in college about doing my homework? You said the main principle is *"do it now."* Before deadlines, you moved your desk in front of the door of our room and wouldn't let me out until I had done my assignment. Karl, you look like shit and need some help. I didn't come here all the way from California to put this off.

Almost physically, Happy "escorted" Karl, with Ellen in tow, into the awaiting limousine that brought them to my office. I saw them together in my office in a 2-hour session. My recommendations were as follows:

Dr. Y.: From the information that you, Ellen, and Happy have so generously shared with me, I believe that you are suffering from two psychiatric disorders. First, you fully meet the American Psychiatric Association's DSM diagnostic criteria for major depression. Depression is a serious brain illness that affects mood, behavior, performance, and relationships—usually for the worse. The good news is that it is highly amenable to treatment with medications and psychotherapy, and, contingent on your willingness to engage in treatment, you should be better soon.

Karl Adler: I agree that I meet the criteria for depression that you gave us. You said this is a brain illness. How do you know that?

Dr. Y.: Wonderful question, Karl. Before you leave my office today, I will give you a packet of scientific papers that review what has been discovered about the brain biology of depression from genetic and epidemiological studies, from brain imaging studies, and from other research sources. I will also provide you a good bit of information substantiating the importance of antidepressants in the treatment of this condition.

Karl: I can assure you that I will read all of this information carefully before taking a drug that affects my brain. Also, doctor, you said I have two illnesses. I agree that I have depression, but what's the other condition that you think I have?

Dr. Y.: It is called a personality disorder. However, with your permission, I would like to wait until after the depression has improved before working with you to confirm this diagnostic suspicion.

Karl: I think you'll find, doctor, that I am a great believer in coaches and specialists—once I manage to find the right one. If I determine that what you say makes sense and is helpful, I will work with you as hard as any patient that you have ever had.

Dr. Y.: Good. Let's start then with my explaining a bit more about depression and your medication. I would also like to meet with you twice a week for at least the time it takes for your depression to abate. With your permission, I would also like for Ellen to attend several of these meetings.

I met regularly with Karl over the next 6 weeks. During that time I took a careful history from him and from Ellen. In the second week of treatment, I recommended that he add an intensive physical activity component to his schedule. The patient agreed with me that for almost all of his life he had worked out vigorously and that his mood disorder could be in part a reaction to his physical inactivity over the previous 3 months. I also communicated to him that I was now confident that he

---

TABLE 8–1. Diagnostic criteria for obsessive-compulsive personality disorder (slightly modified from DSM-IV-TR)

A pervasive pattern of preoccupation with orderliness, perfectionism, and mental and interpersonal control at the expense of flexibility, openness, and efficiency, beginning by early adulthood and present in a variety of contexts, as indicated by four (or more) of the following:

1. The person is preoccupied with details, rules, lists, order, organization, or schedules to the extent that the major point of the activity is lost.

2. The person shows perfectionism that interferes with task completion (e.g., is unable to complete a project because his or her strict standards are not met).

3. The person is excessively devoted to work and productivity to the exclusion of leisure activities and friendships (not accounted for by obvious economic necessity).

4. The person is overly conscientious, scrupulous, and inflexible about matters of morality, ethics, or values (not accounted for by cultural or religious identification).

5. The person is unable to discard worn-out or worthless objects even when they have no sentimental value.

6. The person is reluctant to delegate tasks or to work with others unless they submit to exactly his or her way of doing things.

7. The person adopts a miserly spending style toward both self and others; money is viewed as something to be hoarded for future catastrophes.

8. The person shows rigidity and stubbornness.

Source. Adapted from American Psychiatric Association: *Diagnostic and Statistical Manual of Mental Disorders,* 4th Edition, Text Revision. Washington, DC, American Psychiatric Association, 2000, p. 729. Used with permission.

---

met DSM diagnostic criteria for obsessive-compulsive personality disorder (American Psychiatric Association 2000), as reviewed in the following sections of this chapter and outlined in Table 8–1.

About Obsessive-Compulsive Personality Disorder

Diagnostic Features of Obsessive-Compulsive Personality Disorder

(Slightly Modified From DSM-IV-TR, pp. 725–727)

Individuals with obsessive-compulsive personality disorder attempt to maintain a sense of control through painstaking attention to rules, trivial details, procedures, lists, schedules, or forms to the extent that the major point of the activity is lost. Such people are excessively careful and prone to repetition, pay extraordinary attention to detail, and repeatedly check for possible mistakes. They are oblivious to the fact that other people tend to become very annoyed at the delays and inconveniences that result from this behavior. For example, when such individuals misplace a list of things to be done, they will spend an inordinate amount of time looking for the list rather than spending a few moments recreating it from memory and proceeding to accomplish the tasks. Time is poorly allocated, with the most important tasks being left to the last moment. The perfectionism and self-imposed high standards of performance cause significant dysfunction and distress for these people. They may become so involved in making every detail of a project absolutely perfect that the project is never finished. For example, the completion of a written report might be delayed by numerous time-consuming rewrites that in the mind of the author all come up short of perfection. Deadlines are missed, and aspects of the individual's life that are not the current focus of activity may fall into disarray.

Individuals with obsessive-compulsive personality disorder display excessive devotion to work and productivity, to the exclusion of family obligations, leisure activities, and friendships. This behavior is not accounted for by economic necessity. Rather, they feel that they do not have time to take an evening or a weekend day off to go on an outing or to just relax. They may keep postponing a pleasurable activity, such as a vacation, so that it may never occur. When they do take time for leisure activities or vacations, they are uncomfortable unless they have taken along some work so they do not waste time. If they spend time with friends, it is likely to be in some kind of formally organized activity (e.g., sports). Hobbies or recreational activities are approached as serious tasks requiring careful organization and extreme effort and hard work to master. The emphasis is on perfect performance. These people turn play into a structured task (e.g., correcting an infant for not putting the plastic rings on the toy post in the right order; telling a toddler to ride his or her tricycle in a straight line; turning a game into a harsh lesson about acquiring the fundamental skills of the sport).

People with obsessive-compulsive personality disorder may be excessively conscientious, scrupulous, and inflexible about matters of morality, ethics, or values. They force themselves and others to follow rigid moral principles and very strict standards of performance. They are also mercilessly self-critical about their own mistakes. Individuals with this disorder are rigidly deferential to authority and rules and insist on quite literal compliance, with no rule-bending for extenuating circumstances. An example would be the person who will not lend a quarter to a friend who needs one to make a telephone call, because it would be bad for the person's character: "neither a borrower nor a lender be." People with this condition may be unable to discard worn-out or worthless objects, even when they have no sentimental value. They regard discarding objects as wasteful and risky because "you never know when you might need something." They become upset if someone tries to discard the things they have saved. Their spouses or roommates complain about the amount of space taken up by old equipment, outdated magazines, broken appliances, and so on. People with this personality disorder are reluctant to delegate tasks or to work with others. They stubbornly and unreasonably insist that others conform to their way of doing things, and they often give very detailed instructions about how they demand things should be done. For example, they would believe that there is only one way to mow the lawn, wash the dishes, or assemble a bicycle, and they are irritated if others suggest creative alternatives. At other times they may reject offers of help, even when they are behind schedule or don't know how to accomplish the task. They believe that no one else can do it right.

People with this condition are miserly and stingy and maintain a standard of living far below that which they can afford. They believe that spending must be tightly controlled to prepare and to provide for future catastrophes. They are also rigid and stubborn. They are concerned about having things done the one "correct" way and are unwilling to go along with the ideas of others. Planning ahead with meticulous detail, they are unwilling to consider changes. They overvalue their own perspective and have difficulty acknowledging the viewpoints of others. Friends and colleagues may become frustrated by this constant rigidity. Even when people with obsessive-compulsive personality disorder recognize that it may be in their interest to compromise, they often stubbornly refuse to do so, giving the argument that it is "the principle of the thing."

Psychology of Obsessive-Compulsive Personality Disorder

Sigmund Freud and many other pioneer psychoanalysts posited that the characteristic traits that currently constitute the criteria for obsessive-compulsive personality disorder—such as oppositionalism, perfectionism, orderliness, inflexibility, and frugality—can be traced to problems of the young child during critical developmental stages. As their theory goes, the infant is born in a state of self-attachment and self-involvement, called *autoeroticism.* The infant begins to explore and experience the world through oral modalities until it is approximately 18 months old. If all goes well during this period and if the child is not traumatized or severely frustrated, he or she will move from what is termed its *oral stage* to what is called the *anal stage* of development. However, if there are problems such as neglect or abuse, the infant might not move smoothly from the oral stage to the anal stage, giving rise to what is termed *arrested oral development* (Freud 1908/1959). Adult consequences of arrested oral development can include overdependence on others, problems with trust, paranoia, narcissism, and depression. In the anal stage of development (extending approximately from age 18 months to 30 months), the child becomes preoccupied with bodily functions, particularly those involved with the elimination of waste. Issues around toilet training become increasingly important as the child learns that he or she can control this process. The child is also aware that his or her parents are pleased when elimination is under control and will be disturbed when it is not. Competitions of will can occur between parent and child during this period, and the child learns the meaning and power of "no." The social implications of this process involve future relationships with authority and the development of such concepts as being a "good" or a "bad" person. If problems occur with the child during this stage, the child is said to have *arrested anal development* or *anal fixations.* The characteristic features of obsessive-compulsive personality disorder—opposition to others while rigidly deferential to authority, perfectionism, inflexibility, parsimony, and the excessive need to control others—have been postulated to stem from arrested anal development. Through controlling themselves and others, people with this condition try to earn the favor of others, and they become confused, frustrated, and enraged when it has the opposite result. Freud also believed that there was an erotic aspect to fecal elimination and retention, with pleasurable sensations being mediated by the sensitive soft tissues of the anus. He hypothesized that problems that occurred during this developmental stage could lead to so-called anal sadism, which is often associated with sexual arousal derived from inflicting pain and withholding pleasure from others. Two excellent reviews of Freudian developmental psychology as well as the work of later theoreticians can be found in textbook chapters by gifted psychoanalysts Glen Gabbard (1999) and Stephen Marmer (2003).

Differentiating Between Obsessive-Compulsive Personality Disorder and Obsessive-Compulsive Disorder

In DSM-IV-TR a diagnostic distinction is drawn between obsessive-compulsive personality disorder and obsessive-compulsive disorder

(OCD). Given the similarity of the names and some overlap in the symptoms, this nomenclature has been the source of considerable confusion among patients and controversy among professionals. Approximately one-third of patients with OCD also meet criteria for obsessive-compulsive personality disorder (Bejerot et al. 1998). Notwithstanding the many similarities of these two disorders, there are also important differences between OCD and obsessive-compulsive personality disorder in their presentation, clinical course, and treatment. In summary, although obsessive-compulsive personality disorder, as its name suggests, is a *personality* disorder, OCD is categorized as an *anxiety* disorder, which is in the group of illnesses that includes conditions such as panic disorder, phobias, generalized anxiety disorder, and posttraumatic stress disorder. Although anxiety is certainly a commonplace feature in people with obsessive-compulsive personality disorder, its intensity and persistence form the hallmark symptoms of OCD. Also differentiating OCD from obsessive-compulsive personality disorder is that the characteristic symptoms in the former condition are experienced as being troublesome problems that need to be "fixed" (termed *ego dystonic*), whereas those with obsessive-compulsive personality disorder usually regard their characteristic behavioral patterns as being acceptable and even desirable (*ego syntonic*). Thus, people with this personality disorder are not particularly bothered by their personality traits and are often bewildered that these qualities are so troublesome to others.

The essence of OCD is intrusive, distracting, distressing, and time-consuming mental preoccupations, called *obsessions,* and repetitive behaviors, or *compulsions,* the purpose of which is to reduce the stress of the obsessions and to avoid the related anxiety and fears. Thus, obsessions are thoughts and compulsions are behaviors. An example of an obsession would be a person's preoccupation with being dangerously contaminated by his or her environment. Everywhere he goes he sees potentially lethal sources of infection, such as door handles; banisters; eating utensils; bathroom facilities; and public transportation, including buses, cabs, and airplanes. He spends many hours a day worrying about contamination and figuring out ways to avoid it. Despite great attempts to put his fears and ruminations out of his mind, he is unsuccessful. In his unsuccessful effort to allay his painful preoccupations he engages in many repetitive behaviors, or compulsions. Examples might include washing his hands hundreds of times each day, scrubbing the doorknobs in his apartment with disinfectants every time they are touched by another person, and throwing away towels and sheets that have been used by other people. If he tries to resist a compulsion, he experiences intense anxiety that can be relieved only by relenting to that compulsion.

Once thought to be a rare condition, OCD is now estimated to afflict approximately 2.5% of the population in their lifetimes (Regier et al. 1988). The condition has been found to occur slightly more commonly in women than in men. However, the symptoms of OCD appear earlier in males—often by adolescence—than in females, for whom the onset is commonly in their 20s (Weissman et al. 1994). About 90% of people with OCD have both obsessions and compulsions, and among this group, 28% are most troubled by obsessions, 20% by compulsions, and 50% by both (Foa et al. 1995). Presented in Table 8–2 is a summary of DSM-IV-TR diagnostic criteria for OCD (American Psychiatric Association 2000).

Biology of Obsessive-Compulsive Personality Disorder

Obsessive-compulsive personality disorder is prevalent in about 1% of the population and can be diagnosed in about 3%–10% of people receiving outpatient psychiatric care. The condition occurs twice as commonly in men as in women. Unfortunately, few reliable and valid studies have been conducted on the biology of obsessive-compulsive personality disorder, and no valid studies are available on the genetics that might contribute to the occurrence of this condition. Because an unusually high proportion of patients with OCD (about one-third) also meet diagnostic criteria for obsessive-compulsive personality disorder and because far more has been discovered about the neurobiology and genetics of OCD, I believe it will be useful to briefly review what is known about the biology of OCD. It is likely that some of these facts about OCD also apply to obsessive-compulsive personality disorder.

Biology of OCD

Evidence from twin studies indicates, but does not prove conclusively, that OCD has a hereditary component. There is a greater concordance for the disorder among monozygotic twins than among dizygotic twins (Andrews et al. 1990; Carey and Gottesman 1981). Family studies show that OCD occurs four times more frequently in the close relatives of those with the condition than in the relatives of people who do not have the disorder (Nestadt et al. 2000). I was not able to find a single adoption study to determine the role of inheritance in OCD. In a subset of people with OCD there is a possible relationship between OCD and movement disorders, especially tic-type syndromes such as Tourette's disorder. Higher rates of OCD are present in relatives of people with

---

TABLE 8–2. Diagnostic criteria for obsessive-compulsive disorder (slightly modified from DSM-IV-TR)

A. Either obsessions or compulsions are present:

1. The person experiences recurrent and persistent thoughts, impulses, or images that are perceived as being intrusive and inappropriate and that cause marked anxiety or distress.

2. The thoughts, impulses, or images are not simply excessive worries about real-life problems.

3. The person attempts to ignore or suppress such thoughts, impulses, or images or to neutralize them with some other thought or by taking some type of action.

4. The person recognizes that his or her persistent thoughts, impulses, or images are a product of his or her own mind and are not imposed from without by some magical force.

5. The person exhibits repetitive behaviors (e.g., hand washing, ordering, checking) or mental acts (e.g., praying, counting, repeating words silently), and he or she feels driven to perform these behaviors in response to an obsession according to rules that must be applied rigidly.

6. The behaviors or mental acts are aimed at reducing anxiety and distress as well as preventing some dreaded event or situation. These behaviors or mental acts are excessive and are not connected in a realistic way with what they are designed to neutralize or prevent.

B. At some point during the course of the disorder, the person *recognizes* that the obsessions and/or compulsions are excessive or unreasonable. *Note:* This does not apply to children.

C. The obsessions or compulsions cause marked distress, are time consuming (take more than 1 hour a day), or significantly interfere with the person's normal routine, occupational (or academic) functioning, or usual social activities or relationships.

Source. Adapted from American Psychiatric Association: *Diagnostic and Statistical Manual of Mental Disorders,* 4th Edition, Text Revision. Washington, DC, American Psychiatric Association, 2000, pp. 462–463. Used with permission.

Tourette's disorder than in control groups. In addition, elevated rates of Tourette's disorder and other types of motor tics occur in some categories of patients with OCD (Fyer 1999).

Recent research involving functional brain imaging has convincingly implicated abnormal functioning in the brains of people with OCD. Brain systems involving portions of the ventromedial cortex, the basal ganglia, and the thalamus have been shown to have increased activity in people with OCD (Rauch and Baxter 1998). Other studies have shown diminutions in total white matter and increases in cortical volume in people with OCD compared with control subjects. Readers who are interested in more information on this subject are referred to an excellent chapter by Drs. Stein and Hugo (2003) and a review article by Fitzgerald and colleagues (1999).

Brain biochemical abnormalities have been documented in people with OCD, and these abnormalities prominently involve serotonergic, dopaminergic, and other brain transmitter systems (Russell et al. 2003; Stein and Hugo 2003, pp. 1054–1055). Because of the robust response of many people with OCD to treatment with antidepressants affecting the serotonin systems of the brain (selective serotonin reuptake inhibitors, or SSRIs) and because of other findings, altered brain serotonin levels have been implicated in this disorder. As reviewed below (see "Evidence-Based Treatments of People with Obsessive-Compulsive Personality Disorder"), treatment of patients with OCD most often combines the use of a serotonergic antidepressant and a form of psychotherapy—often cognitive-behavioral therapy.

Table 8–3 summarizes key principles about obsessive-compulsive personality disorder as exemplified by the case of Karl Adler.

Treatment of People With Obsessive-Compulsive Personality Disorder

Resistance to Accepting Treatment

For many reasons, people with obsessive-compulsive personality disorder are reluctant to seek or accept professional help for their condition. First and foremost they equate treatment with loss of control, because they view psychotherapy as turning over control of their lives to another person. They conceptualize psychiatric treatment as being a hierarchical system, with the professional totally empowered and the patient powerless. For these reasons, early in the treatment of a person with obsessive-compulsive personality disorder, it is imperative for the clinician to explain that therapy is a collaborative, advocational process over which the patient assumes much of the control. Underpinning their need to be in complete control is their deep, unexplored reservoir of painful feelings. Intuitively, people with this disorder also avoid circumstances and interactions—such as psychotherapy—that can lead to their gaining access to these repressed feelings. Presented in Table 8–4 is a summary of excuses commonly used by people with obsessive-

TABLE 8–3. Key principles of obsessive-compulsive personality disorder as exemplified by the case of Karl Adler, part I: psychiatric history

Historical fact	Key principle	Interpretation
Despite providing him with material comforts, Karl's parents deprived him emotionally.	People with obsessive-compulsive personality disorder often value things more than relationships.	The hurt and anger associated with real and perceived rejections of childhood impair the formation of intimate adult relationships.
Karl became preoccupied with performance in sports.	People with obsessive-compulsive personality disorder overvalue things that can be quantified.	Despairing of being loved for who they are, people with obsessive-compulsive personality disorder seek love for what they have accomplished.
Karl became an outstanding basketball player.	People with obsessive-compulsive personality disorder often achieve success in school, sports, and vocations.	Intense focus on goals, tasks, preparation, organization, and productivity can lead to successful outcomes for some people with obsessive-compulsive personality disorder—at a cost.
Karl did not experience pleasure or satisfaction from his sports accomplishments.	People with obsessive-compulsive personality disorder most often are anxious, unhappy, and unfulfilled.	Fundamentally, people want to feel loved for who they are rather than for what they have done.
Karl became enraged with others who seemed unmotivated or made mistakes.	People with obsessive-compulsive personality disorder are hard on themselves and others.	People who deprive themselves have difficulties being generous to others.

TABLE 8–3. Key principles of obsessive-compulsive personality disorder as exemplified by the case of Karl Adler, part I: psychiatric history *(continued)*

Historical fact	Key principle	Interpretation
Although Karl became an outstanding college and professional basketball player, he nonetheless perennially felt vulnerable to failure and rejection.	People with obsessive-compulsive personality disorder set lofty and difficult-to-achieve goals for themselves and others.	The mistaken premise of people with obsessive-compulsive personality disorder is, "I accomplish my goals." They thus set impossible goals, so that this mistaken premise will never be disproved.
Ellen was attracted to Karl for his many good qualities, including his intelligence, modesty, hard work ethic, and honesty.	People with obsessive-compulsive personality disorder frequently have positive and attractive personality traits.	When Ellen first met Karl, she looked at the glass as being "half full." During her marriage she came to understand the unfortunate implications of the "empty part" of the glass.
Ellen was a caring and supportive wife, and she grew to have closer relationships with members of Karl's family than he did.	People with obsessive-compulsive personality disorder often choose wonderful people for spouses.	Their careful attention to details and their scrupulosity can result in people with obsessive-compulsive personality disorder marrying people with fine character, mature values, and winning personality traits.

TABLE 8–3. Key principles of obsessive-compulsive personality disorder as exemplified by the case of Karl Adler, part I: psychiatric history (*continued*)

Historical fact	Key principle	Interpretation
Karl rarely expressed warm or appreciative feelings to Ellen.	People with obsessive-compulsive personality disorder are often cold, insensitive, and unappreciative toward people who love them.	People who do not feel loved have problems loving themselves and others.
Karl demeaned recreation, relaxation, socialization, vacations, and other pleasurable activities.	People with obsessive-compulsive personality disorder have problems rewarding themselves and others.	Hard work with no reward results in a vicious cycle of anger, insecurity, and the punishment of self and others.
For almost a decade, Karl resisted Ellen's pleas to have children.	People with obsessive-compulsive personality disorder are rigid, oppositional, and withholding.	By saying "no," people with obsessive-compulsive personality disorder maintain control, avoid risks, and sadistically punish others.
Karl was emotionally detached from and uninvolved with his young son.	People with obsessive-compulsive personality disorder can be cruelly self-centered and insensitive to those who depend on them.	Hard work, constant suffering, and little reward can be a smokescreen concealing selfishness.
Karl became depressed when he was cut from the professional basketball team.	People with obsessive-compulsive personality disorder often develop major depression.	When they have to accept being imperfect and when their ambitions are unmet, people with obsessive-compulsive personality disorder often become depressed.

TABLE 8–4.   Common excuses used by people with obsessive-compulsive personality disorder to resist seeking professional care

---

1. "Psychiatric/psychological treatment costs too much."

2. "I don't have the time to waste on therapy."

3. "Psychiatry is an imprecise science."

4. "Who's to say that there is something wrong with me?"

5. "What are they going to tell me about myself that I don't already know?"

6. "Shrinks all believe that feelings are more important than logic."

7. "What psychiatrists do is teach their patients how to make excuses and blame other people for their problems."

8. "The therapist is far from being perfect herself; so how can I expect her to help me?"

9. "If I want to pay for a friend who thinks I'm OK, I'll buy a dog."

10. I don't need anyone's help; I can solve my own problems."

11. "The last thing I need is to become dependent on some shrink and addicted to their drugs."

12. "I'm not turning control of my life over to anyone."

---

compulsive personality disorder to resist seeking professional help for their condition.

The Treatment of Karl Adler

Prioritizing the Elements of Care

At the time he began treatment, Karl Adler was barely functioning, a state that contrasted sharply with his previous, almost frenetic level of activity and high achievement. He was sleeping less than 3 or 4 hours a night, was not hungry, had lost almost 25 pounds from his playing weight, and was deeply pessimistic about his future. He gave little attention to his personal hygiene and in fact had not bathed in several weeks. Mr. Adler revealed that he had little hope for the future and that he had thought many times in the past month about killing himself. He fully met DSM-IV-TR criteria for two psychiatric conditions, major depression and obsessive-compulsive personality disorder. My preliminary treatment plan was to prioritize the treatment of his major depression by the use of antidepressants, frequent visits to me for supportive psychotherapy, exercise, and proper nutrition. I did not believe that a meaningful treatment plan addressing his personality disorder could be crafted until after he had sufficiently recovered from depression to be hopeful and motivated to evaluate the full range of his therapeutic options. Therefore, not only would his capacity to *participate* in effective treatment choices be severely limited by his depression, but his ability to make informed decisions about these options would also be compromised. *A general and wise treatment principle for people with depression is to discourage them from making important life decisions until their depression has remitted.* At some point in each of his sessions during this period, I questioned him about suicidal thoughts and intentions. During the fourth week of his treatment, Mr. Adler responded to this query as follows:

> **Karl Adler:** Why shouldn't I do myself in? I'm all washed up as a ball player, and don't know how to do anything else. What's the point of hanging around being a burden to everyone?
>
> **Dr. Y.:** I believe that when your depression lifts, you will find that there will be an abundance of vocational and avocational opportunities for you to consider.
>
> **Karl:** Haven't you figured out yet that I am pretty much a one-dimensional person? I spent my whole life learning how to play basketball; I really don't know how to do anything else. I can't even do that anymore.
>
> **Dr. Y.:** That's not at all the way I perceive you, Mr. Adler. I believe that you have never taken the opportunity to understand yourself and discover the full range of your abilities and options.
>
> **Karl:** I have two questions for you, Doc. How long is all of this supposed to take; and how much do you think it's going to cost me?
>
> **Dr. Y.:** I can't answer either question right now. It depends on what you want out of treatment. But I'm glad to hear that you care about money again; it's a sign that the medications must be starting to help you.
>
> **Karl (with a smile):** Well you're right about that, I worry that I will go broke paying for my treatment. It must be the medications, because you haven't told me much I didn't already know. In my entire life, I never once imagined that I'd end up talking to a shrink.
>
> **Dr. Y.:** Well I guess we're also going to have to do some hard work on upgrading your imagination. That is really going to cost you a pretty penny.

Mr. Adler had an excellent response to the initial treatment regimen: his sleep and eating patterns returned to normal, his energy and motivation increased, and he had no further thoughts of suicide. At that point he was able to discuss and consider future treatment options.

> **Karl Adler:** You're supposed to be the expert, what do you recommend that I do now?

Dr. Y.: Since I know a bit about your life history, my principal concern is that you would jump right into another demanding, job-related activity without taking the time to understand yourself better and choose from a more diverse menu of options.

Karl: You have to remember, Doc, you are talking to a jock. Would you mind repeating what you just said in plain English?

Dr. Y.: I'm not falling for your "head fake," Mr. Adler. You are plenty smart and know just what I mean. Although you have believed that basketball has been a way of defining and proving yourself, it has also been your way of running away from your feelings and your basic conflicts.

Karl: Like what?

Dr. Y.: Like deeply rooted feelings of insecurity; dislike and distrust of most people; difficulties with intimacy; inability to relax and have fun; and problems accepting and reciprocating the love of your wife and son.

Karl: You don't pull your punches, do you? Remind me never to try another head fake on you. But back to my original question, What do you recommend that I do about all of this stuff?

Dr. Y.: I recommend that you take about a year off from work to get your life in balance. During this time, I believe you should engage actively in psychotherapy and family counseling to help understand yourself better and learn how to forge a meaningful involvement with your wife and son, which you have not done up to this point.

Karl: You got to the point, so I'll get to the point. I don't know a thing about how psychotherapy is supposed to work. I would like you to provide me some information about the various types of treatment and their rationales, so that I can know what we're talking about when I see you next time.

Dr. Y.: I will prepare a packet of information about diagnosis and treatment options for your conditions that will be ready for you to pick up by the end of the day.

Developing a Long-Range Treatment Plan for Karl Adler

Individual psychotherapies.   Karl Adler carefully read the published material on treatment options for depression and personality disorders. He understood and accepted the justifications for and scientific validations of the use of antidepressants for the treatment of his mood disorder. However, he had many questions regarding obsessive-compulsive personality disorder and its treatments.

Karl Adler: I shared the material on obsessive-compulsive personality disorder with Ellen, and she was blown away. She thinks that it all applies to me and suspects that you have been following me around with a video camera.

Dr. Y.: Like any other medical condition, the fundamental signs and symptoms fall together in recognizable patterns for most people

who have this personality disorder. That being said, the personality disorders affect each person, and their families, differently—
because each person and situation is unique. My own philosophy
is that there is no "one-size-fits all" formula when it comes to
planning treatment.

Karl: I was attracted to the cognitive-behavioral therapy approach. It
seems a more direct approach to solving problems and appears to
work faster. Ellen thinks that psychodynamically informed psychotherapy would work better for me. She thinks that all of my
problems come from my unhappy childhood and dysfunctional
family situation.

Dr. Y.: It doesn't have to be either/or. We can use both forms of therapy
as they are indicated.

Even after his major depression had resolved, I recommended to Mr.
Adler that he continue taking his antidepressant medication. Recurrences of depression are less common when people with severe forms
of this mood disorder continue taking their medication. In addition,
both he and his wife, Ellen, had noticed that since he had begun taking
the antidepressant, he was neither worrying nor ruminating so much
about minor problems.

Hoping to make rapid progress in his treatment, Mr. Adler chose a
three-times-a-week regimen of psychotherapy. An example of how *cognitive-behavioral therapy* was combined with *psychodynamically
informed psychotherapy* arose when he was deliberating about whether
or not to buy a new house.

Karl Adler: Ellen has been driving me crazy about getting a new house.
We already have a wonderful two-bedroom rented townhouse that
costs us about $1,500 a month. Not even taking into account the initial cost of a new home and what that money could be earning as
an investment, I would have to pay almost $700 a month in taxes
alone. I calculate that my costs for utilities and upkeep would add
at least another $700 a month. To me this is like burning money, because you get nothing back from these expenditures.

Dr. Y.: What is your biggest concern? Are you afraid of running out of
money if you buy a house?

Karl: I don't really know what I am afraid of. I know I won't go broke
from buying a house. I think it is just my nature not to want to
waste money.

Dr. Y.: I believe that it would be worthwhile to explore in explicit detail
what might happen to you financially if you were to buy a house.
This might help us understand better why you worry so much
abut money.

Using the techniques of *cognitive-behavioral psychotherapy,*
I asked Mr. Adler to imagine "the worst possible financial conse-

quences" associated with his buying a house for his family. After a long discussion, he came to recognize that buying a home held little risk with regard to his overall fiscal circumstances. In fact, he finally trusted me sufficiently to reveal that as a result of his many years of earning a high salary as a professional basketball player, his excellent investments, and his frugality, he was a multimillionaire. Interestingly, he also confided that Ellen had no idea of their high net worth, because he had been fearful that should she become aware of their wealth she might become less thrifty. He also came to understand that his emotional response to the implications of buying a home was at a catastrophic level, with little realistic possibility of a financial catastrophe. Although he prided himself on being a very clear thinker, Mr. Adler confused his financial concerns about home ownership with other dangerous possibilities. For example, one of his fears was that a fire could occur in the home that would injure his family and others, and that this would lead to financial disaster. On closer examination, he recognized that his liability for fire and injury in home ownership were comparable to that incurred while living in an apartment and that this concern could be reasonably addressed with insurance. He also erroneously believed that his family would be excessively endangered by fire if they lived in their own home, as opposed to living in an apartment. I asked him to confirm this supposition with valid data, but he was unable to do so. The bottom line was that through the techniques of cognitive-behavioral therapy, Mr. Adler realized that much of his worry and anxiety associated with purchasing a home was excessive or unjustified.

Through the use of a psychodynamic approach, Mr. Adler discovered that he had been emotionally neglected by his parents during his childhood and had been psychologically abused by his older brother. Although his parents did not spend much time with him and displayed little interest or involvement in his day-to-day life, they were fairly generous to him with money and gifts. Over time he began to equate money with love, self-esteem, and emotional security. As a result he became reluctant to spend his money, because his net worth was his measure of his value and self-worth. He felt inferior to those whom he believed had greater wealth than he and felt superior to those he believed had less money.

Psychotherapy and change. I continued with Mr. Adler for 18 months in the supportive psychotherapy described above under "Individual psychotherapies." He and his wife also participated in regular couple counseling. He became much more involved in the lives of Ellen and his son, became more flexible, and was able to make important decisions without excessive deliberation and anxiety. He purchased a new home, agreed to try to conceive a second child, and began to entertain novel vocational considerations. Ultimately, he decided to accept an offer to be an assistant coach for the basketball team at a local university. A lifelong student and practitioner of the science of basketball, Mr. Adler was uniquely qualified for many aspects of his new position. However, he was also, for the first time, working in complex interpersonal and social matrices with young athletes, with other coaches who were his peers, and with the high school coaches and families of the players he was trying to recruit. He also was assigned to the job of interfacing with university alumni who were avid basketball fans. Mr. Adler came to understand that his unparalleled knowledge of the fundamentals and strategies of the game was only one component of his job; the other part was motivating and working effectively with individuals and groups of people. Improving his interpersonal skills became a central goal during the third year of his psychiatric care.

In his therapy sessions, Mr. Adler would discuss specific examples from his job in which he had particular difficulties in dealing with people. We soon discovered two patterns in the types of personalities of the people with whom he was having recurrent problems. Paradoxically, Coach Adler often became angered by and impatient with players who seemed to be underachieving because of diminished or inconsistent effort, as well as with the high-achieving, arrogant, overconfident, know-it-all types. His reflexive response was to demean, intimidate, or threaten the underperforming players by saying things as, "By not making an effort, you are disappointing me and letting down the team"; or "If I don't see more effort on your part, you won't see any playing time. You know full well you are in danger of losing your scholarship." From our discussions he came to realize that a significant responsibility of being a coach in a university setting is to be an exemplary educator of those who are not achieving their potential. Coach Adler had been devoting most of his time and effort to the gifted and motivated athletes on his team. We traced his extreme reactions to underperforming players to his older brother's cruelty to him when he was very young. His brother belittled and teased him for being small and unable to compete at the level of the older boys. Karl had adapted by developing himself into a superior athlete, but he was frustrated and felt betrayed when he received little attention and credit from his brother and parents for his achievements. From his psychotherapy he came to understand that he was treating his underachieving players similarly to the ways in which he had been treated by his brother and was displacing his unexpressed anger for his family onto his most vulnerable players. This understanding helped him change not only his unsupportive and intimidating treatment of his basketball players but also his similar treatment of his son, Mitchell.

Valuable insights also emerged from our exploration of Coach Adler's extreme emotional response to arrogant athletes. In our psychotherapeutic work, we discovered that he not only intensely disliked egotistical players, but he distrusted almost all people who acted authoritatively or who were in fact authorities. The origins of these feelings were not obscure but were clearly related to his relationship with his father. Successful in business and well known and highly respected in the Indianapolis community, Karl Adler's father spent almost no time with any of his children. As a child and young adult, Karl struggled heroically, but in vain, to gain his father's attention and approval. His father rarely attended his son's important high school, college, or professional basketball games, and this included state championship games, the NCAA finals, and the NBA finals. Poignantly, Karl recalled all of his teammates hugging their parents in the exuberant celebration that followed his team's winning the NCAA championship game, while he stood by himself—without a single member of his family in attendance. Over the years Karl had motivated himself to accomplish athletic goals to defy and disprove the so-called experts and authorities who said he was too small or too slow. However, when Karl achieved his far-reaching goals, he did not derive pleasure, satisfaction, or enhanced self-esteem from his accomplishments. In his treatment he came to understand that what he really wanted was the approval and prioritization of his father, which never came despite his impressive accomplishments. Through his work in treatment, Karl gained two other important insights: 1) His unfulfilling experience with his father led him not only to resent most authority figures but also to undermine his own assumption of adult leadership roles. He became able to identify and change many types of self-defeating behavior in his job as a basketball coach in the complex and highly political university setting. 2) His lifelong belief that he had to work and perform to gain his parents' love led him to be distrustful of and unreceptive to the genuine expressions of love and intimacy from his wife and son. He worked hard to learn how to accept and reciprocate their love and to how prioritize them in his life.

Evidence-Based Treatments of People With Obsessive-Compulsive Personality Disorder

The history of medicine is replete with examples of treatments that were ultimately found not only to be ineffective but also to be danger-

ous to patients. For this reason, physicians from all specialties of medicine strive to recommend treatments that have been demonstrated by
rigorously controlled clinical trials to be both effective and safe. This approach is currently called *evidence-based medicine.* Unfortunately,
many medical disorders exist that can be painful, disabling, and disruptive to a person's personal and professional life but for which there are
no treatments that been *proven* to be effective. Nonetheless, until clinical
research uncovers new knowledge—supported by evidence—to guide
care, health care professionals must do their best to help these people,
even in the absence of substantiated treatments.

In psychiatry, we frequently use treatments that have been proved
to be effective for one type of disorder to treat people with related conditions for which there are no evidence-based therapies. An example
would be the early use of antidepressants to treat panic disorder. In the
1970s and 1980s, there were convincing data from carefully controlled
clinical research studies that antidepressants were safe and highly effective in the treatment of major depression. Donald Klein and other research psychiatrists noted an overlap in the signs and symptoms of
depression and panic disorder, and they further believed that the underlying neurobiology of the two conditions might also be related. For
these reasons and because there was at the time no proven treatment for
panic disorder, Dr. Klein and other physicians began to use antidepressants to treat patients with this extraordinarily distressing and disabling condition (Klein and Fink 1962). After the early results proved to
be encouraging, I and many other psychiatrists began prescribing antidepressants to treat our many patients with panic disorder while controlled trials of their use for this purpose were being conducted. Even
though many patients with panic disorder demonstrated dramatic responses to antidepressants, it took more than a decade for the U.S. Food
and Drug Administration (FDA) to approve antidepressants for that
purpose. Using a medication that has been approved by the FDA for
treatment of one illness to treat another condition is called *off-label* prescribing. Although it is legal, this practice must be conducted with complete disclosure to patients and with the highest levels of caution and
monitoring for safety. As a neuropsychiatrist and pharmacologist,
I commonly provide consultations to patients who either have not responded to traditional, evidence-based treatments or who have conditions for which there are no FDA-approved drug treatments.
Consequently, *most* of the patients whom I treat are taking medications
for off-label purposes.

Unfortunately, no evidence-based treatments specifically for obsessive-compulsive personality disorder currently exist. However, re-

search has proved that two types of treatments are effective for the treatment of people with OCD: medications in the antidepressant category and cognitive-behavioral psychotherapy. Accordingly, many clinicians are currently using both antidepressants and cognitive-behavioral psychotherapy to treat their patients with obsessive-compulsive personality disorder and are achieving excellent results.

Psychotherapeutic Treatments

Cognitive-behavioral therapy.   This form of psychotherapy helps the patient reformulate perceptions of being vulnerable to impending catastrophes or other sources of anxiety. The therapist frequently begins by helping the patient explore his or her thoughts and feelings immediately before, during, and after performing an action such as making a decision, or a behavior such as a compulsive ritual. Usually the patient ruminates about the repercussions—past and future—of decisions, and the clinician helps the patient explore the extremities of the consequences of his or her preoccupations. Thinking illogically and taking excessive responsibility are issues that are commonly explored. Although this form of treatment has been found by well-designed research studies to be effective in the treatment of OCD, there are no data related to its effectiveness in treating patients with obsessive-compulsive personality disorder. Nonetheless, cognitive-behavioral therapy is currently being used, with probable success, to help patients with obsessive-compulsive personality disorder.

Insight-oriented psychotherapy.   Although little scientific evidence supports this form of treatment for people with obsessive-compulsive personality disorder, psychodynamically informed psychotherapy is likely the most commonly utilized form of therapy for this condition. *The theory underlying psychodynamically informed treatment is that feelings that are not perceived or acknowledged by the patient will take the form of symptoms, and that the access by the patient to his or her feelings will reduce the symptomatology of the personality disorder.* Freud's observations and writings form the theoretical basis of this form of treatment, with special attention being placed on the patient's transference to the therapist and on the defense mechanisms of the patient. Common defense mechanisms of patients with this condition include *isolation of affect,* in which feelings are separated or removed from troubling thoughts; *undoing,* in which a symbolic behavior is believed by the patient to remove an upsetting thought or act; *reaction formation,* in which an unacceptable thought, wish, or feeling is countered by the assumption of an opposing idea, thought, feeling, or character trait.

These defense mechanisms are more easily understood by example than by definition. An example of the defense of isolation of affect in the treatment setting would be when a patient with obsessive-compulsive personality disorder describes a disturbing event from his or her past—such as being abused or neglected by a parent—without any expression of the associated feelings of sadness or anger. In this circumstance, the therapist would encourage and support the patient in connecting with his or her feelings while describing the historical events. An example of undoing would be if a patient were to engage in certain rituals to avoid a feared event—such as never stepping on a sidewalk crack to ensure his father's safety. The therapist might view the behavior as a reaction to the patient's unconscious wishes to harm the father. In this case, the psychotherapist may help the patient connect deep-seated feelings of anger for his father with the ritualized behavior of not stepping on cracks.

Transference issues in the treatment of a patient with obsessive-compulsive personality disorder often involve the patient's attempts to overcontrol the direction of treatment and confine the interventions of the therapist. Often the clinician is experienced by the patient as being hostile, judgmental, exploitive, and vindictive. For example, the patient might unconsciously create power struggles by "forgetting" to pay bills or by making "mistakes" with appointment times to distract from and deter the therapist's efforts to help the patient gain access to repressed feelings and to have insights into the other sources and meanings of his or her symptoms. The patient might directly resist reviewing childhood events by saying, "I don't want to keep reliving the past. All that does is make me upset, and it never changes anything." As in his or her personal life, the power of "no" controls the course of events in treatment. The following encounter in my treatment of Karl Adler illustrates our work with his transference to me:

> **Karl Adler:** Why did you look at your watch? Can't you wait to get me out of here?
> **Dr. Y.:** What makes you think I want to get rid of you?
> **Karl:** That's what I hate most about the racket you are in. You guys never give anybody a straight answer. All you do is answer questions with more questions.
> **Dr. Y.:** I looked at my watch to see what time it is and how much time we have left in our session. I still don't know how you came to the conclusion that I want to get away from you. You could have just as easily concluded that I was hoping to have a lot more time to spend with you.

Karl: Give me a break, Doctor. I pay you good money for you to be in the same room with me. You and I both know that you wouldn't put up with me for a single second, if it weren't for the money.

Dr. Y.: I don't know that at all. You seem to be condemning my values and questioning my commitment to you just because I looked at my watch.

Karl: What other conclusion do you think I could draw when you stare at your watch during my session?

Dr. Y.: It is certainly not my place to tell you what to feel or conclude. I would like you to explore your feelings of being rejected and exploited by me, and where possible to indicate what I have done or not done to make you feel this way.

Karl: I'll try to do that, Doctor. However, I really don't think that you take advantage of me or even dislike me. When your own mother and father didn't seem to be interested in you, it's hard to believe that a stranger would care very much about you, either.

Ultimately, this discussion and many others like it that derived from Mr. Adler's powerful transferential feelings for me led to his gaining insights about his intense resentment for his parents as a result of their neglect of and disinterest in him. For an excellent summary of the use of psychodynamically informed psychotherapy in the treatment of patients with obsessive-compulsive personality disorder, the reader is referred to a textbook chapter by Drs. Philip K. McCullough and John T. Maltsberger (2001).

Pharmacological Treatment

As with psychotherapy for people with obsessive-compulsive personality disorder, evidence-based knowledge about the use of medications to treat this condition is derived from experience with patients with OCD. Although there are no FDA-approved medications for the treatment of patients with obsessive-compulsive personality disorder, several drugs from the antidepressant category have been demonstrated to be effective and are approved for treating people with OCD. Antidepressants with serotonergic qualities are the most commonly used. The tricyclic antidepressant clomipramine (Anafranil) was the first medication proved by valid experimental trials to be effective. Currently, antidepressants from the SSRI category, prescribed in much higher doses than for the treatment of depression, are the pharmacological treatments most commonly used for patients with OCD or obsessive-compulsive personality disorder. Although high doses of SSRIs are recommended for the treatment of the acute symptoms of OCD, much lower doses seem to be effective in maintaining remission from this condition (Mundo et al. 1997). As with other personality disorders, pharmacotherapy for major depression and generalized anxiety disorder—two conditions often present in patients with obsessive-compulsive personality disorder—is essential. Medications may also be useful in treating comorbid alcoholism and other addictive conditions that might also be diagnosed.

Fifteen-Year Follow-up of Karl Adler

Coach Adler had initially planned to remain in treatment with me for about 2 years, during which time he averaged approximately two visits a week. To his great surprise, he found psychiatric treatment interesting, enjoyable, and useful to him both personally and professionally. He decided to continue his psychotherapy beyond 2 years, and he began to approach his therapy with the same intensity and energy that he had formerly reserved solely for his basketball career. He worked assiduously to translate insights and discoveries that occurred during his treatment into meaningful changes in the way he perceived and treated others, particularly his family, the players whom he coached, and his colleagues in the university. As a result, his life changed on nearly every front. He became able to accept and reciprocate the loving feelings of Ellen and his two children. He allocated ample time to being with his family, and he learned to relax and enjoy recreational activities such as golf and to take vacations. At work he was more tolerant, nurturing, and supportive of the young athletes whom he coached. As the hard edge of his personality softened, he became more successful in transmitting to his players his incomparable technical and strategic understanding of basketball. Karl Adler became head coach and built an extraordinary record of victories and championships over the next decade. He became far better known and respected as a coach than he had been as a player. Even more important to him than the perennially high ranking of his team were the personal growth, maturity, and long-term success in life of his players. Although he became nationally recognized as a "coach's coach," he preferred to regard himself as a good teacher of young people. Summarized in Table 8–5 are key principles in the treatment of people with obsessive-compulsive personality disorder as revealed by the case of Karl Adler.

Special Issues Regarding Obsessive-Compulsive Personality Disorder

Many special situations and types of relationships are made especially difficult by people with obsessive-compulsive personality disorder. One purpose of this section is to help the reader recognize and be

TABLE 8–5. Key principles about obsessive-compulsive personality disorder as exemplified by the case of Karl Adler, part II: treatment

Historical fact	Key principle	Interpretation
Karl Adler initially resisted seeking professional help to treat his serious depression.	For people with obsessive-compulsive personality disorder, psychiatric treatment is synonymous with loss of control and admission of being imperfect.	Fears of gaining access to repressed feelings and becoming dependent on the therapist discourage people with obsessive-compulsive personality disorder from seeking or accepting care from mental health professionals.
The initial focus of Karl Adler's psychiatric care was the treatment of his depression.	People with obsessive-compulsive personality disorder are highly vulnerable to depression and anxiety disorders.	The "silver lining" of Karl Adler's depression was that it provided a gateway to the treatment of his personality disorder.
Dr. Y. recommended that Karl Adler not take on a new job for a year so that he could focus on his psychiatric care.	For many people with severe obsessive-compulsive personality disorder, work is an escape from their personal lives and themselves.	For Karl Adler, "jumping right back on the horse after he fell off" would have ensured that he would never change his personality or behavior.
Dr. Y. informed Karl Adler about the full range of his treatment options and encouraged him to participate actively in choosing the type of treatment.	Issues of trust, dependency, and control must be addressed early in the treatment of people with obsessive-compulsive personality disorder.	Effective psychotherapy involves the assumption of control (i.e., understanding self, freedom of thoughts and feelings, overcoming dysfunctional behavior) by the patient rather than turning control over to the therapist.

TABLE 8–5. Key principles about obsessive-compulsive personality disorder as exemplified by the case of Karl Adler, part II: treatment (*continued*)

Historical fact	Key principle	Interpretation
Karl Adler distrusted and resisted authority figures.	People with obsessive-compulsive personality disorder frequently engage in self-defeating, oppositional behaviors with people in positions of authority and power.	Karl Adler so hated and distrusted authorities that he would not permit himself to take on adult leadership roles, including being a devoted husband and parent.
Antidepressant treatment ameliorated Karl Adler's major depression and may have helped treat his obsessive-compulsive personality disorder.	Antidepressants have been proved to be effective in the treatment of major depression and obsessive-compulsive disorder.	Although it has not been proved, it is possible that antidepressants might be effective in the treatment of obsessive-compulsive personality disorder. At minimum, by treating comorbid depression, antidepressants enhance psychotherapeutic treatments of the condition.
Once engaged in psychotherapy, Karl Adler worked hard and made positive changes in his personal life and career.	The assets of many people with obsessive-compulsive personality disorder—high intelligence, strong work ethic, attention to details, and honesty—contribute to the process and beneficial results of psychotherapy.	The art of psychotherapy is to help patients learn to use their intellectual assets and energy to understand and improve themselves—rather than to deceive and defeat themselves.

TABLE 8–5. Key principles about obsessive-compulsive personality disorder as exemplified by the case of Karl Adler, part II: treatment *(continued)*

Historical fact	Key principle	Interpretation
Karl Adler chose to remain in treatment for many years.	Some people with severe personality disorders learn to utilize treatment as a constructive tool throughout their lives.	Spending many years in psychotherapy does not necessarily indicate a dependency on treatment or a use of therapy as a "crutch." It can mean just the opposite: a willingness to confront and solve problems with hard work.

TABLE 8–6.   Three phases of marriage to a person with obsessive-compulsive personality disorder

---

A. Idealization/courtship phase

- Recognition of spouse's admirable personal qualities, such as intelligence, honesty, ambition, hard work, and organizational skills
- Appreciation of spouse's performance orientation and vocational achievement
- Sharing of spouse's scrupulous values and lofty goals for the future

B. Self-doubt phase

- Becoming challenged and unsettled by spouse's unrealistic expectations
- Deepening anxiety and insecurity as a result of spouse's unrelenting criticism and failure to express appreciation
- Isolation and loneliness as a result of spouse's prioritization of work, accumulation of wealth, and productivity over marital and family relationships
- Diminution of self-esteem as the result of having to give in to spouse on each occasion when there is a difference of opinion
- Becoming fatigued and demoralized by spouse's endless task-driven demands and refusal to permit fun and leisure
- Deflation and depression resulting from feeling unappreciated and unloved

C. Enlightenment/disappointment phase

- Recognition that spouse will never be satisfied with himself or with her
- Realization that spouse is rigid, oppositional, controlling, and withholding
- Awareness that spouse is cold, insensitive, sadistic, and unloving
- Frustration that spouse refuses to acknowledge personal problems, try to change, or accept professional help
- Understanding and acceptance that spouse is selfish and self-centered
- Concern and fear that decision to marry spouse may have been a big mistake

---

alerted to the more common relationship problems and patterns in which people with this condition are involved.

Being Married to Someone With Obsessive-Compulsive Personality Disorder

People who are married to someone with obsessive-compulsive personality disorder often have troubled and troubling relationships with that individual. In Table 8–6, marital patterns are illustrated from the perspective of the spouse of a person with this condition.

The Boss or Business Leader With Obsessive-Compulsive Personality Disorder

People with obsessive-compulsive personality disorder create special problems at all levels in the workplace: as employees, as supervisors, and even as customers or clients. Presented in Table 8–7 are common problems associated with working for a person with obsessive-compulsive personality disorder.

A review of Table 8–7 reveals why people with obsessive-compulsive personality disorder make ineffective institutional and business leaders and poor bosses. Their indecisiveness, pessimism, inflexibility, and lack of vision hamper creative development and expansion of the company, and their controlling, sour, non-nurturing, and ungrateful nature is destructive to teamwork and employee morale.

The Customer or Client with Obsessive-Compulsive Personality Disorder

Presented in Table 8–8 is a summary of common business problems associated with customers or clients with obsessive-compulsive personality disorder.

As is apparent from Table 8–8, commercial interactions with people with obsessive-compulsive personality disorder are generally frustrating and money-losing propositions. An understanding of the characteristic features of people with this condition will help you avoid entering into a business relationship with them. Prevention is the best strategy for avoiding a circumstance in which the customer is always right—at your expense.

Pointers on How Best to Deal With People With Obsessive-Compulsive Personality Disorder

In our professional and personal lives, all of us will encounter people with obsessive-compulsive personality disorder. On occasion these encounters will develop into important relationships, and problems will invariably arise. For those who find themselves in this circumstance, Table 8–9 presents advice on dealing with people with this condition.

Afterword

Your relationship with a person with obsessive-compulsive personality disorder will be difficult and devoid of much pleasure. The person's in-

---

TABLE 8–7.   Dysfunctional personality traits of the boss with obsessive-compulsive personality disorder

---

1. **Controlling:** Does not delegate tasks and therefore is inefficient.

2. **Perfectionistic:** Sets unrealistic and unachievable goals for the organization and for employees.

3. **Inflexible:** Is reluctant to listen, accept advice, and modify plans.

4. **Indecisive:** Deliberates endlessly before making decision, then changes his or her mind.

5. **Myopic:** Focuses excessively on details. Misses the big picture.

6. **Unimaginative:** Emphasizes the quantitative at the expense of the creative.

7. **Miserly:** Hoards resources; is not generous with employees or charitable with the community.

8. **Obstinate:** Opposes the initiative of others.

9. **Retentive:** Does not share information, resources, or rewards.

10. **Inconsiderate:** Does not accept that employees have personal lives and responsibilities outside of work.

11. **Unappreciative:** Rarely give compliments; believes that the only tasks that count are those done by him or her.

12. **Critical:** Is quick to find flaws with and point out mistakes of others.

13. **Resentful:** Believes that employees are indolent and not sufficiently devoted to their work.

14. **Nongenerative:** Is a poor mentor; is uninterested in advancing the careers of employees.

15. **Self-centered:** Is unconcerned about the needs of employees and takes credit for their accomplishments.

16. **Pessimistic:** Is preoccupied with risks and catastrophic consequences; fails to consider the up side of opportunities.

17. **Unfulfilled:** Although preoccupied with goals and results, does not derive or express (to others) satisfaction when they are achieved.

18. **Unhappy:** Is uninterested in fun or pleasure for self or others.

19. **Isolated:** Does not understand a team approach; pushes others away.

20. **Ineffective:** The ultimate result for a leader with traits 1–19.

---

flexibility and obstinacy will lead you to having to choose between two negatives: either fighting all of the time to be listened to and to have some say in the relationship, or giving over your power completely to another person. Should you choose to stand up for your right to be

TABLE 8–8. Common characteristics of the customer or client with obsessive-compulsive personality disorder

1. **Time consuming:** Endlessly questions sales personnel about minute, irrelevant details of products or services to be rendered. Requires reassurance about every potential problem that might arise. Cannot make a decision to move forward on a purchase.

2. **Cheap:** Resents paying reasonable costs for items or services rendered. Argues about and is unhappy with standard prices. Expects special consideration and does not understand that the business must make a profit. Is late in paying bills.

3. **Impossible to please:** Has unrealistic expectations about products purchased or services provided. Expects perfection when perfection is not possible. Changes orders and returns products.

4. **Litigious:** Is angry and inflexible on concluding that expectations (no matter how unrealistic or unreasonable) have not been met. Will not consider compromise and is quick to bully, intimidate, and sue.

5. **Vindictive:** Believing that he or she has been taken advantage of and exploited, will take actions to harm business—such as by alarming current or potential customers and reporting "problems" to consumer protection agencies.

heard and to be a person, you will be perennially embattled. Every time that you disagree with him or her, a power struggle will ensue. Your life will become much like the brief but elegant phrase in T.S. Eliot's "Love Song of J. Alfred Prufrock": "a tedious argument of insidious intent." Should you choose the course of appeasement, you will still be criticized, devalued, and unappreciated. Ultimately you will grow tired of being around someone who is preoccupied with tedious details, endless work, hoarding of money, and aspirations to be perfect. You will wonder what happened to the spontaneity, fun, creativity, and optimism in your life. Thoughts of ending the relationship will be bittersweet, because you are also aware of his many good qualities that have been obscured, if not buried, by his personality flaws.

The case of Karl Adler demonstrates that if a person with obsessive-compulsive personality disorder is honest and willing to accept treatment, remarkable change is possible. However, if the person in your life in effect says, "Take me as I am or not at all," he qualifies as having a "fatal flaw." Your seeds of happiness and hope will not bear fruit but will be milled by him into a gray, bitter powder that will poison your future. At this point it is probably time for you to consider moving on.

TABLE 8–9. Tips for dealing with people with obsessive-compulsive personality disorder

1. **Avoid power struggles.**

   Try to avoid confrontations by being clear and quantitative about expectations before engaging in any enterprise with a person with obsessive-compulsive personality disorder. Preparing explicit parameters, in writing, with quantifiable measurements—such as a detailed, task-specific job description—will help avoid misunderstandings and disputes in the long run. Otherwise their rigidity, inflexibility, and obstinacy will transform disagreements into battles and conflicts into wars. Compromise for people with this condition is not an option, because it will be mistaken by them for loss of control and experienced as defeat.

2. **Lower your emotional expectations.**

   People with obsessive-compulsive personality disorder do not tend to be empathic, appreciative, or loving. They can be as retentive with affection as they are with money. Do not expect reciprocity for your emotional investment, or you will be perennially disappointed with the dividends.

3. **Define and grade yourself.**

   People with obsessive-compulsive personality disorder tend to overvalue their own assets and abilities—often involving details, quantification, and organization—and undervalue the contributions of others including creativity, vision, and interpersonal skills. They will expect you to be perfect and to anticipate and meet all of their needs. When you are found to be imperfect and unable to anticipate or fulfill all of their needs and expectations of you, you will be criticized, chastised, and devalued. Do not be lured into a relationship or situation in which your self-esteem, self-worth, and self-definition are based on the unrealistic expectations of another person.

4. **Do not become parent or therapist.**

   In a prolonged relationship with a person with obsessive-compulsive personality disorder, you may perceive that many of their problems stem from trauma and unmet needs from childhood caregivers. Be careful about assuming the "reparative role" of a nurturing parent or psychotherapist. You will be resented for not being able to "fill the hole" and for the person's feeling dependent on and infantilized by you. Rather, encourage the person to seek psychotherapy from an experienced clinician who can help him or her deal with and learn from the powerful transferential feelings that are indelibly connected with insight, dependency, and meaningful change.

References and Suggested Readings

American Psychiatric Association: Diagnostic and Statistical Manual of Mental Disorders, 4th Edition, Text Revision (DSM-IV-TR). Washington, DC, American Psychiatric Association, 2000

Andrews G, Stewart G, Allen R, et al: The genetics of six neurotic disorders: a twin study. J Affect Disord 19:23–29, 1990

Bejerot S, Ekselius L, von Konorring L: Comorbidity between obsessive-compulsive disorder (OCD) and personality disorders. Acta Psychiatr Scand 97:398–402, 1998

Carey G, Gottesman II: Twin and family studies of anxiety, phobic, and obsessive disorders, in Anxiety: New Research and Changing Concepts, edited by Klein DF, Rabkin J. New York, Raven, 1981, pp 117–136

Fitzgerald KD, MacMaster FP, Paulson LD, et al: Neurobiology of childhood obsessive-compulsive disorder. Child Adolesc Psychiatr Clin N Am 8:533–575, 1999

Foa EB, Kozak MJ, Goodman WK, et al: DSM-IV field trial: obsessive compulsive disorder. Am J Psychiatry 152:90–96, 1995

Freud S: Character and anal eroticism (1908), in The Standard Edition of the Complete Psychological Works of Sigmund Freud, Vol 9. Translated and edited by Strachey J. London, Hogarth Press, 1959, pp 169–175

Fyer AJ: Anxiety disorders, genetics, in Comprehensive Textbook of Psychiatry, 7th Edition. Edited by Sadock BJ, Sadock VA. Philadelphia, PA, Lippincott Williams & Wilkins, 1999, pp 1457–1464

Gabbard GO: Theories of personality and psychopathology: psychoanalysis, in Comprehensive Textbook of Psychiatry, 7th Edition. Edited by Sadock BJ, Sadock VA. Philadelphia, PA, Lippincott Williams & Wilkins, 1999, pp 563–607

Klein DF, Fink M: Psychiatric reaction patterns to imipramine. Am J Psychiatry 119:4324–4338, 1962

Marmer S: Theories of the mind and psychopathology, in American Psychiatric Publishing Textbook of Clinical Psychiatry, 4th Edition. Edited by Hales RE, Yudofsky SC. Washington, DC, American Psychiatric Publishing, 2003, pp 107–152

McCullough MD, Maltsberger JT: Obsessive-compulsive personality disorder, in Treatments of Psychiatric Disorders, 3rd Edition. Edited by Gabbard GO. Washington, DC, American Psychiatric Publishing, 2001, pp 2341–2351

Mundo E, Bareggi SR, Pirola R, et al: Long-term pharmacotherapy of obsessive-compulsive disorder: a double-blind controlled study. J Clin Psychopharmacol 17:4–10, 1997

Nestadt G, Samuels J, Riddle M, et al: A family study of obsessive-compulsive disorder. Arch Gen Psychiatry 57:358–363, 2000

Rauch SL, Baxter LR: Neuroimaging in obsessive-compulsive and related disorders, in Obsessive-Compulsive Disorders: Practical Management, 3rd Edition. Edited by Jenike MA, Baer L, Minichiello WE. St. Louis, CV Mosby, 1998, pp 289–316

Regier DA, Boyd JH, Burke JD Jr, et al: One-month prevalence of mental disorders in the United States, based on five Epidemiologic Catchment Area sites. Arch Gen Psychiatry 45:977–986, 1988

Russell A, Cortese B, Lorch E, et al: Localized functional neurochemical marker abnormalities in dorsolateral prefrontal cortex in pediatric obsessive-compulsive disorder. J Child Adolesc Psychopharmacol 13 (suppl 1):S31–S38, 2003

Stein DJ, Hugo FJ: Neuropsychiatric aspects of anxiety disorders, in American Psychiatric Publishing Textbook of Neuropsychiatry and Clinical Neurosciences, 4th Edition. Edited by Yudofsky SC, Hales RE. Washington, DC, American Psychiatric Publishing, 2003, pp 1049–1068

Weissman MM, Bland RC, Canino GJ, et al: The cross national epidemiology of obsessive-compulsive disorder: the Cross National Collaborative Group. J Clin Psychiatry 55 (suppl):5–10, 1994

Chapter

9

PARANOID PERSONALITY DISORDER

> Yond Cassius hath a lean and hungry look;
> He thinks too much: such men are dangerous.
>
> —William Shakespeare, *Julius Caesar*

Essence

Out of the blue he tells you, "I know what's been going on between you and my wife. If the two of you think you're going to get away with it, you both are sadly mistaken. I'm not the fool that you think I am." For an instant, you are not sure whether or not he is playing some type of joke on you. His angry stare vaporizes any doubt that you may have entertained about his seriousness. Frantically, you dredge your memory for exactly what you may have said or done that could have led to his disturbing conclusion. You cannot think of anything specific, other than the fact that his wife is physically attractive and has a pleasing personality. Grudgingly, you admit to yourself that you have always liked her, but nothing untoward has ever occurred between the two of you. You now feel uneasy and vulnerable just because you like her and find her pretty. You manage to stammer, "I really don't know what you're talking about." This response enrages him further. He replies, "I won't stoop down to your disgraceful level by telling you what you already know. I already told you not to play me for a sucker. Don't underestimate me, either. Stay away from my wife, or the next time we meet won't be very pretty." With that, he turns abruptly and walks away. Bewildered and profoundly upset, you consider telling your wife about this interchange, but you decide to let it go and hope that it goes away.

It does not go away. A week later, he sends you a certified letter demanding that you relinquish your family membership in the health and fitness club where he and his wife are also members. You ask one of your attorney friends what you should do. He says, "Don't do a damn thing, he's nuts. Leave him alone and he'll go away." He does not go away. You come home one evening to find your wife looking pale and distraught. When you ask her what is bothering her, she says, "Nothing." Finally you pry out of her the reason that she is distressed. He had called her and asked her, "Did you know that your husband is having an involvement with my wife?" You spend several days trying to reassure your wife, but find yourself skating on thin ice. She points out, "You never told me before that you found her attractive. Is that why you decided not to tell me that her husband confronted you? What else aren't you telling me about?" Afterward, you try to gain some perspective. You ask yourself how you got into this mess in the first place. And where is it going to lead? Sadly, this is just the beginning.

The Case of Wilma Warren

Help From Professor Edith Brooke

For very good reason, Edith Brooke is one of the most admired women in America. Having spent almost her entire career on the faculty of a northeastern university with the highest academic standards, she has made fundamental discoveries in genetics. Hardworking, innovative, productive, constructive, collegial, and affable, Professor Brooke is beloved both by her students and by fellow faculty members. She was the first woman to become the chairperson of a major science department at her university, and she proved to be as fine a leader as she is a scientist. She recruited outstanding faculty members to her department, which soon became acknowledged as among the best in the nation. Professor Brooke took justifiable pride in how well her faculty collaborated with one other and with other scientists in the university and around the world. Competing with her stellar accomplishments as a research scientist is her gift for mentoring both graduate students and faculty members. She takes a personal and abiding interest in advancing the careers of all those under her charge, and she worries about them and works with them to help them resolve the personal and professional issues that might impede their academic progress. Not surprisingly, Professor Brooke became a role model for female graduate students and young women on the faculty, both in the science and the humanities divisions. One such faculty member was Wilma Warren, Ph.D., who was a 27-year-old instructor in the physics department when she first called on Professor Brooke. Their initial conversation went as follows:

> **Dr. Warren:** Thank you for agreeing to see me. I know how busy you are. I will be brief.
>
> **Professor Brooke:** It is my privilege to meet with you, and there is no need whatsoever to rush. Take as much time as you need. Invariably, I learn far more from my meetings with bright young faculty members such as you than I could ever impart to them.
>
> **Dr. Warren:** I have come to ask if you will be an informal advisor to me regarding my career. As you know, there are very few women in the physics department, and, quite frankly, they have had less than stellar careers. I truly need a mentor who is a woman.
>
> **Professor Brooke:** I don't believe I would describe Elizabeth Koster's career as "less than stellar." She is a full professor, with tenure. More important, she is an excellent teacher. For years her survey course in physics has been among the most popular and highly rated in the undergraduate school. Her textbook is used in universities throughout the world. She also has a fine record as faculty advisor to graduate students.
>
> **Dr. Warren:** I don't disagree. However, I have aspirations in research, an area in which Elizabeth has not excelled. I am a single parent with a young daughter. I need your advice about how to balance my family life with an academic career. You are the university's most successful female scientist, and I know that from time to time I will need your help related to my career. If you're too busy, I will of course understand.
>
> **Professor Brooke:** I confess that I don't know much about physics, but I do know how to write a grant proposal. First, let me speak with Lester, your chairman, to see if it is OK with him. If he supports my involvement, I will be pleased to serve as one of your advisors.
>
> **Dr. Warren:** I already asked Lester if I could approach you, and he approved.
>
> **Professor Brooke:** Nonetheless, I would like to run this by him, just to make sure we are all on the same page. I'll get back to you by the end of this week.

As she had promised, Professor Brooke spoke that week with Lester Ballard, Ph.D., chairperson of the department of physics.

> **Professor Brooke:** I believe you know, Lester, that Dr. Wilma Warren from your department has approached me to be one of her advisors.
>
> **Professor Ballard:** She told me that she was going to ask to meet with you. What do you think of her, Edith?
>
> **Professor Brooke:** I only met with her for a couple of minutes. She seems quite serious about having a productive research career in physics.

Professor Ballard: Without question, Wilma is one of the brightest
graduate students who has come through our program in the last
several years. She wrote a wonderful doctoral thesis, a mathematical refutation of string theory, that received a great deal of favorable attention. She was recruited heavily by some very good
departments, but she ultimately decided to accept our offer to
stay here. On the other hand, I fear that she is a bit rough around
the edges.

Professor Brooke: What exactly do you mean by "rough around the
edges"?

Professor Ballard: First, the good news. She is adored by many of the
most senior people in our department and at other physics departments around the country. They find her knowledge about
their work and ideas most captivating. Others, however, find her
to be a bit prickly. She does not have much patience for people
who are less intelligent than she, including some of the college
students in her study section when she was a teaching assistant.
She also seems to have a problem with other bright women. In
fact, she is not on speaking terms with the other brilliant female
faculty member in the department who is at her level. That is too
bad, because it makes it quite tense in the laboratory. Come to
think of it, Edith, she really could use your help in learning how
to get along with people.

Professor Brooke: With your permission, Lester, I will work with
Wilma. As you know, we never seem to have enough women scientists in the university, particularly at the higher ranks. I think
that if we support women at the earliest stages of their careers, it
should prepare them for the difficult and somewhat elusive requirements for advancement in our system. I will try to do just
that with Wilma Warren.

Professor Brooke took Wilma Warren under her wing. She scheduled biweekly meetings with her to review and help advance her scientific work. She introduced her to important colleagues within the
university and in the wider academic community and recommended
her for positions on key committees. Professor Brooke encouraged Dr.
Warren's first grant application to the National Science Foundation,
spent innumerable hours helping her write and rewrite the grant, and
agreed to serve as the senior scientific advisor on the project. When the
proposal was funded, a highly unusual feat for a first-time submission
from a young scientist, they both celebrated. On numerous occasions,
Professor Brooke attended Dr. Warren's presentations at scientific meetings—quite a sacrifice, given the time involved and the fact that physics
was not her primary area of interest. Under Professor Brooke's tutelage,
Wilma Warren's career flourished, and she reveled in the role of a bright
and rising star in science. Soon Dr. Warren was proposed for advance-

ment from instructor to assistant professor, and she was awarded this rank without qualification by the university's notoriously stringent promotions committee. At Dr. Warren's next meeting with Professor Brooke, the following exchange took place:

> **Dr. Warren:** I am so thrilled that I am now a professor. Words cannot express my thanks for your mentorship and help. I could have never gotten so far so fast without your help.
>
> **Professor Brooke:** Let's not get carried away with self-congratulation. The next phase is the most difficult. According to university rules, you now have a maximum of 7 years to move on to associate professor, which is a tenured rank. The standards are much higher for this promotion, and this is where most people fall down. You know very well, Wilma, that we have an "up or out" policy, which means that if you are not promoted to the next stage you must leave the university. Let's get going; there is not a moment to waste.
>
> **Dr. Warren:** Given that I have 7 years, I think we at least have time for a celebratory lunch.

Things Turn Sour

Over the next 5 years, Professor Brooke continued to support Dr. Warren, who became increasingly involved in university committees and in national associations of physicists. Dr. Warren was particularly adept at developing special relationships with academics in positions of leadership and responsibility. During one of their meetings, Professor Brooke expressed concern to Dr. Warren that her research and academic productivity were being compromised by her many trips and "important relationships."

> **Professor Brooke:** Wilma, I am worried that you are getting behind on your academic timetable. You have only 2 more years until your tenure review, and that is not a lot of time.
>
> **Dr. Warren:** I don't believe you are saying this to me. You know very well that no one works harder and longer hours than I do.
>
> **Professor Brooke:** The tenure and promotions committees don't count hours or care about time sheets. What count to them are results. It is very simple: the number of papers in excellent, peer-reviewed journals of which you are first author, the quality and national impact of these papers, and your success in research funding is how they keep score. And from what I can tell, Wilma, we are not doing so well by these standards. You haven't submitted an application for renewal of your first and only grant, and you have published only three papers. You should be publishing at least three papers per year. I fear all of your other activities and commitments are distracting you.

Dr. Warren (with intense rage): Edith, you have really overstepped your bounds this time. I am truly offended. Who gave you permission to investigate my private files to check on how many papers I have published?

Professor Brooke: We've been meeting for over 5 years. I don't need to check up on you to know about your grants and publication. They are also public records instantly available to anyone on the Internet from a search engine. Let's not wait until it is too late to catch up with the basic requirements for academic advancement. I apologize for seeming to be frantic, but Wilma, I am only trying to help you.

Dr. Warren: Are you now telling me that you have gone behind my back to check up on me? Did you ever think of asking me to my face about my grants and papers? And that you of all people should attack me for going to scientific symposia and being on important committees in the university. You know everybody and seem to be on all the university's important committees.

Professor Brooke: First things first, Wilma. The core of your career must be your academic productivity, which in your case means research, publishing, and teaching. Going to committee meetings and getting to know famous people are secondary and for much later in your career. I had three large research grants when I was an assistant professor, and these were my priority. The rest are just decorations on the cake.

Dr. Warren: What I want to know right now is whether you have had this discussion with anyone in my department. Have you said anything to Lester?

Professor Brooke: No, I haven't. But as a serious scientist and an experienced department chairman, he certainly would understand the problem and share my concerns.

Dr. Warren: Don't be so sure. All the feedback that I have been getting about my career from distinguished faculty in physics, both in our university and around the country, is quite different from your accusations. Perhaps you are handicapped by not knowing a thing about our field. Now, if you have finished berating me, I'd like to leave.

Professor Brooke was left feeling confused, frustrated, and shaken. In her entire experience as a university professor, she could not recall an interaction of such bitterness with another faculty member. Believing it to be her responsibility to inform Professor Ballard of her concerns about Dr. Warren's academic progress, she telephoned him that day.

Professor Brooke: I just had a rather unsettling meeting with Wilma Warren. As you know and have approved, I have served as a mentor and faculty advisor to her for the past 5 years. Today when we met, I shared with her my concerns about her academic progress to date, and she did not take it very well at all.

Professor Ballard: If you're referring to the fact that she has only one entry-level grant and virtually no first-author publications, I told her 2 years ago that she was far behind schedule for her tenure.

Professor Brooke: How did she take your critique?

Professor Ballard: Not well at all. In fact, she was quite defensive, and offensive. She said that the physics department—meaning me, of course—had let her down by not making clear to her the criteria for academic progression or by adequately supporting her work. I told her that was hogwash. Every graduate student knows that you need grants and papers to be promoted to a tenured professor at this and other rigorous universities. The specific requirements are also on the dean's Web site. I also told her that she was living in a fool's paradise if she thought that she would be awarded tenure just because she was smart and had impressed a lot of important people. I told her that our tenure and promotions committee is product based. No product, no tenure.

Professor Brooke: I'm afraid that she is not listening to either of us.

Professor Ballard: I can assure you that she's not listening to me, because she hardly talks to me anymore. When she does need to speak with me, her tone is suspicious, angry, and sarcastic.

Several days later, Professor Brooke received the following e-mail from Dr. Warren.

I am putting you on notice that your meeting with me last week constituted harassment. I also have learned from undisclosed sources that you did not heed my admonition that you not speak with my chairman, Professor Ballard. I have solid information that you have poisoned his mind about my abilities and my work. This constitutes slander. It goes without saying that I hereby cancel all future scheduled meetings with you, and ask that you not call me or contact me in any way. I also prohibit you from further violating my rights to confidentiality by discussing my work or me with anyone. You have already seriously taken advantage of me and damaged my career.

Professor Brooke immediately called the university's director of risk management. The risk manager, an attorney, advised Professor Brooke to make a file note of her recollections of her most recent discussion with Dr. Warren and include any other pertinent information from previous meetings. Although he stated that he did not see any justification for a formal complaint, Professor Brooke was not reassured. She understood full well that facts might not carry the day in this situation. Over the next year she had no contact whatsoever with Dr. Warren.

An Offer That Professor Brooke Could Not Refuse

A year later, Professor Brooke was summoned to meet with Mr. Clyde Foster, the chairman of the board of trustees of the university.

Mr. Foster: Edith, I want to ask you for a favor. As you know, President Butler is retiring after an illustrious career leading our university. We have established a search committee to identify a new president. This committee of faculty and board members is advisory to me, as I am authorized by the board of trustees and by policy of the university to make the ultimate decision. The search committee has sent out letters to academicians around the country for recommendations of candidates. Guess what? Your name leads the list by a good margin of those most frequently and highly recommended—both from inside and outside our campus. Everyone seems to be telling us that the best choice is right under our noses: you. We have also gotten numerous responses from "outside" informing us that they have tried, to no avail, to lure you to become president of their universities. You never told us about these solicitations, Edith.

Professor Brooke: Clyde, I never spoke about these offers because I never took any of them seriously. I'm very happy here. I don't want to leave our university, and I wouldn't give up my research to do anything else. I've always said that I have the perfect job.

Mr. Foster: Which brings us to the very reason that I asked you to come see me today. The search committee would like to invite you to be considered one of the candidates for president of the university. The committee understands that you are committed to your research and teaching, and those are the very values that we most respect and that make you such a strong candidate. You embody the mission and ideals of our university.

Professor Brooke: Being president of this university is a full-time commitment for even the most capable administrator and leader. Being a committed scientist and teacher is also a full-time vocation.

Mr. Foster: Clearly there would have to be some "give and take." But we are getting way ahead of ourselves. All that I am asking is that you consider becoming a candidate for the position.

Professor Brooke: I will do exactly as you have asked—consider this very flattering request. Please understand in advance that I don't believe that I am at all qualified for this position. I'll call you tomorrow with my decision.

Mr. Foster: Edith, I ask that you think about this for a bit longer than a day. Why don't you get back to me in a week?

Professor Brooke left Mr. Foster's office with the certainty that she would decline this offer. Over the course of the next week, however, she received calls from nearly every member of the search committee encouraging her to accept the offer to be a candidate. A modest person, Professor Brooke was both surprised and moved by their arguments about her suitability for the role and by the deep reservoir of good feelings toward her. In addition to pointing to her superior intelligence, high energy, stellar reputation as a scientist, and distinguished record of service to the university, they all emphasized her values, integrity, and

collegiality as credentials for the position. Professor Brooke was particularly taken by the expressions of strong support from the committee
members from the university's humanities departments, and she began
to realize that the position would offer her opportunities to learn about
new fields of knowledge and to grow. The next week she called Mr. Foster to accept his offer to be a candidate for the presidency of the university.

The Accusation

Although the activities of the search committee for the university president were supposed to be conducted in strict confidence, it was not
long before word got out among the faculty that Professor Edith Brooke
was among the top candidates for the position. The consensus of the
faculty was that the university would be fortunate and well served if it
could manage to lure Professor Brooke away from her laboratory to become their president. The search committee was far down the road to
making just that recommendation to Mr. Foster when the chairperson
of the search committee, Professor Anita Weiss, received the following
note:

> Dear Professor Weiss,
> I have been asked to represent and convey the conviction shared by
> many faculty that Edith Brooke is unfit to serve as president of the uni-
> versity. I formally request a private and confidential meeting with you
> to present facts that you must know and consider prior to making a final
> determination.
>
> Yours truly,
> Wilma Warren, Ph.D.
> Assistant Professor
> Department of Physical Sciences

Many aspects of this note troubled Professor Weiss. First and foremost, the letter was vague regarding the nature of her charges and who
else among the faculty shared this concern. Nonetheless, Professor
Weiss called Mr. Foster about the communication, and he said: "It
doesn't seem very likely that this young faculty member will tell us
much about an esteemed professor who has been in the university for
nearly 25 years, but we should give her a hearing anyway. She will be
the first person to say something negative about Edith during this entire
process." Professor Weiss scheduled the meeting for later that day:

Professor Weiss: I received your letter 2 days ago, and I am very inter-
    ested in hearing what you have to say.

Dr. Warren: First of all, I want you to know that I am acting solely in the best interest of the university. I have nothing to gain and everything to lose by this meeting. Do I have your assurance that everything that I say will be held in complete confidence?

Professor Weiss: You certainly do not have that assurance. I have no idea what you will or will not say. If what you disclose is sufficiently relevant to the deliberations of the members of the search committee, I am obliged to share that information with them.

Dr. Warren: I understand, but I would hope that you would leave my name out of that discussion. You will understand that it could lead to retribution.

Professor Weiss: Let me be very clear. I make no promises to you whatsoever regarding what you are going to tell me. It is you who contacted me, and if you have something that you want to say about Professor Brooke, let's hear it.

Dr. Warren: I did not come here to engage in an adversarial dialogue with you. I just want to be of help to your committee and my university. Please understand that this is very difficult for me. First let me ask you this question: are you aware of Edith's sexual preference?

Professor Weiss: I have no knowledge of or interest in Professor Brooke's private life. If that's what you want to divulge, we have nothing to discuss.

Dr. Warren: It is my understanding that when a senior faculty member abuses her power and influence to take advantage of a junior faculty member, that is a matter worthy of discussion. Edith Brooke sought me out under the pretense of helping to advance my career in science. Rather than helping me, she came on to me sexually at every opportunity. When I refused to acknowledge her advances, she turned on me, threatened me, and tried to get me to leave the university.

Professor Weiss: How did she threaten you?

Dr. Warren: She told me directly that she would oppose my tenure application. She also called my chairman, Professor Ballard, and tried to influence him against me. This was exceedingly vicious, because I had confided in her that my relationship with Professor Ballard was already strained. I have also been told, in confidence, that she tried to undermine my reputation nationally.

Professor Weiss: Have you filed a formal grievance against Professor Brooke?

Dr. Warren: Not yet, but I am now strongly considering it. Now that Edith seems to be a serious candidate for the presidency of the university, I believe it is my duty to step forward. My fear that she will continue to sabotage my career must now be set aside for the good of the university.

Professor Weiss: As you know, Dr. Warren, there are always two sides to every story. Without your having filed a formal complaint to the university grievance committee, I don't feel comfortable bringing your allegations before the search committee. You must recognize that they are completely unsubstantiated.

Dr. Warren: Since you seem to be encouraging me to file a formal complaint against Edith, I will consider that option and get back to you.

Professor Weiss: You misunderstand me. I am not encouraging you to do anything of the sort. I only indicated to you that I would not bring unsubstantiated charges before our search committee. It is not the role of this committee to adjudicate the veracity of such allegations.

Dr. Warren: I must confess that I'm not surprised that you would stand up for Edith in this fashion. In fact, others warned me that the tenured professors and other interest groups and insiders would close ranks to protect one of their own. I now feel very vulnerable just because I tried to do the right thing.

Professor Weiss: I really don't follow what you are talking about. However, I believe that I have made my point clear to you and do not see any reason for me to take this one step further at this time. I will report to Mr. Foster and the search committee that you have made an unsubstantiated claim against Professor Brooke, and that until such time as this claim is formally substantiated, I will not discuss it or its nature with anyone, including Professor Brooke.

Several days later, President Butler called Professor Brooke to his office and told her that Dr. Warren had filed a formal grievance against her. President Butler explained that she had been charged with sexual harassment and unfair and retaliatory practices against a junior faculty member.

President Butler: I don't have to tell you, Edith, about the seriousness and potential implications of these charges. I have appointed an ad hoc committee of the faculty to look in depth into the matter. Professor Marshall King, an ethicist, will chair the committee.

Professor Brooke: Richard, I am shocked by these allegations. I can assure you right now that they have no factual basis. Wilma Warren must be emotionally unstable.

President Butler: Perhaps so, Edith. But let me give you one piece of advice. You now must respond to a formal complaint and be involved in an investigation. Please be careful not to complicate matters by being careless in what you say, such as accusing Dr. Warren of having an emotional problem. My second piece of advice is for you to obtain legal counsel to help you prepare for this investigation and to see that all of your rights are being protected.

Professor Brooke could not help but note an unusual degree of formality and pique in her colleague and friend of many years. Her state of shock and disbelief was rapidly changing into one of fear and anger.

Professor Brooke: How do you think this will affect my candidacy for the presidency of the university?

President Butler: I have spoken today with both Professor Weiss and Mr. Foster. We have all agreed that it is best for the university and all concerned to place your candidacy on hold until such time as these allegations are resolved. Should the ad hoc committee determine that Dr. Warren's allegations against you are unfounded and should the search committee not have recommended another candidate to Mr. Foster by that time, your candidacy will be reinstated.

Professor Brooke: In other words, with regard to my personal and professional reputation and my career, I am considered guilty until proven innocent.

President Butler: I have asked the ad hoc committee to move rapidly with its fact finding, interviews, and recommendations. No one other than those on the two committees involved needs to be made aware of your situation.

Professor Brooke: Finally, Richard, we have found some common ground. No faculty member needs to be told that I am "under indictment" and that my consideration for your job has been put on hold for this reason, because they probably already know. As you know, faculty committees at any university—including ours—have less than a 100% record for maintaining confidentiality; and do you not believe that Dr. Warren is spreading the word as we speak? This has all the potential to turn into a witch hunt.

About Edith Brooke

Her First Sexual Experience

At the time of this conversation with President Butler, Edith Brooke was 52 years old. An only child, she had been born to formal, stiff, and distracted parents. Both had serious health problems. Her father died from early-onset Parkinson's disease when Edith was 7, and her mother became ill with terminal breast cancer when Edith was a teenager. Edith had come to the university when she was 17 and felt that she had found a home for the first time in her life. Other than her 4 years as a graduate student in cellular biology at Cambridge University in England, she had spent her entire adult life in this university. Immersed in studies, she had based her personal relationships on academics and scholarship, not sexuality. Although she was aware as a teenager that she was attracted to females, Edith did not understand the implications of these feelings until many years afterward. In the era in which she attended college, homosexual relationships were rarely expressed in the open. Even in academic settings, acceptance and trust of people with homosexual orientation was inconsistent. Edith had her first sexual encounter when she was 22, while pursuing her postgraduate degree at Cambridge. For more than 2 years she engaged in an intense sexual and emotional relationship with one her professors, who was married and had two young children. Eventually the husband of her lover learned of the affair and issued an ultimatum to his wife: either break off the affair or get a divorce. For months, Edith's lover contemplated moving to the United States to live with Edith, but she ultimately decided, largely because of her children, to remain in England with her husband.

The Aftermath of Her First Sexual Experience

Edith was not prepared for the psychological repercussions of breaking off the 2-year relationship with her lover and leaving England. Her intense grief reaction developed into clinical depression of paralytic proportions. Even worse than her sadness, loneliness, and unbearable longing for her former lover was her sense of emptiness and self-loathing. She felt hopeless and seriously contemplated suicide. On her return to the university as an assistant professor, she was unable to concentrate on her work and avoided interactions with her colleagues. The chairman of her department recognized the profound change in Edith and referred her to me for psychiatric evaluation. Edith Brooke was 25 years old at the time of our initial meeting.

> **Professor Brooke:** Thank you for agreeing to see me, Doctor, but I don't think you can help me. The truth is that I don't want to be helped, or deserve to be helped.
>
> **Dr. Y.:** Perhaps we can start by your telling me why you don't want to be helped.
>
> **Professor Brooke:** There is only one thing in this world that would make me want to go on living, and that is not going to happen. There is really no point in my discussing this, as it only makes me hurt worse to talk about it. And there is nothing that you or anybody else can do.
>
> **Dr. Y.:** Have you lost someone very important to you? If so, it can help to talk with another person about this loss.
>
> **Professor Brooke:** Even though it doesn't change anything?
>
> **Dr. Y.:** Even though the ultimate outcome of the relationship might not change, how you feel about the loss can change. You can change.
>
> **Professor Brooke:** I confess that I don't believe you, Dr. Y., but I don't have many options. Either I try treatment with you, or I kill myself. I can't bear this pain much longer.

Professor Brooke agreed to meet with me three times a week for as long as she was feeling suicidal. I asked that she call me on the days that we did not have therapeutic sessions to tell me how she was feeling. I also advised that she begin taking an antidepressant medication, a recommendation that she would not accept.

Professor Brooke: As painful as my feelings are, they still belong to me. They are me! I don't want to cover up how I feel with a blanket of drugs.

Dr. Y.: You are correct, Dr. Brooke, that some drugs do cover up or deaden feelings. I don't prescribe such drugs, as they are usually addictive and make depression much worse. Antidepressants treat an underlying brain disorder called major depression, an illness that prevents you from being yourself.

Professor Brooke: You are saying that I have a "sick brain." However, for me to care enough about myself to make a rational decision about taking a medication, my brain has to be well. And it won't be well unless I take a drug. You have a very tough job, Dr. Y.

Dr. Y.: I am happy to work with you, whether or not you decide to take a medication.

Even without taking an antidepressant, Professor Brooke gradually began to feel better. She developed a new understanding of herself and new points of view about the relationship that had ended. She came to understand that her current feelings of despair and desperation could be traced to the paucity and poverty of her personal relationships. She felt that she was drowning and that her lover had served as a life raft to her in an ocean barren of intimacies. Professor Brooke had felt desperate because she did not know how to go about developing close relationships, a skill that became a prioritized goal of her treatment. Several months into treatment, she posed the following question about her sexual orientation:

Professor Brooke: How much of my problem relates to my sexual orientation?

Dr. Y.: You are shy and have a low level of confidence about all close relationships.

Professor Brooke: It doesn't help my confidence or self-esteem to know that many people whom I know would not like me or accept me if they were aware that I have a homosexual orientation. Wouldn't it be easier to change my sexual orientation than to change society?

Dr. Y.: I don't know very much about changing society. Do you really want to change your sexual orientation?

Professor Brooke: You picked up that I was testing you, didn't you? I just wanted to see if you thought I should try to change my sexual orientation.

Dr. Y.: Your sexual orientation is your business, not mine. If you are asking me if I accept you just the way you are, the answer is "yes." However, the only relevant question is whether or not you accept yourself.

Professor Brooke: I don't understand a whole lot about myself, Dr. Y. But there is one thing I know for sure: There is no way that I could ever change my sexual feelings for women.

Professor Brooke made steady progress in therapy, as reflected by her many successes in academic life and her increasing confidence in her personal relationships. She no longer believed that her world had ended with the breakup of her first affair. In fact, she came to accept that she had learned several valuable lessons from this experience. Most important to her, she understood that she could obtain happiness, fulfillment, and enhanced self-worth by loving another woman, feelings that were quite unlike—perhaps even superior to—her other source of self-definition and satisfaction, her academic work. A second valuable lesson was how deeply she could be hurt when an involvement ended. She vowed never again to allow herself to become involved with a woman who was unavailable, for whatever reason, to sustain an enduring relationship. Third, given the conventional standards of the time, she had decided that she would be discreet in future relationships. To Professor Brooke, being discreet meant not mixing her professional life with her personal life or discussing her personal life with her academic colleagues. These three principles guided the course of her adult life and led to many gratifying relationships, including one with Kristin Nolan.

Professor Brooke Finds a Family

At the time of Dr. Warren's accusation, Professor Brooke had for many years been in a committed and fulfilling relationship with Kristin Nolan. Unlike Edith, Kristin came from a large and involved family, to which Edith was a welcome addition. Edith and Kristin spent most religious holidays with Kristin's parents, while they were still living. Edith was closely involved with Kristin's three nieces and nephew, whom she and Kristin regarded almost as their own children. Kristin Nolan worked with her brother in the family business, a real estate development and management firm, of which Kristin was president. The firm had grown and prospered under three generations of Nolans, and Kristin was as successful in the business sphere as Edith was in the academic world. The following conversation took place after Edith told Kristin about Dr. Warren's charges against her and the university's response:

> **Kristin Nolan:** There is really no way of knowing, at this point, where this will lead.
> **Edith Brooke:** My main concern is that I don't want you to be drawn into the middle of this mess.
> **Kristin:** I don't understand this concern, Edith. I've never hidden our relationship from my friends and business associates. If they can't deal with it, I don't regard it as my problem. On the other hand, we are not open with any of your colleagues. It's like we live two

separate lives. The real question is how you are gong to respond
to the spotlight being shone on your personal life. I love you and
trust you and will support you in any direction that this leads.

Edith: Would you mind very much if I went back to see my psychiatrist
while all of this is going on? I'm feeling anxious and a bit depressed, and I don't want to get sick again. Although I haven't
seen him in many years, he knows me well.

Kristin: You also trust him. I strongly support your going back to see
him.

Professor Brooke made the appointment and spent several hours
bringing me up to date on her relationship with Kristin Nolan and the
current situation involving Dr. Warren, about whom she asked the following:

Professor Brooke: What do you think is wrong with her, psychologically?

Dr. Y.: If you are asking about her diagnosis, I can't be sure without
evaluating her in person. However, it does seem that she has paranoid traits, and that she conceivably could have paranoid personality disorder. Please understand that this is purely speculation.

Professor Brooke: Let's assume that she is paranoid, what is the best
way for me to deal with her?

Dr. Y.: If she has paranoid personality disorder, she will not be that
amenable to reason. She will have the conviction that what she believes happened is what actually occurred. There are no gray areas with people with this condition. If this is her diagnosis, there
will be no reasoning with her.

Professor Brooke: If she believes her own fantasies, how do I best protect myself from her accusations?

Dr. Y.: What I am about to say might surprise you. I don't believe that
in the many years we worked together I ever gave you much direct advice, other than to take an antidepressant. And on that occasion, you didn't listen to me, and you got better anyway. Would
you mind if I now give you some direct advice?

Professor Brooke: Don't worry, Stuart. I now have sufficient confidence to reject your advice if I don't believe it is any good. Shoot
away!

Dr. Y.: I agree completely with President Butler's suggestion that you
arrange to have your own attorney to represent you in the committee hearings. I believe that the best way to protect yourself is
to hire Robert Kelly. He is a brilliant, savvy, and confident advocate. He won't be intimidated by the professors on the so-called
ad hoc committee.

Professor Brooke: I know who he is. He's a well-respected lawyer.
I seem to recall that his law partner is an alumnus of the university. I am also pretty sure that his partner is a member of the university's board of trustees. That connection might be helpful in

case academic politics rears its ugly head and things get unfair. I think you are indeed guilty of still trying to look after me, old friend.

Dr. Y.: Your personal life is about to become very public. Let's meet together a few times to explore the implications that this change might have in store for you. I believe that many people's minds have changed since we first worked together many years ago. Perhaps the silver lining in this dreadful cloud could be a reconsideration of your decision to conceal your personal life from your many close friends at work.

Dr. Warren Meets With the Ad Hoc Committee

Dr. Warren met first with the committee and presented a 30-page timeline of her relationship with Edith Brooke. In this document she detailed events and conversations between the two parties and gave her interpretation of how Professor Brooke had established the relationship for the purpose of entering a sexual liaison with her. She also offered printouts of detailed file notes that she had made about these meetings over 5 years and a series of e-mail exchanges between her and a friend at another university. In those e-mails she wrote of her suspicions about Professor Brooke's motives toward her. Dr. Warren presented to the committee the ways in which she believed that Professor Brooke had undermined her career as a result of her rejection of the professor's sexual advances. She also provided the report of a private investigator whom she had hired to check up on Professor Brooke. The investigator had done a thorough job and gave a detailed account of Professor Brooke's relationship with Kristin Nolan. The following interchange then took place between Dr. Warren and Professor King, the chairman of the ad hoc committee that was investigating her charges against Professor Brooke.

> **Professor King:** The committee has read and discussed the materials that you have provided us. We have listened carefully to the statement that you have just made to us. Professor Brooke has asked that her counsel, Mr. Robert Kelly, be present for this meeting. He will only listen and take notes, but he is not permitted to ask questions or make comments at this time. My first question is, did any sexual activity ever take place between the two of you?
>
> **Dr. Warren:** Of course not; but only because I would not allow it to happen.
>
> **Professor King:** Did Professor Brooke ever explicitly proposition you?
>
> **Dr. Warren:** Many times.
>
> **Professor King:** Please give us an example.
>
> **Dr. Warren:** She was always trying to arrange for us to go away together to scientific meetings. She would ask if I wished to save ex-

penses by sharing a room with her. Please understand that this is a woman who, outside of the university, lives a completely gay lifestyle. If Professor Brooke were a male senior faculty member who suggested that we go on a trip together and share a room, would the committee consider that to be appropriate?

Professor King: Did Professor Brooke ever make any physical advances toward you?

Dr. Warren: Just about every time we met together. She was always trying to put her hands on my body. Often in very private places. And when I moved away from her, she would become furious and threaten me.

Professor King: Please give the committee an example of how she would threaten you.

Dr. Warren: She would tell me that I wasn't a good scientist; that I didn't have a chance to be promoted to associate professor; that there was no way that she would support me for tenure. Believe me; I could put two and two together to make four.

The ad hoc search committee questioned Dr. Warren for more than an hour. She maintained her composure and made a convincing case. She also appeared quite rational and extremely intelligent. By the end of her testimony, things did not look very good for Professor Brooke. The university recently had adopted a zero-tolerance policy for matters related to sexual abuse by faculty members. What that meant was that if the ad hoc committee found Professor Brooke guilty of sexual exploitation or sexual harassment, she would lose her job and most likely her career.

The Defense of Professor Brooke

About Wilma Warren

Attorney Robert Kelly is a professional who does his homework, and he is very tough. First he performed a thorough background check on Dr. Warren, and what he found out was very interesting. He learned that her accusation of Professor Brooke was not the first occasion when Wilma Warren had been in a hostile disagreement with professional associates. While working on her master's degree at another university, she engaged in a bitter fight with a supervisor over the authorship of a paper. She accused him of plagiarism and for taking credit for research work that she had done. The chairman of the department tried to intervene by pointing out that it was the accepted standard to include senior investigators as authors on the papers of graduate students who were working in their laboratories. Wilma Warren countered by insisting that she had done all the research work that was being reported in the paper and had written most of the paper. She threatened to write a letter to the leading journal of physics to complain of her exploitation as a graduate student should the professor's name be included on the paper. In the end, the professor relented. Highly published, funded, and tenured, he decided that it wasn't worth the time or trouble to fight just to have his name on another paper. In addition, Mr. Kelly learned that while she was a graduate student Wilma Warren also became embroiled in a dispute with several of her peers over laboratory space and access time to research equipment, a pattern that continued when she transferred to her current position in the university.

E-Mail Evidence

Because Dr. Warren had introduced information about Professor Brooke's personal life, Mr. Kelly believed it fair play to learn what he could about the personal life of Wilma Warren. He learned that she was well liked and highly respected by many people and in many spheres. For a young faculty member, she had an unusually large number of friends in high places. She used her intelligence and abundant energy to achieve leadership positions in many professional and civic organizations. There were abundant examples of her completing innovative and relevant tasks for these organizations. He also learned that Dr. Warren had engaged in many battles, and she seemed to have prevailed in all of them. From court records Mr. Kelly learned that her divorce had been unusually bitter. She accused her husband of being unfaithful to her throughout their 5 years of marriage. Although she was unable to come up with firm evidence, she also brought more serious allegations about her husband: "He is a pervert who was always touching my daughter, wanting to spy on her when she was undressed. She is not safe in his presence without supervision." Dr. Warren's husband contested that although he had never been unfaithful, his wife was perennially accusing him of having affairs with her friends and with others. He challenged the court or his wife to provide one shred of evidence of his infidelity. None was ever produced. He stated, "Living with Wilma is exactly like what I am going through at this very moment. She is always accusing me of committing some crime. I am always on the defensive. I feel that I am living on the witness stand and that she is the prosecuting attorney, judge, and jury. In our entire marriage, she has never admitted being wrong about anything. On the other hand, according to her, I am almost never right." The result of the divorce hearings was a total victory for Dr. Warren: she won sole custody of her daughter, absolute control over the visiting rights of the father, and an unusually generous award for child support and alimony.

Mr. Kelly also learned that Wilma Warren does not shy away from fights. When the flood control commission in her county wanted to run new drainage pipes through her property, she organized a massive community protest. Not only did succeed in changing the route of the drainage system, but thereafter she launched a relentless political vendetta against the county commissioner who had contested her position in the battle. Working closely with the local press and television news media, she accused the commissioner of conflicts of interest and self-dealing in the awarding of high-dollar contracts. Although none of these charges was ever substantiated, the bad press resulted in his failure to be reelected. Finally, Dr. Warren had an unusually high number of disputes over the payment of bills. On numerous occasions, she would contest the bills of contractors by stating that they had caused more damage to her house and property than the amount for which they were billing her. The result was always the same: she did not pay for the services rendered. On two occasions she had gone to court with car dealerships over having been sold a "lemon." In each case the dealership had to replace the automobile after many miles of use. Although attorney Kelly believed that he could establish that Dr. Warren had a history of contentiousness, he did not feel that this information was sufficiently relevant to the current charges to exonerate Professor Brooke. He believed that a bold step was required, and he met with Professor Brooke to obtain her permission to move forward.

> **Robert Kelly:** In Dr. Warren's testimony, she presented e-mail records in support of her case. She used the university's e-mail system for all of these correspondences. I have carefully checked the university policy regarding e-mails produced on their system, and what I found out is most interesting. The university owns this information. They have the right to read e-mails at any time that they determine it is in the best interest of the university to do so. There have been numerous precedents in which the university has inspected the e-mails of faculty members without their permission (or even their knowledge). Dr. Warren might not know that although you can burn up letters written on paper, it is almost impossible to destroy e-mails. My first question to you, Edith, is whether or not you have anything to hide in your e-mail correspondences.
>
> **Professor Brooke:** I am not sure where you are going with this, Robert. However, I use my university e-mail exclusively for academic business. I don't believe that there is anything in my e-mails that anyone else couldn't read.
>
> **Mr. Kelly:** Edith, is there anything that you have written in your e-mails about Dr. Warren that would be damaging to your defense?
>
> **Professor Brooke:** On the contrary. I believe that all my correspon-

dences to her and about her over the years would show how hard I worked to help advance her career. They will reveal how much I cared about her, in respectful and constructive ways. Also, with the exception of her last accusatory missive to me, Wilma's many e-mails to me were uniformly friendly and positive.

Mr. Kelly: I noted that all of the copies of e-mails that Dr. Warren presented to the committee had been sent in the last year. I believe that the ad hoc committee should have every e-mail correspondence in which Dr. Warren makes reference to you. This information can be dug out from the university's database, and I want your permission to move forward.

Professor Brooke: I don't know if I can go along with that. My academic colleagues would be very uncomfortable with such an intrusion. On the surface, it has the appearance of violating her privacy and academic freedom.

Mr. Kelly: I know that you are a highly principled person, Edith. However, I believe that you are now in great danger of being found guilty of this complaint from Dr. Warren. If so, your career will be over. Do not underestimate your adversary in this dispute. We need to fight fire with fire.

With the help of Kristin Nolan, Mr. Kelly finally convinced Professor Brooke to let him try to gain access to all the pertinent e-mails. When he informed the ad hoc committee of his intention, a firestorm ensued. Almost to a person, the members of the committee objected for the reasons that Professor Brooke had anticipated. The committee delegated Professor King to meet privately with Robert Kelly to try to dissuade him from taking this tack.

Professor King: I would like you to reconsider your request of the university for the e-mails of Dr. Warren. Certainly, the committee will be pleased to carefully review any and all of Professor Brooke's e-mails that she provides to us of her own free will. We would never dream of violating her rights to privacy by asking for all of her correspondences.

Mr. Kelly: As you know perfectly well, Professor, according to university policy, no faculty member using university computer systems has such rights.

Professor King: Legalistically, you are correct. However, I can assure you that what you are proposing will anger the committee and will compromise Professor Brooke's case if you persist in this direction.

Mr. Kelly: I want to be very clear with you. Dr. Warren has presented e-mails in support of her case. I have every right to ascertain whether she has presented the complete picture to the committee. Either the university provides me with this information, or this will cease to be an in-house action. Should my request be denied, I will immediately take the university to court for violation of Pro-

fessor Brooke's right to due process. It will then take me about
5 minutes to get a judge to retrieve those e-mail records, as I am
sure you know.
Professor King: Is Professor Brooke willing to air her dirty laundry
publicly?
Mr. Kelly: With all due respect, sir, Professor Brooke has no dirty laundry to air. I hope you are not referring to her personal life and personal choices. I would also like to remind you that even though
this proceeding is—for now—taking place in a university, we still
live in America. Just like any private citizen or institution, universities must abide by the laws of the land. Right now, it's the university's laundry that would appear to the public to be less fresh
than an ocean breeze. If I do not have those records in my hands
in 48 hours, I am prepared to take the university to court.

Professor King promptly spoke with the university's general counsel
about Mr. Kelly's demand. The general counsel knew Mr. Kelly well and
understood that he was not bluffing. He quickly grasped that Mr. Kelly
would prevail in a lawsuit to obtain Dr. Warren's e-mails. To prevent such
an action from getting out of hand and damaging the university, he advised Professor King to release the pertinent e-mails to both parties and
move forward with the committee's adjudications as rapidly as possible.
After consulting with President Butler, Professor King authorized the
university to release all e-mails of each party in which the name of the
other party was mentioned. A computer program accomplished this task
almost instantly, and the e-mails were made available to Professor
Brooke, Dr. Warren, and all the members of the ad hoc committee. When
Dr. Warren learned that the complete record of her e-mails concerning
Professor Brooke had been distributed, she could barely contain her rage.
At first she could not seem to comprehend the fact that the e-mails that
she had sent were not her own private property, but that of the university.
Second, she was totally caught off guard when she found out that e-mails
that she had deleted from her personal computer could be retrieved cen-
trally by the university. Third, she was furious that her counsel did not
foresee this possibility, and promptly fired her.

Robert Kelly carefully reviewed both Dr. Warren's and Professor
Brooke's e-mails. The sheer volume of communications that Dr. Warren
had produced in which Professor Brooke's name was mentioned surprised the attorney and the committee. Mr. Kelly discovered that every
one of Dr. Warren's e-mails that had been written during the first 5 years
of their professional relationship had presented the professor in a favorable light. Most of the letters were technical in nature and revealed Professor Brooke's industry in helping Dr. Warren to conceptualize and
carry out her research. Rarely was anything of a personal nature ex-

pressed, and nothing that gave any hint of a boundary violation. Mr. Kelly was also able to discover that Dr. Warren had only recently deleted these favorable e-mails from her personal computer. No other e-mails that she had written during the same period were deleted. The e-mails that were accusatory of Professor Brooke had all been written during the past year, and Dr. Warren had circulated all of these to the ad hoc committee. There were also communications that provided a window into how deliberately and carefully Dr. Warren had planned her attack against Professor Brooke. Over the Internet, she had reviewed the procedures and results of similar charges made against faculty members at other universities and had discussed her strategy with a trusted friend from a different city. It appeared to Mr. Kelly from these correspondences that Dr. Warren had modeled her charges against Professor Brooke after successful actions taken at other universities. Most disturbing was her correspondence with a member of the board of trustees of the university who was well known for his support of conservative political views. Dr. Warren had informed the trustee of Professor Brooke's sexual orientation and had raised questions to him about "her suitability as the single most visible representative of our university and principal role model for women students." In an e-mail to Dr. Warren this trustee wrote, "I had a long and pointed discussion with President Butler about Professor Brooke's lifestyle, and told him in no uncertain terms that I would vehemently oppose the board's ratification of her appointment, if it comes to that."

On the other hand, Professor Brooke's e-mails to Dr. Warren were brief, to the point, and "all business" from a person who was obviously very busy. Although her e-mails were friendly and supportive, there was not the slightest suggestion of any impropriety. Importantly, over 6 years of their relationship, on many occasions Dr. Warren had invited Professor Brooke to accompany her to out-of-town symposia. Most times Professor Brooke had politely declined because of other pressing commitments. An e-mail from Dr. Warren inviting Professor Brooke to join her at a conference in Hawaii especially caught the attention of Mr. Kelly. It had been written several months *after* many of Dr. Warren's correspondences with her friend about "Professor Brooke's coming on to me." Professor Brooke wrote back that she was unable to get away at that time, and Dr. Warren never registered for the conference in Hawaii. Mr. Kelly strongly suspected that Dr. Warren, in some way, was planning to set up Professor Brooke. Because he was not permitted to speak before the ad hoc committee, Mr. Kelly prepared a summary for the committee of the key evidence that he had gleaned and the conclusions that he had drawn from the e-mails.

Professor Brooke Meets With the Committee

Professor King: The committee has noted that you have made only a very brief response to Dr. Warren's charges, essentially saying that her allegations are unfounded. Do you have any preliminary remarks before we begin the questions?

Professor Brooke: No.

Professor King: Let me begin then. Dr. Warren maintains that your interest in her is a personal one and not a professional one. Is this true?

Professor Brooke: It was both. I admire her intelligence and hoped to help her with her science and her career.

Professor King: She has alleged that your personal interest in her was improper. Is their any truth to this?

Professor Brooke: Let's not mince words or waste valuable time, Marshall. Richard Butler has told me what Dr. Warren has accused me of, and it is entirely unfounded. I have very little to say beyond that. I have spent most of my adult life working in this university, and my record speaks for itself. I do have a question for the committee, however. Can you give me one piece of evidence in support of her allegations? If so, I'd like to hear about it. If not, I'd like to go back to my laboratory and get on with my work.

Professor King: What you are implying is that it comes down to her word against yours. Why on earth do you think Dr. Warren would make up something like this?

For the first time in the proceedings, Norma Person, a professor in the engineering school, spoke:

Professor Person: I disagree, Marshall. What it really comes down to is Professor Brooke's work against Dr. Warren's non-work! Edith is too modest and too fine a person to blow her own horn. I will do so for her. She has written over 300 scientific papers and is the author of six books. She has made genuine discoveries in her field. She has also been the primary supervisor for more than 40 Ph.D.'s, each one of whom adores her. Although Dr. Warren writes a ton of e-mails and seems to know a lot of important people, she can't seem to find the time to write grants or publish papers, much less books. In 7 months she will be up for review for advancement to associate professor with tenure. She doesn't have a legitimate shot at success, based on her non-work. As we all know, it's "up or out." If she is not approved, she has to leave the university. Her only prayer is to try to get an extension of the review, based on this trumped-up charge against Dr. Brooke. If our committee determines that Dr. Warren's grievance against Edith has merit, I can assure you that her next move will be to sue the university. Why? Because, even with an extension on her tenure review, she is too far behind to ever catch up. I think that we know enough at this point to make a decision. I, for one, don't want to waste any more of our time—or Edith's—on this farce.

Outcome

No further questions were asked of Professor Brooke after Professor Person's remarks, and Professor Brooke and Robert Kelly were excused from the meeting. After a brief discussion, the committee voted unanimously to deny Dr. Warren's grievance against Professor Brooke because of the lack of substantiating evidence. Four weeks later, the search committee recommended Edith Brooke as their sole choice for president of the university, and the board of trustees unanimously confirmed her. Her life partner, Kristin Nolan, was at her side at the inauguration ceremony and for every other important university function during her long and successful term as president.

Dr. Warren responded to the ad hoc committee's decision by filing a $10 million lawsuit against the university for a multiplicity of charges, including sexual discrimination and covering up evidence to protect Professor Brooke. No judge believed there was sufficient merit in the case to allow it to go to court. Dr. Warren quit her job prior to her tenure review. In the letter informing President Butler of her decision to leave the university, she wrote the following:

> Through painful experience, I now understand that this university is presently corrupted to serve the special interests of its few privileged full professors at the expense of its students and struggling young faculty. I refuse to submit to an academic review that I know will be biased against me and vindictive for blowing the whistle on an abusive and exploitive faculty member. I hereby submit my resignation with the understanding that I reserve the right to sue the university for damaging my reputation, my career, and my health.

Dr. Warren moved to the West Coast, where she tried unsuccessfully to obtain a position in other universities. The inevitable background checks and requests to the university for recommendations had little positive to report. One can speculate that Dr. Warren truly believes that her reputation was spoiled as the result of her own integrity in taking on a conspiratorial and corrupt academic system. Although there is no evidence that Dr. Warren ever sought treatment, had she done so, she would likely have been found to meet DSM-IV-TR criteria for paranoid personality disorder (American Psychiatric Association 2000, pp. 690–694), as summarized in Table 9–1.

TABLE 9–1.   Diagnostic criteria for paranoid personality disorder (slightly modified from DSM-IV-TR)

A. A pervasive distrust and suspiciousness of others, such that their motives are interpreted as malevolent. The disorder begins by early adulthood and presents in a variety of contexts, as indicated by four (or more) of the following:

1. Suspects, without sufficient basis, that others are exploiting, harming, or deceiving him or her.

2. Is preoccupied with unjustified doubts about the loyalty or trustworthiness of friends or associates.

3. Is reluctant to confide in others because of unwarranted fear that the information will be used maliciously against him or her.

4. Reads hidden demeaning or threatening meanings into benign remarks or events.

5. Persistently bears grudges and is unforgiving of insults, injuries, or slights.

6. Perceives attacks on his or her character or reputation that are not apparent to others and is quick to react angrily or to counterattack.

7. Has recurrent suspicions, without justification, regarding the fidelity of spouse or sexual partner.

B. The symptoms do not occur exclusively during the course of schizophrenia, a mood disorder with psychotic features, or another psychotic disorder and are not due to the direct physiological effects of a general medical condition.

Source.   Adapted from American Psychiatric Association: *Diagnostic and Statistical Manual of Mental Disorders,* 4th Edition, Text Revision. Washington, DC, American Psychiatric Association, 2000, p. 694. Used with permission.

Features of Paranoid Personality Disorder
(Slightly Modified From DSM-IV-TR, pp. 690–692)

Diagnostic Features

The essential feature of paranoid personality disorder is a pattern of pervasive distrust and suspiciousness of others such that their motives are interpreted as malevolent. This pattern begins by early adulthood and is present in a variety of contexts. Individuals with this disorder assume that other people will exploit, harm, or deceive them, even if no evidence exists to support this suspicion. They suspect on the basis of little or no evidence that others are plotting against them and may attack them suddenly at any time and without reason. They often feel that other persons have deeply and irreversibly injured them, even when there is no objective evidence for this. They are preoccupied with unjustified doubts about the loyalty or trustworthiness of their friends and associates, whose actions they minutely scrutinize for evidence of hostile intentions. Any perceived deviation from trustworthiness or loyalty serves to support their underlying assumptions. They are so amazed when a friend or associate shows loyalty that they cannot trust or believe it. If they get into trouble, they expect that friends and associates will either attack or ignore them when they are vulnerable.

People with this disorder are reluctant to confide in or become close to others because they fear that the information they share will be used against them. They often refuse to answer personal questions, saying that the information is "nobody's business." They read hidden meanings that are demeaning and threatening into benign remarks or events. For example, people with this disorder may misinterpret an honest mistake by a store clerk as a deliberate attempt to shortchange them, or they may view a casual humorous remark by a co-worker as a vicious character attack. Compliments are often misinterpreted (e.g., a compliment on a new acquisition is misinterpreted as a criticism for selfishness; a compliment on an accomplishment is misinterpreted as an attempt to coerce more and better performance). They may view an offer of help as a criticism that they are not doing well enough on their own.

People with this disorder persistently bear grudges and are unwilling to forgive the insults, injuries, or slights that they think they have received. Minor slights arouse major hostility, and the hostile feelings persist for a long time. Because they are constantly vigilant to the harmful intentions of others, they very often feel that their character or reputation has been attacked or that they have been slighted in some other way. They are quick to counterattack and react with anger to perceived insults.

Individuals with this condition may be pathologically jealous. Often, without justification, they suspect that their spouse or sexual partner is unfaithful to them. They may gather trivial and circumstantial "evidence" to support their jealous beliefs. They want to maintain complete control of intimate relationships to avoid being betrayed and may constantly question and challenge the whereabouts, actions, intentions, and fidelity of their spouse or partner.

Associated Features

It is generally difficulty to get along with people with paranoid personality disorder, and they often have problems with close relationships.

They are excessively suspicious, hostile, argumentative, and aloof. Because they are hypervigilant for potential threats, they may act in a guarded, secretive, or devious manner and appear to be "cold" and lacking in tender feelings. Although they are capable of being objective, rational, and unemotional, they more often are self-centered, stubborn, and sarcastic. Their combative and suspicious nature may elicit a hostile response in others, which then serves to confirm their expectations of being disliked and treated unfairly.

Because individuals with paranoid personality disorder do not trust others, they exhibit an excessive need to be self-sufficient and autonomous. They also need to have a high degree of control over those around them. They are often rigid, critical, and unable to collaborate with others, although they have great difficulty accepting criticism about themselves. They blame others for their own shortcomings. Because of their quickness to counterattack in response to perceived threats, they are litigious and frequently become involved in court battles. People with this personality disorder seek to confirm their preconceived negative notions of others by attributing malevolent motivations to them. These attributions constitute projections of their own feelings, especially anger and fear. They exhibit thinly veiled, grandiose fantasies; are often attuned to issues of power and rank; and tend to develop negative stereotypes of others, particularly those from population groups different from their own. Some are attracted to simplistic formulations of the world. They may be perceived by others as "fanatics" and can form tightly knit "cults" or groups of others who share their paranoid belief systems.

In response to stress, individuals with paranoid personality disorder may experience brief psychotic episodes. People with this disorder commonly have other comorbid conditions such as alcohol and other substance abuse or dependence; schizotypal, narcissistic, and borderline personality disorders are also frequently diagnosed in people with paranoid personality disorder.

About Paranoia

How It Feels to Be Paranoid

During my residency training in psychiatry at Columbia University College of Physicians and Surgeons and at the New York State Psychiatric Institute, it was my great privilege to be taught by psychoanalyst Arnold M. Cooper, M.D. In addition to his extraordinary gifts as an educator and writer, Dr. Cooper has an uncanny ability to understand and

---

TABLE 9–2. What it feels like to be paranoid

---

1. At this very moment, I feel that my life is at stake.

2. I have no time to enjoy myself, because I must be constantly alert to defend myself from imminent attack.

3. Nothing is as it seems. Everything of importance goes on underground and out of sight.

4. My enemies are entirely fraudulent. They disguise their motives, hide their intentions, cover over the true meaning of their actions, and operate in total secrecy.

5. I have many enemies, but what I hate most are my enemies who pretend to be my friends.

6. Although endangered and embattled at every front, I will not be intimidated or passive.

7. My enemies underestimate me. I am smarter than they. I will surely outsmart them.

8. It comes down to either them or me who will be destroyed.

9. I have no choice other than to fight fire with fire. I will defeat my enemies, and they deserve what they will get, and more.

10. I have to accept the fact that I am in this entirely by myself. I won't count on anyone else to help me.

Source. Adapted from Cooper 1994.

clearly describe the mental and emotional lives of his patients. As summarized in Table 9–2, Dr. Cooper's description of what people with paranoid personality disorder experience psychologically (Cooper 1994) is an essential and illuminating complement to the DSM criteria and explanations of this disorder. Presented in Table 9–3 is an outline of the key principles regarding paranoid personality disorder as exemplified by the case of Dr. Wilma Warren.

The Symptomatic Spectrum of Paranoia

Historically, paranoia connoted impaired reality testing of psychotic proportions. Early in the twentieth century all delusional disorders were termed *paranoia*; most of these conditions were later subsumed under the diagnosis of schizophrenia. Because a DSM diagnosis of paranoid personality disorder cannot be made if the patient is delusional, psychiatrist Alistair Munro (1999), an expert on paranoia and delusional disorders, argues cogently that this condition should be renamed.

TABLE 9–3. Key principles of paranoid personality disorder exemplified by the case of Dr. Wilma Warren

Historical fact	Key Principle	Interpretation
Dr. Warren initially idealized Professor Brooke.	People with paranoid personality disorder distort their positive feelings toward others.	It is possible and likely that Dr. Warren's belief that Professor Brooke came on to her was a projection of her own repressed feelings.
Dr. Warren got behind in her academic work.	People with paranoid personality disorder waste vast amounts of time ruminating about the motives of others.	The vast amount of time and effort that Dr. Warren spent on plotting and politicking was no substitute for doing real work.
Dr. Warren became furious with Professor Brooke, who pointed out to her that she was falling behind in her academic work.	People with paranoid personality disorder confuse constructive criticism and honest feedback with personal attacks.	Dr. Warren had no insight into her own role in causing the problems associated with her academic advancement.
Dr. Warren was furious with Professor Brooke for speaking with her department chairman.	People with paranoid personality disorder try to monitor and control all communications about themselves.	There is a direct connection between Dr. Warren's neglect of her work and her fury over Professor Brooke's communication with her chairman.
Dr. Warren got into disputes and power struggles with several of her academic colleagues.	People with paranoid personality disorder feel personally threatened by competent peers.	Dr. Warren expressed her competitive anger with and envy of successful colleagues by engaging in professional disputes and power struggles.

TABLE 9–3. Key principles of paranoid personality disorder exemplified by the case of Dr. Wilma Warren

Historical fact	Key Principle	Interpretation
Dr. Warren suspected her husband of infidelity.	A fundamental flaw of people with paranoid personality disorder is their inability to trust the trustworthy.	Dr. Warren destroyed her marriage through her unfounded suspicions about and relentless attempts to control her spouse.
Dr. Warren disputed and refused to pay bills for services rendered to her.	The rigidity of people with paranoid personality disorder is often patently self-serving.	By demanding perfection and always finding faults, Dr. Warren avoided her responsibility to pay her bills.
Dr. Warren circumvented her chairman to be mentored by Professor Brooke; went around the ad hoc committee to a board member; and tried to dispute the university's decision in civil court.	People with paranoid personality disorder seek to avoid responsibilities and advance their goals through alignments with powerful people and systems.	Dr. Warren became increasingly desperate in her efforts to blame others for her failure to fulfill her academic responsibilities.
Dr. Warren left the university with the belief that it had been corrupted by its senior professors.	People with paranoid personality disorder project their own feelings and motives onto others.	Dr. Warren sought to ruin the reputation and career of Professor Brooke, yet felt that others were out to get her.

I conceptualize paranoia as a symptom, not a diagnosis. Thus, paranoia would be likened to fever, as opposed to pneumococcal pneumonia. First, I define paranoia as a false belief by a person that he or she is
being unjustly persecuted or is in imminent danger of being harmed.
Second, I believe that the level of intensity of the false belief, the extent
to which the mistaken thinking preoccupies the individual, and the
types and degree of emotional and behavioral responses of the person
to the false belief should determine whether or not the paranoid thinking is of delusional (and thereby psychotic) proportions. Third, as with
most psychiatric conditions, there is a continuum of disability associated with this symptom. I view paranoid personality disorder to be at
the milder end of the spectrum and the frank psychosis associated with
paranoid schizophrenia to be at its other extreme. As depicted in the
case of Wilma Warren, people with paranoid personality disorder appear to most others as rational, can carry out job- and family-related responsibilities, and are capable of reasoning clearly in most areas that are
not affected by their paranoid concerns. On the other hand, people with
paranoid schizophrenia are characteristically tormented by terrifying
auditory hallucinations and bizarre delusions that make it impossible
for them to maintain employment or sustain almost any type of normal
personal relationship. An example of the latter would be a person who
believes that her child is the devil incarnate and hears persistent voices
that tell her to sacrifice that child.

Survival, the Human Brain, and Paranoia

My clinical experience has shown me that when the human brain is
compromised by medical or psychiatric illnesses, paranoid symptoms
often occur. I understand this phenomenon as follows. The brain is the
major organ of human survival. Specifically, the regions of the cerebral
cortex that are responsible for our abilities to use logic, to think in ab-
stractions (like using numbers), to conceive and execute plans, to use
reason, and to function in complex social groups enable us to secure
food and to protect ourselves from the dangers in our environments
and from predators. For example, it is the cerebral cortex that enhances
the survival of jungle-dwelling tribespeople by giving them the capacity to figure out and to remember which reptiles or plants are poisonous
and which are not, and to react and make decisions accordingly. In more
technologically advanced societies, it is the cerebral cortex that enables
people to collect and collate complex data that enhance human survival. For example, the human "fight-or-flight" response to sharks is innately stronger than it is to mosquitoes. This emotionally driven

response is mediated by deeper, more primitive structures of our brain, including the limbic system. However, although the shark might appear to be much more formidable and dangerous than a small, delicate insect, sharks are responsible, internationally, for fewer than 100 human deaths each year, whereas mosquitoes transmit microorganisms that lead to the deaths of millions of humans annually. Fortunately, our cerebral cortex overrides our limbic system in the service of our survival. Therefore, advanced societies devote far more time and resources to controlling mosquitoes than to combating sharks. As a consequence, countless lives are spared. If our cerebral cortex is sufficiently compromised—by head trauma, by drugs, by poisons, or by a broad range of diseases—our survival is endangered. When this occurs we respond by becoming paranoid: we are hypervigilant, overly suspicious, and excessively combative.

Among the most common medical conditions that affect the neurons in the cerebral cortex and can lead to paranoia are the following: reactions to alcohol (both intoxication and withdrawal) and other substances of abuse such as cocaine or amphetamines, medication side effects, and postoperative surgical states. Almost any central nervous system disorder can lead to paranoia and paranoid psychosis, including Alzheimer's disease, brain tumors, seizures, multiple sclerosis, and traumatic brain injury. Paranoid psychosis has long been recognized to be a sequel to traumatic brain injury. One study compared a group of 45 patients who had experienced traumatic brain injury and developed psychosis with a matched group of 45 patients with brain injury who did not become psychotic (Sachdev et al. 2001). The investigators determined that the most common form of psychosis was paranoid delusional, that there was a gradual onset, with a mean latency of the psychosis of almost 4.5 years after injury, and that the regions of the brain most commonly affected were in the left temporal and right parietal lobes. Similarly, paranoid psychosis is common in several of the most severe psychiatric illnesses, including schizophrenia, bipolar disorder, and major depression. For both neurological and psychiatric disorders, one cannot be certain whether paranoia results from the direct effects of these conditions on the brain or from the secondary effects of a person's feeling vulnerable and endangered by not being as able to assay and respond effectively to environmental conditions. Finally, it has long been recognized that paranoia can be induced in almost anyone by sensory deprivation. In such circumstances, the subject cannot use his or her senses to monitor the external environment and thus feels exposed and vulnerable.

The Biochemistry and Genetics of Paranoia

As is commonly observed in clinical settings, substances such as co-caine and amphetamines that increase brain dopamine levels are strongly associated with paranoid psychosis. Medications such as chlor-promazine (Thorazine) or haloperidol (Haldol) that block dopamine brain receptors in certain regions of the brain can be highly effective in treating paranoid psychosis. When enzymes (such as β-hydroxylase) that metabolize brain dopamine are reduced, brain dopamine levels are thereby increased, as is the concomitance of paranoid psychosis. Ge-netic conditions that lead to low levels of dopamine β-hydroxylase in the plasma or cerebrospinal fluid have been found to be associated with increased incidence of paranoia, as can occur with cocaine use (Cubells et al. 2000) or in major depression (Wood et al. 2002). This implies that predispositions to becoming paranoid might have a genetic component.

Family studies, adoption studies, and twin studies convincingly dem-onstrate a strong hereditary component to psychiatric conditions such as schizophrenia and bipolar disorder in which paranoid psychosis is com-mon. Because similar studies have not yet been conducted for people who meet DSM criteria for paranoid personality disorder, the role of heredity and genetics remains unknown. Certain investigators have suggested that there may be a genetic relationship between paranoid personality disorder and schizophrenia (Akhtar 1990; Kendler and Gruenberg 1982); however, this has not yet been convincingly substantiated.

The Psychology of Paranoia

The origins of psychological considerations of paranoia are often traced to a 1911 paper by Sigmund Freud (1911/1958) in which he described the psychology of a patient named Judge Schreber. Daniel Paul Schreber was a well-known German judge who had several long psy-chiatric hospitalizations because of severe delusions. In 1903, Schreber published a book entitled *Memoirs of My Nervous Illness* (Schreber 1988) that provided a vivid personal account of his paranoid delusions. Freud further developed and expounded his theories on the unconscious ori-gins of paranoia from the detailed autobiographical portrayal offered in Schreber's book. In his book Schreber detailed his delusional preoccu-pations with one of his psychiatrists, Dr. Flechsig, for whom he had in-tensely ambivalent feelings. Freud believed that Schreber experienced powerfully erotic feelings toward Dr. Flechsig but that these feelings were unacceptable to Judge Schreber and were therefore repressed. Freud posited that Schreber unconsciously "projected" his own homoerotic feelings onto his psychiatrist, whom he then feared would violate him sexually. Thus, Freud believed that a basis for paranoid delusions is an unconscious response to unacceptable homosexual feelings. Nearly a century has passed since Freud's paper about Schreber and paranoia, and many useful amplifications of this theory have been advanced. Noting that not only Schreber but many other people with paranoia experienced abuse or neglect as children, clinicians have theorized that anger, impotence, and a need to be connected to others play important roles in the development of this symptom. The psychological defense of *projection,* in which powerful and unacceptable feelings (especially aggressive and sexual feelings) are unconsciously transferred to the feared, persecuting, other person has weathered the test of time, and it remains a useful concept in understanding and treating people plagued by paranoia. Readers who are interested in an excellent review of psychoanalytic and other psychological theories of paranoia are encouraged to read a small gem of a book, *Paranoia: New Psychoanalytic Perspectives* (Oldham and Bone 1994).

Treatment of People With Paranoid Personality Disorder

Barriers to Treatment

As is emphasized throughout this book, accurate diagnosis must precede effective treatment. A study of patients seeking treatment at the Columbia University Psychoanalytic Center compared the diagnosis and diagnostic report of admitting clinicians with the results of structured diagnostic scales that were administered by research psychiatrists (Oldham and Skodol 1994). What they found was alarming: "It is striking that for all 12 patients who were positive for paranoid personality disorder by ether the PDE or the SCID-II [the rating scales used], the word 'paranoid' does not ever once appear in the routine clinical evaluations recorded by the admissions service" (Oldham and Skodol 1994, p. 158). We can infer from this study that even mental health professionals may not recognize that a patient whom they are evaluating or treating has paranoid personality disorder. Even when the correct diagnosis is made, people with this condition are reluctant to accept treatment. Presented in Table 9–4 is a summary of the barriers to treatment for people with this disorder.

From reviewing Table 9–4, one can understand why people with paranoid personality disorder only rarely seek out treatment and why, when they are in treatment, they can find it threatening. The knowledgeable and experienced therapists who understand the obstacles and

---

TABLE 9–4. Barriers to treatment for people with paranoid personality disorder

---

1. **People with paranoia have fundamental problems with trust.** "How could I be sure that the secret and sensitive information that I would tell a therapist would remain confidential and not be used against me?"

2. **People with paranoia like to believe that they are self-sufficient.** "I don't like the idea of becoming dependent on a professional."

3. **People with paranoia believe they are smarter than others.** "What could some therapist tell me that I don't already know?"

4. **People with paranoia blame others for their problems.** "Why should I have to go see some doctor, when it is really the other person who is sick and needs help?"

5. **People with paranoia are not psychologically minded.** "I don't agree that my angry feelings for him have anything to do with my suspicions about him. I know that he is out to get me."

6. **People with paranoia distort intense feelings.** "I suspect that this therapist has the hots for me."

7. **People with paranoia are inflexible and argumentative.** "I work a hard job, and the most convenient time for me to see you is after 8:00 P.M. Therapists always seem to do what's best for themselves."

8. **People with paranoia are litigious.** "This doctor's advice has made me feel much worse. His terrible advice has caused most of my problems. Not only won't I pay his outrageous bills, but I am going to sue him for malpractice."

9. **People with paranoia can become dangerous.** "I have now put the entire puzzle together. My doctor has been out to get me all along. Because he knows so much about me, I am in great danger. I had better get him before he gets me."

---

very real dangers in treating individuals with paranoia are often reluctant to take them on as patients. As a result, people with this condition commonly do not receive the treatment that they so desperately need. Even worse, when they have therapists who do not have the knowledge, skills, or professional discipline to treat people with paranoid disorders, the therapeutic relationship can become destructive to the patient and unsafe for the practitioner.

Effective Treatment

Because people with paranoid personality disorder are reluctant to acknowledge that they need treatment and are distrustful of caregivers, their first experience with a mental health professional often occurs under duress. An employer may insist that an employee get professional help for his or her constant accusations of co-workers or else be terminated from the job. An exasperated labor attorney may want clarification about a union member's mental status before pursuing a far-fetched unfair-termination lawsuit against an employer. A husband or wife may insist that the spouse get treatment for the persistent jealous tirades and suspicions of infidelity. Thus the patient will often enter treatment both resistant and skeptical. The skilled therapist will straddle a fine and fragile line between avoiding power struggles and being overly solicitous, which the patient would also distrust. An important goal of all treatment of patients with paranoid personality disorder is *insight*, which, in this circumstance means an understanding and acceptance by patients of their own role in their presenting problems. Their tendency in conflicts will be to place all blame on the other party and to insist that the only possible resolution is for that party to be punished or somehow eliminated. The mental health professional must avoid the patient's insistence that he or she become the patient's agent in changing or defeating his or her putative adversaries. Deep psychological interpretations are rarely helpful, because they are perceived by the rigid and inflexible patient to be either ridiculous or threatening: "I can't believe that you are telling me that I am sexually attracted to him. I have never been attracted to another man in my entire life." Rather, the therapist should make simple, helpful interventions such as, "Since neither you nor I can do much to change their behavior, let's work together to find ways so that it doesn't bother you as much."

People with paranoid personality disorder commonly have depression and anxiety. Although medications can be helpful in mitigating these disorders, patients with this condition often refuse to accept this form of treatment. They are fearful that the medications might cause them to lose control. That "something could get inside of me and take over my thoughts and feelings" is a prospect that a person with paranoid tendencies would wish to avoid. Nonetheless, when the skillful psychiatrist is successful in getting the patient to accept a trial of medications, positive results often ensue. Although antipsychotic medications are highly effective in treating paranoid psychosis, they are rarely helpful in treating the unjustified suspicions and hostilities of people with paranoid personality disorder. Dependence on alcohol and illegal substances compounds the disabling symptoms of people with this condition, and treatment of these comorbid conditions constitutes a therapeutic priority. Couple treatment can be useful if it is accepted by the patient, who will be afraid of being "ganged up on" by the spouse and the doctor. Couple treatment should focus on reducing hostilities in the relationship, improving communication, supporting attempts at intimacy, and allaying unwarranted concerns of the patient about the infidelity of the spouse. Most often, group treatment produces too much anxiety for patients with this disorder.

What To Do If You Are in a Relationship With a Person With Paranoid Personality Disorder

First Ensure Your Safety

If you currently have a relationship with or are being harassed by a person whom you suspect has paranoid personality disorder, you must first determine whether or not you are in any danger. The most efficient and effective way of arriving at such a determination is by enlisting the consultation of a mental health professional who is experienced in diagnosing and treating people with this condition. In other words, the clinician must first understand the psychopathology of people with this disorder before being able to advise you meaningfully. Please refer to Table 7–11 ("Questions to Ask When Selecting a Mental Health Professional") in Chapter 7 ("Antisocial Personality Disorder") for recommendations on how to go about finding a qualified clinician when you may be endangered by a person with a personality disorder. If this clinician and you determine that you are in fact endangered, the key decision will be how best to make an intervention. In some cases it is safer for you not to respond directly to the individual, because your attempts at remediation will be misunderstood and become grist for the paranoid mill. This is particularly true if the person has a history of *any* of the following: violence, incarceration, preoccupation with or access to weapons, psychosis. People with paranoid psychosis are prone to misinterpreting efforts to help them or to restrain them, and they are at increased risk of responding to attempted interventions with aggression. If such is possible, it is imperative that you work closely with your knowledgeable and competent mental health professional to determine the most judicious approach to ensure your safety. If police and courts are required to restrain the person in question, close communication among you, your clinician, the police officers, and the court personnel is essential.

Communicate and Respond Effectively

The same elements that are summarized in Table 9–4 as barriers to the treatment of people with paranoid personality disorder are also impediments to communicating with and relating effectively with them. In Table 9–5, suggestions are offered on how to overcome these barriers.

TABLE 9–5. Suggestions for overcoming barriers to communicating and relating effectively to people with paranoid personality disorder

Barrier #1: People with paranoia have fundamental problems with trust.

Suggestion: Take special efforts to communicate your intentions clearly before you embark on any action related to them.

Barrier #2: People with paranoia like to believe that they are self-sufficient.

Suggestion: Reassure the person that you have no intention of controlling or confining them in any way.

Barrier #3: People with paranoia believe they are smarter than others.

Suggestion: Do not acknowledge or try to defend yourself from their continuous condescending devaluation of you.

Barrier #4: People with paranoia blame others for their problems.

Suggestion: Without defensiveness or anger, use simple facts to communicate clearly that you are not responsible for what they are accusing you of.

Barrier #5: People with paranoia are not psychologically minded.

Suggestion: Try to help them understand that appearances may be misleading. Just because a person might seem irritated with them does not mean that this person is dangerous to them or out to get them.

Barrier #6: People with paranoia distort intense feelings.

Suggestion: Refrain from establishing a relationship that will evoke intense feelings—either positive or negative—with a person who has this disorder.

Barrier #7: People with paranoia are inflexible and argumentative.

Suggestion: Avoid arguing and power struggles, if at all possible.

Barrier #8: People with paranoia are litigious.

Suggestion: Avoid doing business and forming contractual relationships with people with this condition. If such a relationship is necessary, be careful to articulate all obligations, potentialities, and understandings *in writing* in advance.

Barrier #9: People with paranoia can become dangerous.

Suggestion: Do not back people with this condition into corners. Offer them safe and face-saving avenues of escape from responsibilities and avoidance of punitive actions, whether deserved or not.

Avoidance Is the Best Medicine

I cannot assure you that every one of the suggestions listed in Table 9–5 will be successful every time in overcoming barriers to your interactions with a person with paranoid personality disorder. All too frequently, nothing seems to help in resolving the endless conflicts and hassles associated with dealing with people with this condition. By now you are probably gaining the impression that relationships with people who have this disorder are most often much more trouble than they are worth. In far too many circumstances, this impression is true. I hope that the information in this chapter will help you confirm or dispel your suspicions that you are dealing with or about to encounter someone who has this illness. Where possible, avoidance of people with this disorder is usually the best course of action.

Afterword

As was revealed in the case of Dr. Wilma Warren, relationships with people with paranoid personality disorder often begin on a very positive note. People with this condition will initially appear considerate, thoughtful, and willing to contribute meaningfully to your relationship with them. However, their fundamental insecurities, self-centeredness, need for total control, and distortions of their own intense feelings will begin to unravel your relationship with them. They will begin to distrust all of your motives, monitor your every move, discover hidden meanings in all of your communications, and seek and find "evidence" that you have harmed them. Their rigidity and inflexibility will inhibit their acceptance of the facts that you provide to contradict their impressions and conclusions. They will grow increasingly resentful, hostile, belligerent, and litigious. They bear enduring grudges and are prone to retaliate. They will not accept help from either mediators or mental health professionals. People who disagree with them or take your side in the dispute will be discounted or regarded by them as being "on the other side"—as enemies like you. Ultimately you will ask yourself, "How did I get myself involved with this person in the first place?", "How can I get disengaged from the relationship at this point?", and "What will it take to protect myself from his retaliations for my imagined transgressions?" Learn from your bitter experience and the information provided in this chapter how to recognize a person with paranoid personality disorder and, if you can, stay away.

References and Suggested Readings

Akhtar S: Paranoid personality disorder: a synthesis of developmental, dynamic, and descriptive features. Am J Psychother 44:5–25, 1990

American Psychiatric Association: Diagnostic and Statistical Manual of Mental Disorders, 4th Edition, Text Revision. Washington, DC, American Psychiatric Association, 2000

Cooper AM: Paranoia: a part of every analysis, in Paranoia: New Psychoanalytic Perspectives. Edited by Oldham JM, Bone S. Madison, CT, International Universities Press, 1994, pp 133–149

Cubells JF, Kranzler HR, McCance-Katz E, et al: A haplotype at the DBH locus, associated with low plasma dopamine beta-hydroxylase activity, also associates with cocaine-induced paranoia. Mol Psychiatry 5:56–63, 2000

Freud S: Psychoanalytic notes on an autobiographical account of a case of paranoia (dementia paranoides) (1911), in The Standard Edition of the Complete Psychological Works of Sigmund Freud, Vol 12. Translated and edited by Strachey J. London, Hogarth Press, 1958, pp 3–82

Kendler KS, Gruenberg AM: Genetic relationship between paranoid personality disorder and the "schizophrenic spectrum" disorders. Am J Psychiatry 139:1185–1186, 1982

Munro A: Delusional Disorder: Paranoia and Related Illnesses. New York, Cambridge University Press, 1999

Oldham JM, Bone S (eds): Paranoia: New Psychoanalytic Perspectives. Madison, CT, International Universities Press, 1994

Oldham JM, Skodol AE: Do patients with paranoid personality disorder seek psychoanalysis? In Paranoia: New Psychoanalytic Perspectives. Edited by Oldham JM, Bone S. Madison, CT, International Universities Press, 1994, pp 151–164

Sachdev P, Smith JS, Cathcart S: Schizophrenia-like psychosis following traumatic brain injury: a chart-based descriptive and case-control study. Psychol Med 31:231–239, 2001

Schreber DP: Memoirs of My Nervous Illness. Translated and edited by Macalpine I, Hunter RA. Cambridge, MA, Harvard University Press, 1988

Wood JG, Joyce PR, Miller AL, et al: A polymorphism in the dopamine beta-hydroxylase gene is associated with "paranoid ideation" in patients with major depression. Biol Psychiatry 51:365–369, 2002

Chapter

10

BORDERLINE PERSONALITY DISORDER

He jests at scars that never felt a wound.

—William Shakespeare, *Romeo and Juliet*

Essence

Have you ever been in a relationship with a person by whom you feel persistently criticized, devalued, and controlled? Does this person, with an incredible level of invective and irritability, accuse and convict you of having caused *all* of the pain and problems in the relationship and in her life? Do you feel that you are always the defendant and that she is prosecuting attorney, judge, and jury? Do you believe that the level of emotion in this relationship is overly intense and that the nature of the feelings fluctuates drastically? On one day are you regarded by that person as the best person in the world, and on the very next day as the very worst person? As a result of the relationship, are your self-esteem and self-confidence continuously being eroded? Although the person attacks you vehemently, is he or she so sensitive that you feel that you can neither defend yourself nor fight back? When you try to withdraw from the relationship, does the person indicate that your "abandonment" will cause irreparable harm to her? Are you concerned that because of your withdrawal she will become self-destructive or suicidal? Have you in fact been told that if something drastic happens to her, it will be *your* fault? Do you feel as if you were perched at one end of a log balanced over a high cliff, with this person at the other end? Are you worried that if you move a muscle, the log will become unbalanced, causing her to fall from the edge of the cliff to the rocks below? Do you feel controlled and trapped in a spider web of intense, ever-shifting emotions and confusing behaviors? If you answer "yes" to many of these questions, it is very possible that the other person in the relationship may have borderline personality disorder. If so, this chapter should be helpful to you in gaining a better understanding of this person, this relationship, the other person's psychiatric condition, and yourself. A careful reading of the chapter should also be helpful in guiding you toward the best course of action to make things better for this person, the relationship, and you.

The Case of Denise Hughes

A Doctor's Dilemma: An Unusual Request

Shortly before I moved to Houston from Chicago, I received a call from my friend Dr. Boswell Hughes, a noted cardiovascular surgeon. Dr. Hughes told me that he was worried about his son and needed my advice. Judging from the uncharacteristic anxiety and urgency in Bo's voice, I was certain that this was not a matter that would be best handled over the telephone, so I asked him to come right over to my office. He told me that he would be there in 15 minutes, the time it would take him to postpone an elective surgical procedure that had been scheduled. Clearly this was a matter of great importance to Dr. Hughes. On arriving at my office, he told me the following:

> **Dr. Hughes:** I think my son, James, has been sort of kidnapped. Either that or he is being brainwashed. Let me try to calm down and start from the beginning.
>
>   James is now 24 years old. He is our youngest son. Since he was a child, he has always been a wonderful person. He is easygoing, sensitive to others, and popular. He was always a fairly good student and very active in extracurricular activities. In his senior year at the University of Michigan, he was president of both his fraternity and the African-American Students Organization. On graduating from college, he was accepted in the Teach for America program in Houston, where he was assigned to teach math and science to inner-city kids in middle school. He loved his job and was doing great. His plans were to come back to the Midwest to get a master's degree in physics and to become a high school teacher. That has all changed now. He hasn't been doing anything for the past 2 years.
>
> **Dr. Y.:** What happened?
>
> **Dr. Hughes:** He met this girl from Texas about a year ago. She has an 11-year old daughter from a previous marriage. James met this woman, whose name is Denise, when her daughter was in his

fifth-grade math class. Denise is 3 years older than James. Somehow, through her daughter, Denise got her hooks into James. Within weeks after she met him, she moved into James's small apartment with her daughter. I understand that this occurred shortly after her divorce from the father of the little girl. The first time my wife and I heard about Denise was when James called me and my wife, Lois, to tell us he was married. In fact, he had been married for almost 6 months before he told us anything about this whole deal. We were stunned! Prior to this, he had always been so open and communicative with us. The reason that he called at that time was that he needed money to pay his rent. In that phone call we also learned that he was no longer employed at his teaching job. For some unknown reason Denise had insisted that he quit his job. We told him we would send the rent money right away and that we wanted to fly to Houston to see him and his new wife. He told us that he would call us back to tell us when would be a good time for us to come. When we didn't hear from James for an entire week, we called him back. He then informed us that we should not come to visit him now, perhaps some time in the near future. We asked if we could speak with his wife, but James said that she was not at home at that time. That disturbed us greatly, because we could hear a woman's voice screaming at him in the background. To our knowledge, James had never lied to us before this. This is all so strange and disturbing, Stuart....Have you ever heard anything like this story before?

Dr. Y.: Actually, Bo, there *are* familiar elements and themes in what you are recounting. But more about that later. Please go on.

Dr. Hughes: Over the next few months, on the rare occasions that we were able to speak with James, we learned bits and pieces about what had happened to him. Not that we understand any of this. He would only call us when "they" needed money, which became pretty regularly. Truth be told, we have been supporting James, Denise, and the daughter since he first called us. James has not gone back to work. He asked us for money so they could move into a larger apartment, which has turned out to be fairly expensive. We could afford it, so we agreed somewhat reluctantly. They moved from their one-bedroom apartment to a large luxury condominium in suburban Houston. We were smart enough to keep the apartment in our name, but we pay $2,800 a month in maintenance fees and taxes. In fact, we pay for everything for them— their food, their clothes, their doctors' fees, the school stuff for the kid, and much more. Before his involvement with Denise, James had always been frugal and for the most part self-sufficient. It is a totally different story now. Of course, I feel he is being used by this Denise person.

About a month ago, Lois and I decided that we would not give them any more money unless we could come to visit them in Houston. James got very upset and excited when we told him this. He told us that Denise did not want to meet us. When we asked why, James told us that Denise believed we were "prejudiced against her and white people in general." We were floored! She doesn't even know us. When I asked James how she came to such a preposterous conclusion, he said that she could tell from what he had told her about us. At that time my wife and I sought some counsel from a psychologist, who talked to us about "tough love." We were advised to hold our ground and not give them any more money unless we could come to see them. I was in favor of doing this, but Lois was fearful that James and the family would starve or that he would never speak to us again. Nonetheless, we held out somewhat and didn't send any money other than to pay the monthly maintenance fees on the condominium apartment, which we own ourselves. After about 2 weeks, James called to tell us that they didn't have any money for food. Just barely, I convinced Lois to hold out a bit longer before sending any more money to Houston.

One week later, James called us with a deal. He would fly home to see us by himself if we would send him a ticket and agree to pay what they owed on their credit cards. With some coaching from our counselor, we said that if he would send us the credit card bill, we would pay the debt directly. We wouldn't send him any more money until he came home to Chicago to meet with us. After greatly protesting and many calls, he sent us the credit card bill. To our shock, James owed over $26,000 on five different credit cards, and he had been paying enormous amounts in interest alone. Some of these credit cards were in Denise's name and were debts that she built up before she even met James. Stuart, this has been an ongoing nightmare that just keeps getting worse and worse the more we find out about what has been going on with them.

Dr. Y.: What happened next, Bo?

Dr. Hughes: At this point we did not trust James. We strategized that if we gave him the $26,000 for his credit card debt directly, he might not keep his end of the bargain. We feared that he and Denise might spend the money on other things and not pay off the credit card loans. Also, we were pretty sure that if we paid in advance he would not come to Chicago as he had agreed. Instead we contacted all the banks from which the credit cards were issued and told them that we would pay the $26,000 on James's and Denise's debit, but we could not be counted on to pay anything more. We advised the banks not to extend them any more credit. Of course the creditors agreed. We told James about our plan: to pay off his debt, but only after he came to visit us. He seemed somewhat relieved by our plan. However, over the phone, we could again hear Denise screaming at him uncontrollably in the background. Nevertheless we held our ground, and James finally flew home to Chicago, without bringing the rest of the family—even though we offered to pay for their tickets, too.

We had not seen our son for more than 2 years, and we were

shocked by what we saw. James had ballooned up to well over 250 pounds, from about 175 pounds the last time we saw him. He had sort of a dazed look about him, like he was on some kind of drug. We even asked him if he were taking drugs, and he said "no." We believed him because he had no history of ever taking drugs. He was never really interested in drinking. Even though he had agreed to stay with us for only 2 days, almost every hour or so he would go into a room to get away from us to call his wife back in Houston.

We were able to learn a bit about Denise and about their life together. First of all, he believes that Denise is the most brilliant and beautiful woman in the world. She comes from a very disadvantaged background, and because of "financial reasons," she left home when she was 17. She certainly did not attend college, and James did not know whether or not she had even graduated from high school. At age 17, she married a man named Larry who was about 24 at the time. James was not sure what Larry does for a living, but he thinks he works as a car mechanic. Larry is the father of the little girl, but according to Denise he was a drunk and was abusive to her. I really am not sure what to believe, however. James has never met him, because Denise believes he is a bad influence on the little girl. James was not able to provide much additional information about Denise's family background, because she is estranged from her entire family. James has never met her parents and has seen one of her two sisters only once. He said that this meeting was very strained and brief because of the negative feelings between Denise and her sister.

Denise convinced James to ask us if we would pay for a lawyer to help James adopt Denise's daughter. We told him we would have to think about this request before committing to anything. When we asked James how they intended to support themselves, James said that he was looking for a job—like working in a bank—but that Denise had no plans to work. Just as James was preparing to go back to Houston, we asked him if he would see a psychiatrist there for some support. His response upset us further. He said that Denise would never agree to such a thing. James knew, somehow, that she hated psychiatrists. James told us that she would become enraged if he even brought up the subject. Oh, by the way, James told us she reacted the same way whenever he would try to call some of his old friends from college.

Dr. Y.: I think I am getting the picture, Bo. How can I be of help to you?

Dr. Hughes: I heard through the rumor mill that you are going to leave the University of Chicago to take the psychiatry chair at Baylor College of Medicine in Houston. If that is true, I want you treat our son. We have no idea what is wrong with him, but we know that it is a serious mental condition of some sort. Of course we will pay for everything.

Dr. Y.: Don't you think it is highly unlikely that James will be willing to see me? Or that Denise will allow him to do so?

Dr. Hughes: We have made up our minds that we will not support him financially one penny further if he refuses to accept help from you. This includes taking our apartment back from him. We fear that by paying for everything without any demands for him to get help, we are just enabling him to stay caught in the most terrible situation.

Dr. Y.: Bo, you must realize that psychiatry by coercion is neither the usual nor the ideal way to establish a productive treatment alliance. But I recognize fully that this is not the usual or ideal circumstance. It is true that we will be moving to Houston in several months, and I will be happy to try to help him if he agrees to see me. I think it is best for James to call me. Two more things, Bo. As a parent myself, I can imagine the personal distress and fear that you and Lois are now experiencing. Second, thank you for you for placing your confidence in me for the care of your son. I will do my very best to be of help.

Setting Up Treatment: Scheduling the First Session

I had been in Houston for about 6 months when I first heard from James Hughes, who told my office staff that his wife, Denise, would be calling for an appointment. At the time that she first called, I was giving a lecture to the full class of second-year medical students (about 180 students). Initially, Mrs. Hughes demanded that my administrative assistant schedule her for an appointment that afternoon. When told that this would not be possible because my afternoon was already filled with appointments that had been scheduled many weeks in advance, Mrs. Hughes became furious.

Mrs. Hughes: I don't think you are getting it. This is a medical emergency! I am the daughter of heart surgeon Dr. Boswell Hughes. If Dr. Yudofsky doesn't know who I am, you can be damn sure he will know who Dr. Hughes is. Now have him paged to me at once if you want to keep your job!

Administrative assistant: He is giving a lecture now. But if this is a true emergency, I can page him. He will get right back to me. Please give me your number, and he will call you back as soon as he is free.

Mrs. Hughes: I have a better idea. I am sure you have more than one line in your office. Page him right now to the other line; and I will stay on this line. As soon as he answers, you can transfer him over to me.

My administrative assistant did page me. She was both apologetic and angry.

Administrative assistant: I am sorry to interrupt your lecture, but a Denise Hughes, who says that you know her, insisted that I do so.

> She says she wants to speak with you urgently about your seeing her as a patient today. I think you should also know, Dr. Y., that she has a very, very rude and entitled attitude.
>
> **Dr. Y.:** I am sorry that you were not treated with respect. That is unacceptable, but it is something that I might have to deal with a bit later. Please connect me to Mrs. Hughes.
>
> **Mrs. Hughes:** First, Dr. Yudofsky, not that it is my business, but I think you should do something with your staff. They seem to me to be incompetent. Second, my husband, James, says that you promised our father, Dr. Boswell Hughes, that you would see us immediately when we called. I want to see you today. James is not feeling well, so he can't come this time.
>
> **Dr. Y.:** I will arrange to see you today in my office at 2:00 P.M. if that is convenient for you.

When I returned to my office, my administrative staff told me the following:

> **Office administrator:** We can't believe you are going to see Mrs. Hughes today. It will take us hours to move your schedule around to make this work out. We believe that she was unbearably rude to us, and it worked. By her abusing us, and you, she is going to get her way. Why do we have office protocols if we are going to break them as soon as someone raises a stink?

Treatment Approach to Denise Hughes, Part One

Frequently, the first data that I use to assess a patient and reach a diagnosis are obtained before I actually meet with that person in my office. These data come from many sources, including the people who refer the patient, such as their physicians, clergy, and concerned family members. In addition, before their first visit patients often have many conversations with my office personnel about such things as directions to the office, whether or not they should bring their medical records, and my billing policies. My office staff will communicate to me any information that they believe is pertinent, particularly if they believe that the patient might be experiencing a high level of psychological distress. Invariably, the administrative staff will let me know if a patient is impolite with them or is unusually nice to them, which of course they appreciate. Occasionally, a patient is demeaning to my staff while showing great respect to me (or vice versa). This information may be useful to help me understand how the patient functions in diverse circumstances. In the case of Denise Hughes, I already had extensive circumstantial information about her from my talk with her father-in-law, Dr. Hughes. From this discussion, I learned many things—especially that she tried to control as many aspects of her husband's life as she was able. That was the "what" regarding her behavior, and I had many speculations about the "why."

I learned even more about Mrs. Hughes from the way she interacted with my office staff and from their reactions to her. My office staff is accustomed to handling psychiatric emergencies, which they always accomplish with efficiency, deep compassion, and respect for the patient. They understand the anxiety, urgency, and vulnerability that is characteristic of people in emergency situations, and these situations do not bother them. However, their brief interaction with Denise Hughes left them furious with her and with me. Essentially, they believed that despite her insulting and intrusive behavior, I *chose Mrs. Hughes over them!*

The powerful reactions of my office staff to Denise Hughes gave me important diagnostic information. What was happening among Denise Hughes, my office staff, and me is a phenomenon known as **splitting.** At the most descriptive level, the term denotes the behavior of a person that results in intense disagreements between and among other people with whom he or she interacts. People who exhibit splitting behaviors often have pervasive fears of being abandoned. By pitting people whom they know against one another, they believe that they will have less competition for their attention and affection. At deeper levels splitting is a primitive defense mechanism—an unconscious process whereby people are divided up into two groups: those who are "all good" and those who are "all bad." This unconscious dynamic often stems from the ways very young children conceptualize themselves and others. Adults who have not advanced to a more mature way of thinking about themselves and others strive to be special by being perceived as being "all good" by people who are important to them. They become precipitously upset if they believe that people do not regard them as being perfect. In such circumstances they often feel rejected, and they react with the most intense anxiety and anger. On feeling rejected, they will perceive the rejecting party as being "all bad" and will communicate their antipathy to that person by their disparaging affect and behavior. This pattern of thinking and behavior is common in people with a diagnosis of borderline personality disorder. After all the commotion that Denise Hughes elicited among my office staff with one telephone call, I speculated that she might have this condition. However, I would never make up my mind about the psychodynamics of a patient before undertaking a thorough evaluation of that individual in person. As in every specialty of medicine, many different types of underlying pathology can lead to similar symptoms.

My speculation about Denise Hughes' possible diagnosis and psychodynamics had a clinical purpose. If indeed she turned out to have borderline personality disorder, it would be critical that I avoid power struggles with her in all phases of her treatment, particularly in the early phases. Patients with borderline personality disorder are adept at engaging in power struggles to manipulate others and to achieve specific goals. To use a boxing image, they are "counter punchers." For example, if I or my staff were to become huffy when Mrs. Hughes demanded to see me that day and were to say, "Who do you think you are to displace another patient who has been waiting several months for their appointment?" Denise might have called her father-in-law, Dr. Hughes, to report the following: "When I called for my appointment, both Dr. Yudofsky and his office staff were rude to me. They kept telling me how important he is and how long it takes to get an appointment with him. It didn't make any difference that you had referred James and me to him; in fact, he and his staff acted as if they had never heard of you. The only thing that they did seem to be interested in was whether or not I had an insurance coverage and when we would pay him. The way I feel now is that I wouldn't see that man if he were the only doctor on earth." As you can see, this type of communication would have misrepresented what had actually happened in order to effect a split between me and Dr. Hughes. Denise's ultimate goal would have been to control the process of treatment, about which she was highly suspicious. A second common characteristic of people with borderline personality disorder is to distort the communications of others in the service of splitting them. This, of course, constitutes a type of misrepresenting of the truth, or lying. Usually, this process of distortion is automatic, and the person has little or no awareness of his or her mendacity.

Knowing full well that the main reason—perhaps the only reason—that Denise Hughes was seeing me was to get money from the Hughes family, I realized that she would use almost any excuse to avoid treatment. At the cost of upsetting my staff and inconveniencing another patient (whom I rescheduled), I saw her that day, and I did not express any objection or irritation. My own understanding of the clinical reasons that I was being so accommodating enabled me to keep my angry feelings under control and to avoid a hostile, unproductive interchange with Mrs. Hughes. I was also intensely aware that *it would be difficult to avoid power struggles with her while at the same time maintaining appropriate boundaries.* This is the prototypical "high-wire balancing act" that is involved in relating with or treating someone with borderline personality disorder. Let me give you an example: As my staff correctly pointed out, I was already treating Mrs. Hughes as if she were a privileged character by changing office protocols to accommodate her

unreasonable demands. I understood that although I was being accommodating to establish a treatment relationship, it was at the cost of creating the expectation that she would continue to get her way in the
future, notwithstanding the rules and the rights of other people. Knowing this, I realized that I had to be very clear with her about the many
other boundaries involved in a clinical relationship. Therefore, even
though Mrs. Hughes had demanded that she see me at 2:00 P.M. on that
day, I requested that my staff call her to explain—and document in a file
note—that, as she requested, I would be ready to see her at *exactly* 2:00
P.M. and that the initial appointment would last until precisely 3:30 P.M.
Although this sounds quite rigid, if she were to show up an hour late
and expect a full 90-minute consultation, a power struggle would ensue. My technique was to provide clear information about therapeutic
rules and boundaries to try to minimize power struggles. When my administrative assistant dutifully conveyed this message to Mrs. Hughes
by telephone, she replied, "Oh great! What if I have a heart attack at
3:29? Will Dr. Yudofsky leave me dying to go to his golf appointment?"

First Therapeutic Session With Denise Hughes

Mrs. Hughes arrived right on time for her first session, which she began
by asking me the following question:

> **Mrs. Hughes:** Tell me, Dr. Yudofsky: Does everything I say in here get
> held against me?
> **Dr. Y.:** Psychiatric treatment is advocational, not adversarial. By that
> I mean that I am here to be helpful to you. However, I am not ex-
> actly sure I understand what you mean by "held against you."
> **Mrs. Hughes:** Will you tell everything I say to you to Dr. Hughes?
> I don't particularly feel that I need your help, thank you very
> much. My father-in-law said that he wouldn't give his son our
> rightful living allowance unless we came to see you. I am asking
> whether or not you need to have my permission to send him a re-
> port on me? I can tell you right now that I am not giving you per-
> mission to say anything about me to anyone. Dr. Hughes wanted
> me to come see you, so here I am.
> **Dr. Y.:** Without your permission, I will not reveal anything you tell me
> to anyone—unless you are a danger to yourself or others. You
> must also understand, however, that all medical records, includ-
> ing my personal notes about our meetings, are subject to the sub-
> poena of a judge.
> **Mrs. Hughes:** What I want to work out with you today is how to tell
> Dr. Hughes I am coming to see you so we can get our money. At
> the same time I don't want you telling him anything else that I say
> to you.

> **Dr. Y.:** I am sure that this can be worked out. By the way, doesn't Dr.
> Hughes expect his son to come see me as well?

For the entirety of the first session, Denise Hughes and I discussed and came to agreement about how communication with Dr. Hughes would be accomplished without violating her confidentiality. We also began a detailed discussion over the structure of treatment. Mrs. Hughes did not want her husband to see any psychiatrist, and she tried to get me to persuade Dr. Hughes to pay them their allowance if she alone came to see me. I told her that her request was unrealistic, because Dr. Hughes mainly wanted his son to be in psychotherapy. Mrs. Hughes was emphatic about not wanting to share her sessions with her husband or for me to see him individually. Finally, we agreed that I would refer him to another psychiatrist, but only if she could have access to that doctor. She assured me that that would be fine with her husband. Mrs. Hughes spent the entirety of her next session with me reviewing boundary issues in psychotherapy. The following exchange captures the tenor of this discussion:

> **Mrs. Hughes:** Not that it will ever happen, but how do I get in touch
> with you in an emergency? All of my other doctors give me their
> home telephone numbers.
> **Dr. Y.:** In case of an emergency, you may call my answering service and
> have me paged.
> **Mrs. Hughes:** Does that mean you don't trust me with your home tele-
> phone number? What do you think will happen—that I will kid-
> nap your children?
> **Dr. Y.:** I can be reached quite reliably through my answering service.
> **Mrs. Hughes:** That's very generous of you. Don't go out of your way to
> help me or anything. By the way, are you a real doctor?
> **Dr. Y.:** I am not exactly sure what you are asking, Mrs. Hughes.
> **Mrs. Hughes:** You know exactly what I mean, Mr. Politically Correct.
> I mean are you a *real* physician who can prescribe *real* drugs?
> **Dr. Y.:** Yes, I am a physician and may prescribe medications when they
> are indicated.
> **Mrs. Hughes:** Great. Then you won't mind refilling my birth control
> prescription and my Percodan [oxycodone/aspirin] prescription
> for my back pain.
> **Dr. Y.:** I will leave the refilling of those prescriptions to the physicians
> who prescribed them to you originally. If it turns out that you re-
> quire a psychiatric medication, I will take care of that.
> **Mrs. Hughes (with an angry and ironic tone):** You are all heart and a
> big help.

Dr. Boswell Hughes agreed to allocate to Denise and James $3,000 a month for family expenses over the next 2 years, on the condition that they both see their psychiatrists once a week, except when the doctors were away on business or on vacation. It was eventually agreed that each would be allowed to miss one session per month. If, for any reason which Dr. Hughes did not approve, either James or Denise missed more than one session during a calendar month, he would not send them a check for the next month. Dr. Hughes also said that he would not repay any of their new debts—no matter what trouble they got into.

Treatment Approach to Denise Hughes, Part Two

Establishing Boundaries

I had never before—nor have I subsequently—conducted treatment under the structure and types of restrictions that were established for Denise and James Hughes. However, I believe that *so long as the established boundaries and ethics of conducting psychiatric care are strictly maintained, there is room and necessity for considerable flexibility in treating patients.* I liken this to the game of basketball, wherein, despite its many rules—prohibitions against walking with the basketball, fouling other players, stepping out of bounds, and the like—there is still great opportunity for individuality and creativity in how the game is played. I strongly believe that clinicians who treat all patients similarly, according to unyielding formulas—usually based on some theory of the causality of the illness—will not be successful in helping many patients. All patients have differing genetics, brains, biochemistries, temperaments, life experiences, and spiritual proclivities, and gifted psychotherapists will make adjustments in how they treat each patient to accommodate these differences. Too many practitioners expect their patients to adapt to their rigid rules for treatment, which is frustrating for the patients. I often tell patients who have not been compliant in taking the medications that I have prescribed, "The pills don't work if you leave them in the bottle." Likewise, I often tell therapists who have been too rigid in treating their patients, "Treatment doesn't work if the patient won't come back to see you." Most importantly, however, *for effective treatment to take place, the establishment and maintenance of clear ethical boundaries between patient and clinician is of prime importance.* How this is accomplished for patients with borderline personality disorder is discussed throughout this chapter.

For the first 4 months of treatment, Denise Hughes squabbled about what she described as "the self-serving rules of psychiatry." For example, she spent an entire session "negotiating" with me about how we should address each other. She wanted to call me Stuart and wanted me

to call her Denise. I was steadfast in calling her Mrs. Hughes and made
it clear that I preferred that she call me Dr. Yudofsky. A sampling of that
interchange is as follows:

> **Mrs. Hughes:** I don't see why you won't call me by my first name, if
> that's what I prefer. Don't I have any rights in treatment?
>
> **Dr. Y.:** I believe that it is more respectful to you and the serious work
> that we are trying to accomplish. Why is it so important to you
> that I call you by your first name?
>
> **Mrs. Hughes:** It makes things more equal and friendly. Why do things
> in here have to be so formal and impersonal? You expect me to
> talk about such personal things, and yet you don't tell me a single
> thing about yourself. How do you expect me to open up to you, if
> you are a complete stranger? I think psychiatry is one big power
> trip. I'm going to call you Stuart, even if you won't call me by my
> first name.

Trust

Although to a casual and uninformed observer, prolonged discussions
about how the doctor and patient should address one another might appear to be a colossal waste of time, this issue is more serious than it
seems. Many people with borderline personality disorder have histories of being physically and sexually abused as children—often by one
of their parents or by other members of their family who were in important positions of responsibility and trust. Understandably, people with
histories of familial abuse have difficulties establishing trusting relationships with other people. For example, why should they trust a
stranger, just because he is a doctor, when they couldn't trust their own
parents? Second, people who have been physically abused or sexually
violated as children have, as adults, great confusion and problems with
the regulation of their own feelings and drives. They are constantly testing the safety of their environment, often by baiting people with angry
remarks and by being seductive.

Repetition Compulsion

Freud introduced the concept of **repetition compulsion** to help explain
why people with painful childhood experiences replicate these experiences though their choices of people for significant adult relationships.
Often they choose abusive people as their spouses, and the key conflicts
of their childhood are continually reenacted in their marriages and with
their children. Tragically, the cycle of abuse continues. In addition, their
provocative behavior with mature, respectful people also invites abusive responses. Mature intimacy is threatening to them, because it
makes them feel out of control and vulnerable. People who have been

abused sexually or physically will behave in a broad range of ways to discourage closeness with others and to replace closeness with hostile and devaluing interactions. The structure and formality of the therapeutic relationship make it inherently protective, and over time the patient may feel sufficiently safe to explore and communicate the strongly repressed feelings and memories that have led to his or her incapacitating psychiatric symptoms. These communications will be associated with the evocation of intimate feelings toward the therapist, feelings that patients are encouraged to speak about in the treatment setting but not to act on. The establishment and maintenance of clear and respectful therapeutic boundaries is required for this healing process of revelation and treatment to take place. Should these boundaries be breached—for example, by the therapist's permitting a personal relationship to occur outside the formal treatment setting—not only will the patient's symptoms become worse, but the therapist will also jeopardize his or her professional integrity and future.

For 6 months I continued to explain to Mrs. Hughes the rules and boundaries of the psychotherapy. For 6 months I refused to reciprocate in kind her angry outbursts or to respond to her seductive behavior. Over time, Mrs. Hughes began to feel sufficiently safe to review a few details of her early life history. At the same time, she did not trust me sufficiently to plumb and communicate her most personal thoughts and feelings. From the beginning of treatment, however, she was quite willing to communicate her angry and devaluing feelings toward me.

Self-Reflection

There were reasons for the confrontational ways in which Denise Hughes treated my staff and me. Realistically, I could never learn about these reasons and help Mrs. Hughes in an informed way until I had established a therapeutic relationship with her. I was quite sure that she treated most other people in her life in a similar fashion, with consequences that were destructive both for her and for them. My ambitious goal was to establish a trusting therapeutic relationship with Mrs. Hughes in which we could assess the following:

- *How and why* she treated other people in a dysfunctional fashion
- *How and why* the results of her behavior with other people hurt her and alienated them
- *Why and how* to change her thinking and behavior

It is important to note that each of these assessments requires that the persons involved have the incentive and capacity to reflect on the meaning of their actions—both for themselves and for others. Difficulties with this type of self-reflection in people with borderline personality disorder has been traced to problems with early-life attachment to critical caregivers, usually their mothers (Fonagy 2000). Termed *reflective functioning,* this capacity refers to the person's ability to consider a broad range of reasons why he or she and other people might feel and react in a certain way in response to a specific situation. For example, early in her treatment with me, Mrs. Hughes arrived in my office in obvious distress:

> **Mrs. Hughes:** I don't want to talk to you about this psychological bullshit; I think I am about to die.
>
> **Dr. Y.:** Why do you think you are about to die?
>
> **Mrs. Hughes:** For the last two months I have been feeling this pain on the left side of my chest. I thought it might be a heart problem until this morning. I felt this lump in my breast. It hurts when I push on it. I am sure it is cancer. If you really want to help me, you will examine it for me and tell me if I am going to die.
>
> **Dr. Y.:** I certainly understand and share your concern. However, it is not appropriate for me to examine your breast. What I will do right away is to refer you to Baylor's Breast Center, where you can be evaluated in a thorough and informed way by experts in this area.
>
> **Mrs. Hughes:** I know that will take at least several days before I am seen. I am frightened out of my mind right now! All I want is your opinion about whether you think that lump is breast cancer. What did you go to medical school for if you can't practice the least bit of medicine? The one time I ask you to do something real for me, you want to dump me off on someone else!
>
> **Dr. Y.:** What I would like you to do is to consider some of the other possible reasons for my decision not to examine your breast.
>
> **Mrs. Hughes:** Well, probably because you think that my body is disgusting, and you don't want to touch me. Another reason is that it's too much trouble for you to get out of your goddamn chair, walk over here and examine me.
>
> **Dr. Y.:** You are implying that I don't believe that you are worth helping. In fact, the very opposite is true. First, I believe that it is important for me to respect your boundaries: I am your psychiatrist, not your general physician. It is not appropriate for me to do physical examinations of you. Second, I believe that you are best served by a true expert in breast cancer. Such an expert will be in the best position to evaluate your breast lump and to advise you what to do. I believe that you deserve to receive the best possible care for this concern.

What I was trying to accomplish in this interchange was to teach Mrs. Hughes, when she feels upset and rejected, to consider many alternatives before arriving at a firm conclusion. As a result of her low self-esteem and pervasive feelings of worthlessness, Mrs. Hughes felt rejected and abandoned by my unwillingness to examine her breast. By encouraging her to reflect on other possible reasons for my decision, I hoped that she would understand that my responses to her in a given situation might be quite different from those that she might expect from her mother or from others whom she felt had abused, rejected, or abandoned her. Mrs. Hughes's pattern of explosive reactions to her perception of being rejected or abandoned was most often the result of her refusal to reflect on what the other person was feeling or thinking. This episode highlights two fundamental goals of my therapeutic strategy for Mrs. Hughes:

1. To help Mrs. Hughes learn to consider a full range of potential reasons—including both her own feelings and actions and those of the other party—when she feels abandoned or rejected.
2. To help her learn to recognize people who are likely to exploit and reject her and to avoid having relationships with them.

People with borderline personality disorder repeat the most painful patterns of their childhood by choosing, for their significant relationships, other people who devalue and take advantage of them. A significant part of their therapy is helping them learn to identify such people and helping them end these relationships. People with borderline personality disorder also identify with abusive and exploitive parental figures by exhibiting such behaviors themselves, as Mrs. Hughes did in her relationships with her husband, James, and his parents.

Psychiatric History of Denise Hughes: Parental and Sibling Relationships

It took many months in treatment before Mrs. Hughes felt sufficiently secure to reveal her personal history and the feelings that were associated with her important life events. The middle child of three sisters, she recalled constant criticism from her mother:

> **Mrs. Hughes:** My mother hated everything about me. Unlike my sisters, she thought I favored my father's side of the family, all of whom she also despised. One of my earliest memories is of her telling me that I had narrow-set, sneaky eyes—like the devil's. Now, what could I do about that? At night in bed, I used to spend hours pulling at the skin on the corners of my eye sockets, hoping I could spread my eyes apart. Mom adored both of my sisters,

whom she thought were beautiful in every way. She recruited
them in her war against me. They would join up to tease and torture me. If they made me cry, mother would punish me for being
"a pathetic whiner"; if I fought back and hurt one of them, she
would beat me with a belt.

Dr. Y.: What was the role of your father in all of this?

Mrs. Hughes: I think Daddy favored me, which made things much
worse. Mother criticized him all the time for not making enough
money. Things were a little better when he was around, but he
was almost never around. The worst thing of all is that mother
had constant affairs with all sorts of men when he was away. She
lied to us about who these guys were. She often told us that they
were her relatives, like uncles and cousins. When I was 11 years
old, she threw Daddy out of the house, and some guy she knew
named Jake moved in about a week later. Jake never worked, so he
was around the house all the time. It wasn't long until he started
bugging me, but I don't want to talk about it.

Treatment Approach to Denise Hughes, Part Three

Although I immediately suspected that Denise Hughes had been sexually abused by Jake, I did not press Denise to explain just what she
meant by saying that Jake had started "bugging" her. Unconsciously,
Denise would experience my pushing her to disclose painful memories
of sexual abuse as *my being abusive.* In treating people with borderline
personality disorder, one must have patience and must at all times respect what the patients consider to be their private matters. After first
speaking about Jake, Denise missed the next two sessions for reasons
that Dr. Hughes believed were "spurious." As he had warned he would
do, he did not send the next month's check. Even though I believed that
she missed her sessions because of the strong feelings evoked by recall-
ing Jake's abuses and her conflicted feelings about sharing this information with me, I did not intervene on her behalf with Dr. Hughes. This
would have made the treatment too complicated, even though Mrs.
Hughes thought that I was being disloyal to her by not intervening on
her behalf. I believed that she had unconsciously set up a situation (by
missing treatment and violating her agreement with Dr. Hughes) in
which she wanted me to be her father and to intervene on her behalf.
I fully expected her to be furious with me, as she unconsciously transferred her angry feelings about the failure of her father to protect her
from Jake onto me. (For a review of the concept of transference, see
"Psychotherapeutic Techniques" in Chapter 6, "Narcissistic Personality
Disorder, Part II: Treated Narcissism.") My strategy was to work back-
wards by gently probing Mrs. Hughes about the source of her overflow-

ing anger toward me. Because I had been so careful in avoiding power struggles and in being sensitive to her boundary issues (e.g., by not taking advantage of her despite her many concealed invitations to do so), eventually I expected her to look inwardly for the sources of her rage and paranoia.

I detail this discussion of my treatment strategies toward Mrs. Hughes for four primary purposes:

1. To help the reader understand the complex life experiences and specific unconscious processes that lead to the emotional symptoms and behavioral patterns of people with borderline personality disorder.
2. To provide the reader an insider's view of the deliberate and painstaking process of psychotherapy for a person with borderline personality disorder: how it's done and why it works.
3. To help the reader who is in a relationship—clinical or otherwise—with someone with borderline personality disorder to gain insight into the reasons for the way that he or she is being treated by the person with this condition. In many situations, *although it affects you intensely and personally, you should learn how not take it so intensely or personally.*
4. To offer a model of behavior for the reader who is in a relationship with someone with borderline personality disorder that might help him or her reduce the level of conflict and misunderstanding.

Psychiatric History of Denise Hughes, Continued

Several months after Mrs. Hughes first mentioned her mother's boyfriend, Jake, she began to talk about his behavior toward her.

> **Mrs. Hughes:** Of course, I felt uncomfortable around all of my mother's boyfriends, but Jake was much, much worse than the rest of them. He was around the house all the time, and I felt that he was always watching me. One day he burst into the bathroom when I was taking a bath. I screamed at him to get out, but he pretended to be looking for his razor. I was completely exposed in the bathtub, and he just kept looking at me and ignoring my insistence that he leave. Finally, he found his razor and said the most disgusting thing that I have ever heard in my entire life.

Mrs. Hughes then began to sob, and she was unable to speak for about 20 minutes. This was the first time that she had cried in treatment. When she began to speak again she said,

Mrs. Hughes: Jake then pointed to my private parts with his hand that was holding the razor. I had been trying to hide myself under the clear water. Jake finally said, "What I really would like to do is shave that pretty little thing down there." I froze and could not scream or say a word. At that point I wasn't feeling anything. I was completely numb. He finally left the bathroom. When he saw me later that day he acted as if nothing had happened. I felt totally humiliated and violated. I was just 12 years old and felt very sensitive and embarrassed about growing breasts and pubic hair. My sisters teased me all the time about this stuff. I didn't dare tell my mother. Either she wouldn't believe me, or she would blame me for what happened, like she blamed everything else bad on me.

Over the next five sessions, Mrs. Hughes recounted the horrific tale of being sexually abused and threatened by Jake. She revealed how he would arrange for different ways to be alone with her and would molest her during those times. At first he would take Denise on errands and would take advantage of her sexually while they were in the car. When Denise was 13 years old, he began to take her to motel rooms, where he engaged in fully penetrated sex and would make her do "all sorts of disgusting things" to him. Regarding what she was feeling during these episodes, Mrs. Hughes said the following:

Mrs. Hughes: Whenever I was with Jake, I would go completely numb. I didn't feel anything. I was like some rag doll that he was having his way with.

Even though Jake constantly fought with Denise's mother, they managed to stay together for several years, during which time his sexual abuse of Denise continued on a regular basis. At the same time, Denise became uninterested in school and in her relationships with her female peers. She failed the tenth grade and also got into trouble for bringing marijuana to school. She said that she would get stoned on marijuana almost every day and that she would drink "anything that came in a bottle" and take any type of drug that she could get her hands on. Her favorites were alcohol and marijuana.

By the time she was 17 she was being promiscuous with several different older guys, mostly high school dropouts, who would take her to bars. Her mood became highly labile, and she would get into many physical fights with her female friends and even with the boys she was dating. On other occasions she would become deeply depressed and filled with self-loathing. She began to cut herself with Jake's razor blades.

> **Mrs. Hughes:** At first, I would make dozens of cuts on the inside of my arm, just above my wrist. Doing this somehow made me feel better. Because I was numb so much of the time anyway—with drugs or depression or from being with Jake—it didn't hurt at all. What I really liked was seeing my blood ooze out of the cuts. I'm not kidding, it was like a downer to me. Later I learned to cut all over my body, especially in places that couldn't be seen—like under my breasts or around the insides of my upper thighs.

Denise was sent to the local hospital's emergency room on several occasions. Most of the time this would happen when someone discovered that she had been cutting herself. On several occasions she was sent to the hospital after she communicated suicide threats to her high school counselor or to parents of her friends.

When she became pregnant at age 17, she was not sure who the father was. However, she strongly suspected it was Jake, who continued to have sex with her.

> **Mrs. Hughes:** I used my pregnancy as my ticket out of the house, to get away from my sisters, my mother, and Jake. There was nothing there for me, anyway; I hated each one of them more than the next. I convinced Larry, one of the guys I was dating, that he had knocked me up, and I got him to run away and marry me. That's how my daughter, Hope, was born.

Larry Bishop was 23 years old when he married Denise. He also came from a family with significant problems: his father had chronic alcoholism, and his mother was, on and off, addicted to narcotics, including heroin. Larry had gotten into significant trouble involving drugs and fights during high school, and on being convicted for dealing in drugs, he had spent several years in a reformatory institution for youths. At the state reformatory, Larry learned automobile mechanics, and he pursued this vocation on his release at age 18. His occupational pattern was to work for several years in the service department of a large automobile dealer until being fired for missing too much work or for being insubordinate to his supervisors. On the positive side, Larry was a talented mechanic, and he became more proficient with each job experience. His dream was to open a repair shop of his own.

Larry was unexpectedly taken with his new daughter, Hope, and he resolved to be a responsible father, a reliable husband, and a good provider. Toward that purpose, he cleaned up his act somewhat by stopping taking drugs, but he drank several beers every night. He also devoted himself to his work and was soon being assigned supervisory positions in the large service department in which he worked. However, as hard as he tried, he was never able to have a stable relationship with Denise. He was never able to predict the mood she would be in when he would come home from work. She always seemed furious with him for things that he had or had not done, or for who he was and who he was not. For example, one evening he came home and Denise would not speak to him, nor would she reveal why she was angry with him. Finally, Larry was able to pry from Denise the reason she was so furious with him.

> **Larry Bishop:**[1] You haven't spoken to me in a week. All you do is glare hatred at me. I'm getting sick of being treated like this by you.
> **Denise Bishop:** That's a joke. I haven't done anything to you. That's a lot more than I can say about you.
> **Larry:** I don't have a clue what you are talking about.
> **Denise:** Well, did you screw her yet?
> **Larry:** Screw who?
> **Denise:** That new bitch that I heard is working under you at work. You know who I mean. The young chick who replaced Marvin in the parts department.
> **Larry:** You have really lost it this time, Denise. I don't even know that new girl's name. I don't know anything about her.
> **Denise:** You didn't know my name when you screwed me the first time. You were too damn drunk to care. You never said one word to me about this new chick. What would you expect me to think?
> **Larry:** I think you need bigtime help. You have tormented me for a week and are upsetting Hope over something that has never happened. I told you I don't know her name, and I haven't said the first word to her.
> **Denise:** Then why didn't you tell me about her in the first place? Do you have something to hide?
> **Larry:** I might as well try to screw her—whatever her name is. The truth doesn't seem to make any difference to you.

At that, Denise grabbed a pot of pasta and boiling water from the stove and hurled it at Larry. Most of it missed, but his arm was slightly burned. Denise charged toward Larry and began to scream expletives at him. Larry picked up Hope, who was frightened and crying, and ran out of the house. When they returned to their small home several hours later, he was startled to find that the interior of the house was a sham-

---

[1]This dialogue was reconstructed from the detailed hospital record of an interview with Larry Bishop and Denise Bishop by a social worker on the psychiatry inpatient service of a general hospital where Denise had been committed after a suicide attempt.

bles. Furniture was overturned, lamps were thrown on the floor and broken, and Larry's clothes had been taken out of his drawers and closets and scattered about. His only dress suit had been shredded. In the bedroom he found Denise unconscious in a pool of blood. When he looked more closely, he discovered that she was breathing but had made multiple deep cuts into her left wrist, on her left forearm, and on both of her upper thighs. Blood was pouring profusely from all of these wounds.

At the hospital, Denise was revived. It took two surgeons several hours to stop her bleeding and to clean and close the self-inflicted lacerations. Three units of blood were required to replace what had been lost. On regaining consciousness, Denise was combative with the hospital staff. She pulled the intravenous tubes from her arms and screamed that she wanted to go home immediately, that she was being held illegally against her will. The psychiatry team was brought in, and they promptly committed her to the locked psychiatry unit of the general hospital. As a standard part of the legal procedure, Larry was asked to be the petitioner for the commitment, and he agreed.

On the psychiatry unit, Denise was placed on highly sedating antipsychotic medications and was continuously watched by hospital staff to prevent suicidal behavior. Although she was not hallucinating and did not seem to have paranoid delusions, the intensity of her rage and her combativeness with the hospital staff approached psychosis. After 5 days on high doses of the medications, Denise calmed down—to a point. During couples counseling it was determined with certainty that Larry had no relationship whatsoever with the woman over whom Denise had erupted. As he had stated, Larry had never even spoken with her. Denise, however, shifted the reason for her fury to Larry's participation as the petitioner in her legal commitment to the psychiatry locked unit:

Denise Bishop:[2] I will file for divorce as soon as I get out of here. How could you ever expect me to trust a man who turns against his wife and locks her up in a mental hospital? That will be on my record forever. How do I know that he won't try to lock me up again any time that we have the slightest disagreement?

Psychiatric social worker: Larry was trying to get you help and save your life. He was doing what any responsible husband would do after his wife made such a serious suicide attempt. Don't you think that your behavior had any role in his decision to commit you to the hospital?

---

[2]This dialogue was reconstructed from hospital records as described in note 1.

> **Denise:** You are wasting your time and my time. It's all over between us. As soon as I get out of here, I am filing for a divorce and for full custody of Hope.

Denise refused to speak with Larry further. She was discharged from the hospital with the diagnosis of borderline personality disorder. On her discharge, Denise hired an attorney who specialized in family law. Even though Larry had not taken illegal drugs for several years and had cut way down on his drinking since Hope had been born, Denise and her attorney made a major issue of his history of substance abuse and the potential danger to Hope. Denise was successful in securing full custody of Hope, as well as alimony and child support from Larry.

Treatment Approach to Denise Hughes, Part Four: Self-Mutilation and Suicidality in People With Borderline Personality Disorder

Self-Mutilation

Self-mutilation can be differentiated from suicide attempts. Both behaviors occur frequently among people with borderline personality disorder, and both behaviors must be addressed actively and definitively by the patient's clinician. People with this condition self-inflict bodily injuries in a variety of ways and for many reasons. Burning one's skin with matches or cigarettes, making multiple lacerations with sharp objects or even fingernails, and inflicting blunt trauma on parts of the body with the fists or other implements are among the more common means of self-mutilation. Many patients are not able to explain their reasons for injuring themselves, but they are able to describe how they feel during the act. They will say such things as the following:

> I don't know why I cut myself. A strange feeling overcomes me and I find myself cutting on my arms.
> I become overwhelmed with anger and self-hate. When I begin to burn myself, I start to feel more calm and in control.
> I like the feeling of the warm blood on my skin. It makes me feel more alive and less numb.
> I don't feel anything when I bruise my legs. It is as if someone else is hitting me and I am floating above it all, looking down on them doing it to me.

When the clinician asks these patients whether or not they are trying to kill themselves or wish to be dead, they will respond as follows:

> Oh no, Doctor, this has nothing to do with wanting to die. In fact, it is
> much more about my wanting to be alive. When I cut myself
> I have no intention whatsoever of killing myself.

My treatment strategy with Denise Hughes was first to make it clear to her that I construed that her past episodes of self-mutilation were seriously harmful to her and that I wished to work with her to find ways of controlling and stopping this behavior. Please note that I did not feign therapeutic neutrality about this behavior. Rather, I clearly communicated to Mrs. Hughes that as a physician, it was my responsibility to work with her to identify, prevent, and treat anything that would be potentially damaging to her body. Second, I engaged her in the exploration of the situational and psychological precipitants to her cutting herself. It was soon evident to both of us that when she felt abandoned or rejected by people who are important to her, she would feel frantic, furious, vulnerable, and out of control. Third, we developed strategies for her to identify these situations, feelings, and alternatives to dealing with her feelings. When similar feelings and situations would arise in the future, she was encouraged to discuss her feelings with the other party involved. Through such communication she found that she felt safer and more in control. Fourth, I worked with her to understand the life experiences and resultant feelings that led her to react so fiercely to abandonment, such as the psychological abuse by her mother and the sexual abuse by Jake. These insights helped her to relinquish her self-blame for these experiences and to improve her sense of self-worth. Over time, her episodes of cutting herself became progressively fewer.

Suicide

Not only are suicide attempts common among people with borderline personality disorder, but also 8%–10% of people with this diagnosis will ultimately kill themselves (American Psychiatric Association Practice Guidelines 2001). For this reason, mental health professionals must regularly assess the suicidal potential of their patients with this diagnosis and must respond accordingly. Responses can include hospitalization to protect patients from themselves and to provide treatment until it is safe for them to return to an outpatient setting. *All suicide threats must be taken with the utmost seriousness, and the clinician and family should avoid interpretations regarding the manipulative nature of such threats or gestures.* Summarized in Table 10–1 are the guiding principles regarding the suicidal potential of people with borderline personality disorder; presented in Table 10–2 is a summary of key principles

TABLE 10–1. Guiding principles for responding to the suicidality of people with borderline personality disorder

1. Suicide attempts and completed acts are common among people with borderline personality disorder.

2. All threats and so-called gestures must be taken seriously and responded to directly by clinicians and family members.

3. Frequent, regularly scheduled sessions with a qualified, experienced clinician should be arranged, and suicide risk should be monitored routinely in these sessions.

4. Family members and significant others should be educated regarding the identification of suicide risk and should be encouraged to communicate increased risk to the clinician.

5. Identification of precipitants of suicidal behavior—including perceived rejection and abandonment—will help the patient understand, avoid, and deal with these sources of stress.

6. Pharmacological and psychosocial treatment of coexisting major depression, bipolar disorder, alcoholism and substance abuse, and symptoms such as impulsivity and intense anger are powerful measures in the prevention of suicide.

Source. Adapted from "American Psychiatric Association Practice Guidelines: Practice Guideline for the Treatment of Patients With Borderline Personality Disorder." Am J Psychiatry 158 (10 suppl):24, 2001. Used with permission.

regarding the psychiatric history of people with borderline personality disorder as exemplified by the case of Denise Hughes.

Diagnosis in the Case of Denise Hughes

Data From Multiple Sources

From the time that I first learned about Denise Hughes from her father-in-law, Dr. Boswell Hughes, I hypothesized that she might have borderline personality disorder. This was confirmed by her behavior during the early stages of her treatment. Presented in Table 10–3 is a summary of the behaviors of Mrs. Hughes and the responses of others to her behavior that helped support this diagnosis.

DSM-IV-TR Diagnostic Criteria for Borderline Personality Disorder

Listed in Table 10–4 are DSM-IV-TR diagnostic criteria for borderline personality disorder (American Psychiatric Association 2000).

TABLE 10–2. Key principles of borderline personality disorder exemplified by the case of Denise Hughes, part I: initial psychiatric history

Historical fact	Key principle	Interpretation
Denise neither felt close to nor trusted her mother.	The lifelong pattern of intense and unstable interpersonal relationships of people with borderline personality disorder often begins with problematic relationships with a parent or parents.	Not having a positive and nurturing role model as a mother was an early genesis of Denise's low self-esteem and poor self-confidence.
Denise's mother fought constantly with Denise's father and turned Denise's sisters against her.	It is likely that Denise's mother also had borderline personality disorder, which is five times more common among first-degree biological relatives of those with the disorder than in the general population.	From both genetic (i.e., nature) and experiential (i.e., nurture) perspectives, Denise had a high risk of developing borderline personality disorder.
Denise was sexually abused during her childhood and adolescence by her mother's boyfriend, Jake.	Approximately 50% of women with borderline personality disorder were sexually abused as children and/or adolescents; in 25% of cases, they were sexually abused by a primary caregiver such as their father.	Having been psychologically and physically abused by her mother and sexually abused by Jake, Denise was not able to establish close or trusting relationships with either women or men.

TABLE 10–2. Key principles of borderline personality disorder exemplified by the case of Denise Hughes, part I: initial psychiatric history *(continued)*

Historical fact	Key principle	Interpretation
Denise's feelings "went numb" during her repeated episodes of molestation by Jake.	The denial and repression of powerful feelings leads to the development of symptoms.	Denise's deadening of her painful feelings began as an adaptive response to Jake's sexual abuse and persisted as a maladaptive pattern of denial of her important feelings and dissociation as an adult.
On numerous occasions, Denise would make multiple cuts on her body with razor blades.	Self-mutilation can bring transient relief to people with borderline personality disorder in several ways: by reaffirming their ability to feel, by reestablishing a sense of body boundaries, and through self-punishment for their sense of being "bad."	On feeling abandoned by a loved one, Denise would redirect the resulting rage from the other person to herself.
At times of extreme stress, Denise would want to die and would attempt suicide.	8%–10% of people with borderline personality disorder will commit suicide. All gestures and attempts must be taken seriously and constitute medical emergencies.	In addition to her diagnosis of borderline personality disorder, Denise also met DSM criteria for major depression and alcohol abuse. Cumulatively, these diagnoses exponentially increased her risk of suicide.

TABLE 10–2. Key principles of borderline personality disorder exemplified by the case of Denise Hughes, part I: initial psychiatric history (*continued*)

Historical fact	Key principle	Interpretation
Denise became violent and self-destructive when she thought that Larry was interested in another woman.	Overreaction to perceived abandonment and to perceived rejection is a core problem of people with borderline personality disorder.	Denise's fear of abandonment by Larry led to her rejection of him. Her fear became her reality.
In court, Denise was awarded full custody of her daughter and a substantial settlement from Larry on their divorce.	People with borderline personality disorder can rise to the occasion for brief periods of time, during which they appear reasonable and are persuasive.	Although she was on many occasions out of control and appeared psychotic, at other times Denise was able to be calm and convincing. She was also able and willing to distort the truth to get her way.
Denise forced her second husband, James, to cut off all contact with his family and friends.	People with borderline personality disorder try to control the outside interactions and communications of all people who are important to them.	Denise sought to devalue and "excommunicate" James's parents while at the same time soliciting and accepting large amounts of money from them.
James Hughes believed Denise to be "the most brilliant and beautiful woman who has ever lived."	People with borderline personality disorder insist that they be idealized by those with whom they have important relationships.	Denise was fearful that she would be abandoned if James was realistic in his appraisal of her.

TABLE 10–2. Key principles of borderline personality disorder exemplified by the case of Denise Hughes, part I: initial psychiatric history *(continued)*

Historical fact	Key principle	Interpretation
On marrying Denise, James left his job, became obese, and grew progressively dependent on her and his parents.	People with borderline personality disorder are threatened by the success and self-sufficiency of those with whom they have important relationships.	Through her relentless criticism of James, Denise reinforced his weaknesses and dependencies. She feared that if James were successful and self-sufficient, he would have the confidence and wherewithal to leave her.
Denise despised psychiatrists.	People with borderline personality disorder are initially threatened by the impartiality and authority of qualified and ethical mental health professionals.	Denise's experience with mental health professionals in the general hospital after her suicide attempts revealed to her that they were not easily manipulated or controlled.

TABLE 10–3. Data from the history and treatment of Denise Hughes that support a diagnosis of borderline personality disorder

1. Her refusal to allow James to interact freely with his parents while at the same time demanding, expecting, and accepting large amounts of their money

2. Her confrontational interactions with my office staff over the scheduling of her initial appointment

3. The uncharacteristically intense, negative reactions of my office staff to Mrs. Hughes

4. Her continued efforts to coerce me to alter the standard boundaries and rules of psychotherapy

5. Her expressions of anger and devaluation when I would not change the standard boundaries and rules of psychotherapy

6. Her history of being physically and psychologically abused as a child by her mother and sexually abused by Jake

7. Her recurrent episodes of major depression as an adolescent and an adult

8. Her regular use of illicit substances (primarily marijuana) as an adolescent and an adult

9. Her severe rage attacks and suicidal behavior as a reaction to perceived abandonment by her first husband, Larry Bishop

10. Her unfounded beliefs about Larry Bishop's relationships with other women that approached paranoia

11. Her persistent negativity and irritability

12. Her predominant psychological defensive style of splitting, in which she idealized people whom she believed admired her and devalued just about everyone else

13. Her compulsion to control what people think of her by limiting their communication and interactions

14. Her failure to establish a sustained and positive identity, either in her family (e.g., as a daughter, sister, or wife); academically, or vocationally (she did not study in school and never trained for a job nor held a job for a sustained period of time), or spiritually (she did not attend church)

Diagnostic Features of Borderline Personality Disorder
(Slightly Modified From DSM-IV-TR, pp. 706–708)

The essential feature of borderline personality disorder is a pervasive pattern of instability of interpersonal relationships, self-image, and affects, along with marked impulsivity, that begins by early adulthood and is present in a variety of contexts.

TABLE 10–4. Diagnostic criteria for borderline personality disorder (slightly modified from DSM-IV-TR)

A pervasive pattern of instability of interpersonal relationships, self-image, and affects, and marked impulsivity beginning by early adulthood and present in a variety of contexts, as indicated by five (or more) of the following:

(1) frantic efforts to avoid real or imagined abandonment. **Note:** Do not include suicidal or self-mutilating behavior covered in Criterion 5.

(2) a pattern of unstable and intense interpersonal relationships characterized by alternating between extremes of idealization and devaluation

(3) identity disturbance: markedly and persistently unstable self-image or sense of self

(4) impulsivity in at least two areas that are potentially self-damaging (e.g., spending, sex, substance abuse, reckless driving, binge eating).

(5) recurrent suicidal behavior, gestures, or threats, or self-mutilating behavior

(6) affective instability due to a marked reactivity of mood (e.g., intense episodic dysphoria, irritability, or anxiety usually lasting a few hours and only rarely more than a few days)

(7) chronic feelings of emptiness

(8) inappropriate, intense anger or difficulty controlling anger (e.g., frequent displays of temper, constant anger, recurrent physical fights)

(9) transient, stress-related paranoid ideation or severe dissociative symptoms[a]

Source.   Adapted from American Psychiatric Association: *Diagnostic and Statistical Manual of Mental Disorders,* 4th Edition, Text Revision. Washington, DC, American Psychiatric Association, 2000, p 710. Used with permission.

[a]*Dissociative symptoms* refer to psychological disruptions, either temporary or permanent, of a person's consciousness, memory functions, perceptions, and/or identity. People with dissociative disorders can have *dissociative amnesia,* in which they cannot recall important personal information or significant events, or *dissociative fugue,* in which they wander away from their home or workplace and do not recall who they are or how they got to the place where they are. These conditions are usually associated with significant distress secondary to extraordinary physical, sexual, and/or psychological trauma. Although Denise Hughes felt "numb" during the times when Jake was abusing her sexually, she recalled the traumatic events and retained her sense of identity. At the time of my evaluation of Mrs. Hughes, she met all nine criteria for borderline personality disorder. —*S.C.Y.*

People with borderline personality disorder make frantic efforts to avoid real or imagined abandonment. The perception of impending separation or rejection, or the loss of external structure, may lead to profound changes in self-image, affect, thinking, and behavior. These individuals are very sensitive to environmental circumstances. They experience intense abandonment fears and inappropriate anger, even when faced with a realistic time-limited separation or when there are unavoidable changes in plans (e.g., sudden despair in reaction to a clinician's announcing an impending vacation; panic or fury when someone important to them is just a few minutes late or must cancel an appointment). They may believe that this "abandonment" implies that they are "bad." Their frantic efforts to avoid abandonment may include impulsive actions such as self-mutilating or suicidal behaviors.

People with borderline personality disorder have a pattern of unstable and intense relationships. They may idealize potential caregivers or suitors at the first or second meeting, demand to spend a lot of time together, and share the most intimate details early in a relationship. However, they soon switch from idealizing these people to devaluing them, because they feel that the other person does not care enough, does not give enough, or is not "there" enough for them. Some people with borderline personality disorder can empathize with and nurture other people, but usually with the expectation that the other person will "be there" in return to meet their own needs on demand. They are prone to sudden and dramatic shifts in their views of others, who may be viewed by them alternately as beneficent and supportive or as cruelly punitive. Such shifts often reflect disillusionment with a caregiver whose nurturing qualities had been idealized or whose rejection or abandonment is expected.

There may be an identity disturbance characterized by markedly and persistently unstable self-image or sense of self, accompanied by sudden and dramatic shifts in self-image characterized by shifting goals, values, and vocational aspirations. People with this disorder may experience sudden changes in opinions and plans about career, sexual identity, values, and types of friends. They may rapidly change from the role of a needy supplicant for help to a righteous avenger of past mistreatment. Although these individuals usually have a self-image that is based on being bad or evil, people with this disorder may at times have feelings that they do not exist at all. Such existential types of experience usually occur in situations in which they feel the lack of a meaningful relationship or sufficient nurturing and support.

People with borderline personality disorder display impulsivity in at least two areas that are potentially self-damaging. They may gamble, spend money irresponsibly, binge eat, abuse substances, engage in unsafe sex, or drive recklessly. They frequently exhibit recurrent suicidal behavior, gestures, or threats, or self-mutilating behavior. Completed suicide occurs in 8%–10% of such individuals, and self-mutilative acts (e.g., cutting or burning) and suicide threats and attempts are very common. Suicidal acts are often the reason that people with this condition are first evaluated by psychiatrists. Their self-destructive acts are usually precipitated by threats of separation or rejection. Self-mutilation may occur during dissociative experiences and often brings relief by reaffirming the ability to feel or by expiating the individual's sense of being evil.

People with borderline personality disorder may display unstable emotions that stem from a marked reactivity to events in their lives. The basic depressed mood of those with borderline personality disorder is often punctuated by periods of intense anger, panic, or despair. Periods of well-being or satisfaction are rare and brief.

People with borderline personality disorder may be troubled by chronic feelings of emptiness. Easily bored, they may constantly seek something new to do. They frequently express inappropriate, intense anger or have difficulty controlling their anger. Expressions of anger may take the form of extreme sarcasm, enduring bitterness, or verbal outbursts. The anger is often elicited when a caregiver or suitor is regarded as neglectful, withholding, uncaring, or abandoning. Such expressions of anger are often followed by shame and guilt that contribute to their feelings of being a bad or evil person.

During periods of extreme stress, people with borderline personality disorder may experience transient paranoia or dissociative symptoms. These episodes occur most frequently in response to a real or imagined abandonment. The real or perceived return of the caregiver's nurturance may result in a remission of their dissociative or psychotic (most often paranoid) symptoms.

Borderline Personality Disorder as a Medical Illness

Epidemiology

Borderline personality disorder is, by a large measure, the most commonly diagnosed personality disorder. It is estimated that about 2% of the general population has this condition (Clarkin and Sanderson 1993; Swartz et al. 1990), and about 75% of the people with this diagnosis are women. The high proportion of women to men *reported to have this diagnosis* may be the result of cultural factors. It is possible that women with this condition are more often seen in mental health programs, where 10% of outpatients and up to 20% of inpatients carry this diagnosis. Men with borderline personality disorder may go undiagnosed and untreated and are probably overrepresented in prison populations compared with the percentage of people with this condition who are not incarcerated. Note that intense anger, impulsively, and substance abuse combine to form a dangerous brew in men, who are more prone to act violently than are women. On the other hand, childhood sexual abuse—which is highly correlated with the occurrence of borderline personality disorder—is much more common for girls than for boys, which could lead to the higher prevalence of the diagnosis in women. Although several child psychiatrists believe that children can exhibit many of the signs and symptoms that are diagnostic of borderline personality disorder, most mental health professionals believe that this diagnosis cannot and should not be made before adolescence. I fully agree, and in fact I do not believe that diagnosing this disorder in children or adolescents is helpful to them. Right or wrong, the diagnosis of borderline personality disorders carries with it a great stigma, not only among the general population but also with health care providers, who are wary of becoming enmeshed in time-consuming and emotionally draining power struggles with the patients and their families. I also believe that the emotional lability and interpersonal upheavals that are so common among adolescents are easily confused with the symptoms of borderline personality disorder.

Inheritance and Genetics

Many investigators have documented an increased incidence of borderline personality disorder in family members of those with the condition. Dr. Mary C. Zanarini and colleagues (1988) not only found that about 25% of the first-degree relatives of patients with borderline personality disorder also met criteria for this diagnosis (significantly higher than the expected 2% as seen in the general population), but also that these relatives had somewhat higher risks for major depression (31.2%) and for alcoholism (24.3%) than are found in the general population. Twin studies and adoptive studies, however, are needed to separate the "nature versus nurture" aspects of these findings. Although such studies have been conducted and have provided strong evidence for the hereditary transmission of alcoholism, schizotypal personality disorder, and antisocial personality disorder, comparable twin research does not confirm a genetic transmission of borderline personality disorder. The only twin study conducted to date did not confirm greater prevalence of the condition in monozygotic twins with borderline personality disorder than in the dizygotic twins with this diagnosis. However, the sample size for this study was very small (Torgersen 1984). No adoptive studies have been published for patients with this condition. Thus there is a serious deficiency of first-rate genetic research of borderline personality disorder, particularly for a condition that constitutes from 30% to 60% (depending on the specific study and the level—inpatient vs. outpatient—of treatment of the patient) of the diagnoses among clinical populations of people with personality disorders.

The strong association of major depression with borderline personality disorder may be the result of the psychological and physical trauma experienced during childhood by most people with this personality disorder. In other words, the same trauma that in part gave rise to the personality disorder also precipitated the mood disorder. It is also possible that the association of these two serious psychiatric diagnoses is the result of an identical gene or, much more likely, a series of many genes that underlie both conditions. On a positive note, some progress has been made in understanding the genetics of specific dimensions of personality that are common in patients with borderline personality disorder. For example, twin and adoption studies have been conducted on such traits as *reward dependence* (social attachment vs. disgust and isolation) and *novelty seeking* (impulsivity vs. slowness to anger), and the heritability of these traits has been demonstrated at a level 40%–60% greater among twins than in other close family members (Knowles 2003). In the absence of other data, this finding might indicate that certain genetically transmitted brain-based traits or tendencies such as impulsivity, emotional lability, aggression, and even abandonment sensitivity might be the *primary* biological phenomena that lead to the secondary behavioral patterns, or **epiphenomena,** such as self-mutilation and temper outbursts, that make up the criteria for the full-blown syndrome of borderline personality disorder.

Among what I would consider primary biological phenomena of borderline personality disorder, the genetics of aggression is the best studied and understood. I would expand the usual definition of aggression—violence against another person—to also include acts of violence against oneself such as self-mutilation and suicidal behavior. In addition, I would include both physical violence and verbal violence (e.g., threats, virulent criticism, psychological abuse) as conceptualized in the Overt Aggression Scale (Yudofsky et al. 1981). Given these factors, twin and adoption studies derived from more than 20 separate studies indicate that more than 50% of the contribution (technically called *variance* among geneticists) toward aggressive behavior derives from genetic predispositions, as opposed to environmental and experiential factors (Miles and Carey 1997; Tecott and Barondes 1996). I believe that in the future, epidemiological research with twins and adoptees with aggressive disorders will lead to locating sites on genes that are responsible for abnormal human aggression. This will then pave the scientific pathway for further research that will increase the understanding of the brain chemistry behind aggression and violence. Such knowledge will then guide our development of novel genetic and pharmacological treatments for people with the many types of aggressive disorders, including borderline personality disorder, in which hostility and violence toward others and the self are common.

Role of the Brain in Borderline Personality Disorder

Evidence from a variety of disparate sources indicates that patients with borderline personality disorder have increased incidences of brain-based dysfunctions. That being said, the most important principle in linking brain biology to all personality disorders is that *brain and other biological abnormalities relate more closely to abnormal behaviors and emotions than to specific diagnoses.*

Poor Executive Functioning

Neuropsychological tests show that patients with borderline personality disorder have impairments in the type of planning that involves multiple operations—such as moving a business to a new location—and in performance of complex auditory and visual memory tasks (Burgess 1991). The net result is frustration with having to perform several different tasks simultaneously or with having to make plans that require sequencing or staging of activities. These capacities to plan and perform complex, sequenced tasks are called *executive functions,* and they are localized prominently, although not entirely, in the prefrontal cortex of the brain.

Neurological Soft Signs

Neurological testing of people with borderline personality disorder has demonstrated that they exhibit increased involuntary movements such as tics, as well as problems with complex patterned movements, such as rapidly alternating hand movements (Gardner et al. 1987). These functions are coordinated by brain systems and pathways that involve vast networks of neurons and connections in the cortical and deeper brain regions. Such dysfunctions are called *soft signs,* as contrasted with other types of motor and sensory impairments that can be localized to lesions in specific brain areas. The bottom line is that although these soft signs are suggestive of some brain-based impairment, the neurological examination of people with borderline personality disorder is not especially clinically useful at the present time.

Disinhibition

Impulsivity, irritability, affective instability, and low frustration tolerance are core symptoms of borderline personality disorder. These symptoms are characteristic of lesions to specific regions of the brain that are involved in the disinhibition of anger and aggressive behavior. In general, regions in the prefrontal cortex of the brain maintain control of (i.e., inhibit) deeper brain regions such as the limbic system (the amygdala and cortex of the temporal lobe) that are involved in fight-or-flight types of behavior. If any type of lesion—resulting, for example, from birth trauma, head injury, brain infections, or exposure to toxins—were to affect the neurons in the prefrontal cortex, the ability of the frontal cortex to keep the limbic region under check would be compromised, a process called *disinhibition* (Ovsiew and Yudofsky 1993). ***The net result would be an excessive response of rage and aggression to minor stimuli or provocations.*** Investigators have found an increased incidence of brain injuries in certain populations of patients with borderline personality disorder (81%) compared with control subjects (22%) who are matched for age, gender, and life experience (van Reekum et al. 1993).

Brain Biochemistry

The source of the incomparable complexity and potential of the human brain is the system of chemical messengers (called *neurotransmitters*) that connect the billions of neurons, the cells that are the fundamental unit of the brain. In broad overview, human functions are coordinated in the brain by opposing systems and operations—very much like the accelerator and brake of an automobile. The brain coordinates, for example, the flexing of an arm by simultaneously tightening the biceps and relaxing the triceps. Different brain systems use specific chemical transmitters to regulate feelings and behaviors. Prominent symptoms in borderline personality disorder include episodic depression, irritability, violence, self-mutilation, and suicidal behaviors. Psychiatry has learned a great deal about the brain biochemistry that underlies all of these symptoms. We know, for example, that the neurotransmitters serotonin, epinephrine, dopamine, and norepinephrine are involved in this constellation of symptoms. We also know that medications that affect these transmitters can be helpful in the treatment of these syndromes and symptoms. For example, we know that medications called selective serotonin reuptake inhibitors (SSRIs) are not only beneficial in treating the depression of patients with borderline personality disorder but are also effective in mitigating their other symptoms, such irritability, aggression, and self-mutilation.

Fight-or-flight types of behaviors and associated feelings are known to be regulated in part by systems in the brain and the rest of the body called the *sympathetic nervous system.* A category of neurotransmitters involved in *initiating* fight-or-flight behaviors are called *catecholamines,* and these include brain transmitters such as epinephrine, dopamine, and norepinephrine. Prolonged use of certain drugs (such as cocaine and amphetamines) that increase levels of these brain chemicals are strongly associated with increased irritability, paranoia, rage, and violence. Fight-or-flight types of behaviors are inhibited by brain systems that involve neurotransmitters including serotonin and γ-aminobutyric acid (GABA). Medications that increase levels of these neurotransmitters can have a calming effect on feelings and a modulating effect on behavior. Certain investigators have persuasively proposed that people who have impulsive aggression and commit violent suicides (stabbing oneself as opposed to overdosing) have abnormalities in the brain systems that involve serotonin and its receptors, and at the root of these abnormalities are genetic risk factors (Mann et al. 2000, 2001). One excellent study demonstrated that people who have made violent suicide attempts have *lower* levels of the metabolized byproducts of brain serotonin and increased levels of the breakdown product of epinephrine (Traskman-Bendz et al. 1992). This finding would support the theory that serotonin inhibits self-violence and that an overactive sympathetic nervous system heightens this type of behavior. Although there are interesting therapeutic correlations to these theories in the pharmacological treatment of patients with borderline personality disorder, I must emphasize that due to the extraordinary complexity of the human brain, most of these theories will be modified significantly (or disproved) over time.

Necessary Qualifications for a Mental Health Professional Treating a Patient With Borderline Personality Disorder

Basic Educational Requisites

Clinicians who are inexperienced and not specifically trained to treat patients with borderline personality disorder will rapidly find themselves over their heads. What does it take to become an educated and experienced professional in the treatment of people with this condition? Of course, the clinician must first have had formal training in a mental health discipline such as psychiatry (medical school and a psychiatry residency); psychology (graduate school in clinical psychology; psychology internship); or social work (graduate school at the master's level; postgraduate education in psychotherapy or psychoanalysis).

Although such training is a requisite bare minimum, it is insufficient for treating patient patients with borderline personality disorder.

The Essential Role of a Supervisor in the Education of the Clinician

A therapist cannot learn how to treat people with this disorder from books or in the classroom. Similar to the way a young surgeon learns his or her skills in the operating room alongside a master surgeon, an experienced *supervisor* must work, on a regular and ongoing basis, with the novice clinician as he or she cares for a patient with borderline personality disorder. The supervisor will review and guide the clinician on each aspect of the care of a patient with this disorder. Every issue that the patient raises in treatment has important meaning and implications, which the novice clinician must understand to be able to make the correct response and intervention. Supervision is accomplished by the novice clinician taking careful notes during each treatment session documenting as exactly as possible what is said by both the patient and the therapist. Then, in a regular and ongoing fashion, the novice must carefully go over these notes with the supervisor to gain a better understanding of the patient and to learn which responses are helpful and which are not.

Unwarranted Pessimism Regarding the Treatment of People With Borderline Personality Disorder

Many mental health professionals have unwarranted therapeutic pessimism about the benefits of treatment for people with borderline personality disorder. Their pessimism derives from the disastrous treatment experiences that many patients with this condition have as the result of their care by inexperienced therapists. Often such therapists are incapable of establishing therapeutic boundaries with their patients, an essential first step that must be accomplished before any meaningful change can occur. What usually happens is that the patient will find a way to induce the clinician to change the standard rules of treatment. Examples include the therapist's increasing the duration of sessions, giving the patient special access during off hours, or sharing personal information about himself or herself with the patient. Initially there is a "therapeutic honeymoon" during which the patient feels unique and special and idealizes the clinician for being a real and caring person, as opposed to some rigid automaton. Unconsciously, what the patient is usually after is a replication by the therapist of a type of parental prioritization and nurturing that the patient did not receive as a child. Of course, no therapist can or should replace the functions of a parent. If the therapist is seduced into trying to become the "good parent," at some point the patient will make a request or demand that the clinician cannot accommodate. Representative examples include the following: 1) the patient asks to join the clinician on his or her vacation; 2) the patient asks to be allowed to spend the night at the therapist's house during times of high anxiety or stress; 3) the patient demands to know the birthdates of the therapist's children, so that he or she may send them gifts. When the inexperienced clinician is finally pushed too far and refuses to acquiesce to these or similar requests or demands, the patient feels betrayed and abandoned. At that point, the tenor of the relationship changes dramatically as the patient experiences and expresses the full depth of his or her anger that stems from parental deprivation and abuse. The transferential situation is now out of control, because the patient cannot differentiate the therapist from the abusive parent. Often the patient will turn this rage on himself or herself with a self-defeating behavior ranging from missing work and therapy sessions to suicide attempts. The patient's message to the therapist is "Not only haven't you helped me, but you have made me worse!"

The good news is that in many studies scholars have reported that people with borderline personality disorder are profoundly helped and changed when they have the opportunity to be treated by clinicians who are well trained and *experienced* in helping people with this condition (Koenigsberg et al. 2000; Stone 1990, 2000).

Initial Treatment of Denise Hughes: The First Six Months

Setting Limits

Please recall that the initial sessions of my treatment of Mrs. Hughes consisted of seemingly endless discussions of format and formalities, including 1) how we should address each other, 2) why she could not have my home phone number, and 3) why I would not prescribe certain medications for her. Mrs. Hughes expressed, in no uncertain terms, her deep resentment at my unwillingness to be flexible and accommodating. My setting of clear limits for Mrs. Hughes accomplished several important therapeutic ends:

- She learned that I was not promising to fulfill all her needs, as a devoted mother would be responsive to the needs of her baby.
- Her expressions of anger and bitterness toward me early in treatment obviated her idealization of me. Had she idealized me, I would have been raised to a treatment-threatening height—a pedestal from which I was certain to fall.

- She learned that I was an individuated person who could not be controlled by her threats, devaluation, or other types of coercion.

Because I had kept her expectations of me and of treatment modest and realistic by discouraging her idealization of me and by insisting that she respect my boundaries (and that I respect hers), Mrs. Hughes did not feel misled or abandoned when I could not or would not fulfill her unrealistic or unreasonable needs. For the first time in her life, Denise Hughes was in a significant, prolonged relationship that was neither abusive nor exploitive nor one in which she was in complete control. This relationship was to serve as a testing ground and model for more healthy involvements in the future. Very much worth noting about this phase of treatment is that Mrs. Hughes insisted on seeing me individually and agreed to have her husband treated by another psychiatrist. Given her history of demanding total control in her relationship with her husband, I viewed her granting him permission to see a psychiatrist on his own as a positive indication that Mrs. Hughes had some motivation to be helped by psychiatric treatment. I speculated that this motivation derived from the considerable psychological pain from which she chronically suffered, and from her desire not to damage her daughter, Hope, by replicating the abuse that she herself had experienced in childhood.

Taking Inventory of Mrs. Hughes's Current Psychiatric Symptoms

Although Mrs. Hughes initially did not believe that she needed psychiatric treatment, she nonetheless reported a wide range of symptoms. The psychiatric symptoms that Denise Hughes exhibited at the initiation of her treatment are summarized in Table 10–5.

Taking a History of Mrs. Hughes's Important Life Events

The history of Denise Hughes, which included psychological and sexual abuse and severely impaired interpersonal relationships, is presented above under "The Case of Denise Hughes."

Working With Mrs. Hughes to Link Her Aggressive and Self-Destructive Actions to Her Feelings

As obvious as it might be to someone else, Mrs. Hughes was largely unaware of her own angry feelings, the types of events that evoked these

---

TABLE 10–5.   Denise Hughes's psychiatric symptoms at the initial
phase of treatment

---

1. Sadness

2. Feelings of self-loathing, worthlessness, and hopelessness

3. Feelings of emptiness

4. Chronic anxiety

5. Insomnia and frightening dreams

6. Irritability, episodic temper tantrums, and violence

7. Binge drinking of alcohol

8. Episodic marijuana use (approximately once a week)

9. Use of Percodan (oxycodone/aspirin)

10. Suicidal thoughts

11. Episodic self-mutilation by cutting her arms, legs, and upper thighs with
    razor blades

12. Dissociation (alterations in one's state of consciousness or identity that can
    give rise to symptoms including amnesia, fugue, and multiple
    personalities)

13. Social isolation, including hostile relationships with the very few people
    with whom she interacted closely

---

feelings, and the relationship between these feelings and her self-defeating and self-destructive behaviors. I tried to help her identify the
connections between her angry feelings and hostile behaviors with the
current events of her life, including her therapeutic relationship with
me. Given our careful attention to structure and boundaries, Mrs.
Hughes's therapeutic relationship with me provided a much cleaner
field than her outside life for her to examine these connections. One
clinical example occurred after about 6 months of treatment, when it
was necessary for me to miss one of her usually scheduled therapeutic
sessions because of an out-of-town scientific symposium. I had notified
her several months in advance about the trip and encouraged her to discuss her feelings about the disruption of our work. Before my trip, Mrs.
Hughes maintained that she welcomed the opportunity of not being obligated to come to therapy and that she was "glad to have the extra time
to do some things that are really important." However, she forgot to
come to the next session that was scheduled on my return. At her following appointment, she first stated that she had been fine during the
2-week period when we had not seen one another. Much later in that

session, Mrs. Hughes disclosed, without any sign of emotion, that she had had several episodes of self-mutilation during the time that I was away. Chillingly, on the day of the canceled session, she carved in her arm with a razor blade the words "I hate me." Nonetheless, she was reluctant to associate her feelings of abandonment by me with her self-destructive act. When I asked her what she had been feeling when she cut herself, she said, "I wasn't feeling anything. I have no idea why I cut myself. I just felt like doing it."

Long-Term Treatment of Mrs. Hughes

In my experience, meaningful and lasting change for people with borderline personality disorder requires many years of intensive treatment. I do not trust "quick fixes" for people with this condition. Therefore, not only must clinicians be experienced and gifted in treating people with borderline personality disorder, they also must be committed to staying with their patients over the long haul. The patient must also be motivated to work in treatment, which is much different from just showing up for sessions. As stated, boundary and limit setting occur early in treatment, and the patient will invariably test these boundaries and limits throughout the course of treatment. Over time, however, the patient should feel more safe in the treatment setting and with the therapist, who can then explore the more sensitive and threatening life events and issues that lead to the patient's most disabling feelings and behaviors. In this section I summarize several key areas of treatment that took place during the next 3 years of Mrs. Hughes's treatment.

Exploring Mrs. Hughes's Relationship With Her Daughter, Hope

I believe that Mrs. Hughes's principal incentive to participate in treatment with me—beyond even the financial imperatives of Dr. Hughes—was to obtain help in her relationship with her daughter, Hope, who was 12 years old at that time. Bound by professional, legal, and humanitarian mandates to determine and report any form of child abuse, I inquired directly about this possibility during our first session. I noted that Mrs. Hughes was not at all upset or put off by this line of inquiry, as she seemed to be by just about every other issue that I raised regarding her treatment. I learned, and corroborated over subsequent sessions, that Mrs. Hughes was a devoted and attentive mother and that there was no evidence whatsoever of child abuse. This is not to say that she was the perfect mother (as if such a person exists). Mrs. Hughes was having significant difficulties in raising and caring for her daughter. Her primary concern was to protect Hope from experiencing the type of abuse that she herself had suffered as a child. Although it was mostly positive, Mrs. Hughes's priority of protecting Hope had several unintended, deleterious consequences. For example, she did not permit her daughter to spend the night at the homes of any of her friends, nor did she permit Hope to go on school-sponsored, teacher-supervised, overnight field trips with her classmates.

> **Mrs. Hughes:** Haven't you read in the paper about all the teachers who have sexually abused their students? And these are only the ones we know about. How can I be sure that one of them won't abuse Hope on an overnight field trip?
>
> **Dr. Y.:** You are right to be ever-watchful for any type of abuse of Hope. However, we don't want to place Hope in a glass bubble that isolates her from her peers and makes her feel self-conscious. If you will permit me, I will work with you to determine what activities place her at an unacceptable risk of being harmed and what activities are most likely safe. Given your terrible experience as a child with abuse, it is difficult for you to know where to draw this line.
>
> **Mrs. Hughes:** O.K. What would you advise about this 4-day field-trip to the state Capitol in Austin and to the Alamo in San Antonio? Hope has never spent one night away from me in her life. If you have children, would you let one of them go on a trip like this, particularly when I don't even know most of the teachers who will be going?
>
> **Dr. Y.:** First of all, Mrs. Hughes, thank you for your confidence in asking my help regarding Hope's well-being. I know and respect how concerned you are about her safety, particularly related to issues that have affected you so personally. Second, I believe it is safe to permit Hope to go on the field trip with her class. I believe that she will be around other students and several teachers all of the time on this trip. Therefore, the types of abuse about which you are concerned are very unlikely to occur. Third, I believe that it will be good for her to have some experience in being away from home for a brief period of time. This will help her self-confidence and healthful independence. Finally, I recommend that you invest in a cell phone for Hope and ask that she call you at a pre-arranged time, such as 7:30 P.M. This will reduce your anxiety about her well-being, and I also know that Hope will like to touch base with you daily. One caveat, however, Mrs. Hughes. You have to show restraint and call her only at the prearranged time. On the other hand, if there is an emergency, Hope can call you. If you don't hear from her or a teacher, you can assume she is fine. In this fashion, you don't need to be worried about her safety the whole time that she is away.

This interchange demonstrates the types of psychotherapeutic treatment that is recommended for people with borderline personality disorder: The therapist should be empathic and supportive, directive (e.g., offer advice about key issues in their lives), and interpretive (e.g., explore with them the unconscious origins of their self-defeating behaviors) (Gunderson and Links 2001). The therapist should be more active and directive in treating people with this condition than in the care of most other people in outpatient therapy for different types of psychiatric problems. There are several reasons for this approach. First, people with borderline personality disorder can have problems with reality testing, especially when they are under stress. One component of the psychotherapist's job is to advise them on ways to avoid stressful situations, as well as to help them with testing reality. For example, most of the patients whom I treat would not require nor would they seek my advice regarding cellular telephone communication with their children. However, I made this suggestion to Mrs. Hughes to allay her anxiety sufficiently to allow her daughter to begin to make healthy separations from her. The most important part of that advice was to suggest that she not call her daughter during the trip, but allow Hope to control this aspect of their communication by calling at a prearranged time. After the field trip, I reinforced how the anticipation of feelings of separation and planning for ways to deal with them is a successful strategy to avoid stress and anxiety. Second, because of the high incidence of their being abused by parents or parental figures as children, people with this condition do not have good judgment about whom they can trust, nor have they been blessed with appropriate role models for functioning as parents. The therapist serves in and models these roles until such time as the patient has learned to perform these functions for himself or herself. This process, whereby the psychotherapy provides a vital interpersonal experience that the patient was not sufficiently fortunate to have previously and from which the patient can learn more adaptive behaviors, is termed a *corrective emotional experience.*

From what I learned from Mrs. Hughes, Hope seemed to be fairly well adjusted and was earning excellent grades in school. She made good friends in her neighborhood school and excelled in several extracurricular activities, including soccer and playing the flute. From her mother's report I detected no specific target symptoms that would justify a consultation from a child psychiatrist. Having been psychologically and physically abused by her own mother, Mrs. Hughes was fearful that she herself would someday lose control and harm Hope physically. This had never happened. Being a nurturing and supportive mother, however, was a great challenge for Mrs. Hughes. I explained to her that it is hard to give what you didn't get and that she deserved great credit for working so hard to support and sustain Hope. I also realized that there were many intrapsychic conflicts that Mrs. Hughes had to overcome (such as feeling envious of or competitive with Hope for having a more stable and nurturing childhood than she); but I postponed these explorations and insights until later in her treatment, when Mrs. Hughes would be psychologically stronger. My therapeutic strategy was to support Mrs. Hughes for many months until she had sufficient trust in me and adequate self-esteem to approach and (we hoped) to change the unflattering aspects of her personality, behavior, and emotions.

Exploring Mrs. Hughes's Relationship With Her Husband, James Hughes (Family Counseling)

Although James Hughes had consistently been thoughtful and generous to Denise and to Hope, Mrs. Hughes described him as a "weak person." By "weak" she meant that he was for the most part passive, avoided confrontations with everyone, and was easily manipulated. Mrs. Hughes believed that her husband's parents were overbearing, and she had convinced James that the only way he could achieve independence was by cutting off all contact with them. She also believed that he was being exploited in his teaching job by being required to work long hours (6 days a week) for very low pay, so she insisted on his quitting. In addition, Mrs. Hughes believed that James's friends in Houston (mostly other teachers) and from college discriminated against her because she was not college educated, and therefore she discouraged him from having any contact with them. From her descriptions it was clear to me that as a direct result of their relationship, James Hughes had changed from a happy, successful, and independent person to someone who was dependent on and terrorized by his wife. Paradoxically, Mrs. Hughes ceaselessly criticized James for the very behaviors and personality traits that she had encouraged.

> **Dr. Y.:** What do you most admire about your husband, James?
> **Mrs. Hughes:** In all candor there is very little to admire. He is not much of a man. He literally does nothing right, so I end up having to do everything myself. I make all the decisions, while he sits around like a lump eating junk food.
> **Dr. Y.:** What initially attracted you to James?
> **Mrs. Hughes:** I can't say that I have ever been attracted to him in a physical sense—especially not now since he has gotten so fat. What I first liked about him was how kind he was to Hope when

she was his student. She was having trouble in his math class, so he took extra time to help her and always included me in what he was doing and trying to accomplish. For the past 2 years he just gets in the way, like an overstuffed easy chair that takes up too much room and no one wants to sit in.

Dr. Y.: That is not a very flattering image to have of your husband.

Mrs. Hughes: Not flattering, but perfectly accurate.

From the earliest part of her treatment it was obvious to me that Mrs. Hughes had actively cut off all of her husband's contacts with his important past and current relationships so that she could exert complete and unchallenged control over him. Her fundamental fear of abandonment led her to criticize and devalue all of James's assets and personal strengths, lest he use these qualities to seek independence from her. Without seeing her part in his decline, she described the erosion of James's self-esteem, the loss of his self-confidence, and his progressive and paralytic passivity. Initially I chose not to emphasize with Mrs. Hughes the connection between her abandonment fears and her emasculation of her husband, because such a revelation, although accurate, would be too threatening. She would see me as being disloyal to her by my turning the very information that she provided against her in a way that made her feel like a "bad person." To make this connection too soon (technically termed a *premature interpretation*) would likely have resulted in her feeling abandoned by me, which she would counter by withdrawing from therapy: "I'll quit before you fire me." Inexperienced therapists (and friends of patients) often are in a great rush to share with patients (and friends) every insight they discover, most often with disastrous results. Conducting effective therapy is much like hitting a baseball thrown by a great pitcher: the pitches at which you don't swing are often more important than those you try to hit. Rather, I chose to devote the necessary treatment time that it would take for Mrs. Hughes to understand the source of her abandonment fears and pervasive needs to control, and thereafter to demonstrate the debilitating effects of these fears and needs in her present-day life. Over a long period of time, I also helped Mrs. Hughes understand how she confused a person's abusive behavior toward herself with his or her having strength and power. Thus the conflict: If she could get her husband to fight with her and abuse her, Mrs. Hughes would reexperience the devaluation and humiliation of her childhood. When James Hughes refused to be hostile and abusive, she regarded him as being weak and castrated.

I recommended that Mrs. Hughes engage in *family treatment* that was conducted by the psychiatrist who was treating her husband. This recommendation was made for a number of reasons:

- Meeting on a regular basis with her husband's psychiatrist would mitigate her fears and paranoia about what was going on in James's individual treatment. Otherwise she would fear that any growth or change by James would lead to his abandoning her.
- As James progressed in treatment, he would be become less tolerant of his wife's excessive control and criticism of him. Through ongoing family treatment, she could work on and improve her behavior toward him gradually as he progressed. This would prevent a precipitous breakup of the relationship, the result of Mr. Hughes becoming more independent while Mrs. Hughes's fears of abandonment led to the escalation of her outrageous behavior toward her husband.
- Both Mr. and Mrs. Hughes could learn to communicate better about key issues between them and how to work more productively as a team in caring for Hope.
- It was not advisable that I conduct the family treatment for Mr. and Mrs. Hughes. In the initial phases of her treatment with me, Mrs. Hughes would not have been able to tolerate the sharing of my attention with her husband. Sharing her psychiatrist with her husband would certainly have provoked intense transference feelings derived from her mother's favoritism toward her siblings during her childhood. Mrs. Hughes would have experienced me as a depriving parental figure who favored her husband, whom she would perceive as the favored sibling.

Psychopharmacology

Concurrent Psychiatric Disorders

Psychiatric medications can have great value in treating people with borderline personality disorder. I and several other psychopharmacologists advocate the identification of specific concurrent psychiatric disorders (such as depression and alcoholism) and target symptoms (such as irritability, agitation, impulsivity, psychosis, and anxiety) and using the medications that have been proven effective in the treatment of these conditions (Soloff 1993, 1998). For example, if a patient with borderline personality disorder also meets DSM criteria for major depression (which is quite common), antidepressants are indicated. In such circumstances, the medications will not only help relieve the debilitating physical and psychological symptoms of depression but will also— by enhancing the energy level, motivation, self-esteem, and optimism of the patient—greatly facilitate the progress of psychotherapy. When patients become episodically psychotic (e.g., showing paranoid and other types of impaired reality testing), the prompt use of antipsychotic medications is required to help abate self-destructive behaviors and avoid the necessity of hospitalization.

Anger and Aggression

Intense anger, irritability, agitation, impulsivity, and aggression are among the most disabling and disturbing symptoms and behaviors of almost every patient with borderline personality disorder. *Frequently, their hostility and violent outbursts result in precipitous life-changing events such as the loss of their jobs, injuries of themselves or other people, or physical and psychological abuse of family members.* In my treatment of patients with this condition, I pay close attention to this constellation of symptoms and behaviors. I work with these patients in psychotherapy to identify these feelings and related violent acts so that the patients can be aware of and avoid the circumstances in their lives that elicit these responses. I also work with them on a range of techniques that are helpful in anger management. In addition, I have found the knowledgeable, creative, and precise use of medications to be of extraordinary value in this population of patients.

Presented in Table 10–6 is a summary of important principles in the psychopharmacological treatment of anger and aggression in patients with borderline personality disorder.

One of my own research interests involves the use of medications to treat disinhibited anger and aggression that is often associated with neurological conditions such as traumatic brain injury, stroke, or seizure disorders. I and other investigators have demonstrated that medications used for other medical conditions are effective in reducing anger and precipitous, episodic violent behaviors. For example, a class of medications called β-blockers—propranolol (Inderal) is an example—reduces violent outbursts in patients with neurological conditions without sedating them (Yudofsky et al. 1981). Anticonvulsant medications such as carbamazepine (Tegretol) and valproate (Depakote) are also effective in this group of patients. I believe that the principles that have been developed for the "off-label" use of these medications in patients with neurological conditions also apply to treating the anger, irritability, impulsivity, and aggression of patients with borderline personality disorder. Readers who are interested in a review of the use of medications to treat aggression and anger are referred to the chapter on this subject in *The American Psychiatric Press Textbook of Psychopharmacology* (Yudofsky et al. 1998).

TABLE 10–6.   Key principles in the treatment of anger and aggression in patients with borderline personality disorder

---

1.   Self-treatment with alcohol, prescribed sedatives, and illicit substances— such as marijuana and opiates—aggravates their anger and aggression.

2.   Psychopharmacological treatment is rendered ineffective by the simultaneous use of alcohol and other substances of abuse.

3.   Many physicians are inexperienced in treating these symptoms of rage and violent behaviors. They use sedating medications such as benzodiazepines (e.g., Xanax, Valium, Ativan) to cover over the symptoms. Unfortunately, these drugs have no antiaggressive properties, are addictive, will oversedate the patient, and can even elicit violent outbursts.

4.   Currently there are no medications approved by the U.S. Food and Drug Administration to treat agitation, anger, aggression, or violence.

5.   Several studies have shown that medications approved for other purposes can be greatly helpful in the reduction of agitation, anger, irritability, impulsivity, aggression, and violence in patients with borderline personality disorder. This type of medication usage is termed "off-label" prescribing (Yudofsky et al. 1998).

6.   Among the types of medications that have been demonstrated to be helpful in treating anger and aggression (including self-directed aggression) in patients with borderline personality disorder are antidepressants, particularly selective serotonin reuptake inhibitors, and anticonvulsants, particularly carbamazepine (Tegretol) and valproate (Depakote) (Coccaro and Kavoussi 1997; Kavoussi and Coccaro 1998).

7.   These medications facilitate psychotherapy by reducing the patient's hostility toward the clinician and his or her therapeutic interventions.

Use of Medications in the Treatment of Mrs. Hughes

Early in the course of her treatment, I recommended to Mrs. Hughes that she consider taking fluoxetine (Prozac). I believed that this medication would not only treat her major depression, but would also reduce her anger that led her to be chronically irritable, hostile, and hypervigilant. Concurrent with this recommendation was my encouraging her to discontinue her use of alcohol and prescribed pain medications, which intensified her depression and rage. She accused me of pigeonholing her as a drug addict and refused to accept my recommendation of the antidepressant medication. Given her willingness to accept medications from other physicians, I reasoned (but did not interpret to her) that the highly personal nature of psychotherapy (e.g., meeting regularly, discussing intimate subjects) led her to be uncomfortable with the degree of trust of me that would be required to accept a mood-altering medication. I respected her boundaries and did not try to convince her to accept the prescription. Over the next several months, however, without fanfare or discussion, Mrs. Hughes tapered her use of Percodan (oxycodone/aspirin) and also stopped drinking alcohol. I viewed Mrs. Hughes's decision to stop taking addictive substances as a sign of her engagement in and commitment to psychotherapy. In psychiatric treatment, as in most of life, actions speak louder than words.

About a year later, she became greatly upset when Hope, then 14 years old, started to mature physically and emotionally and to attract the attention of the boys in her school. Quite appropriate to her age, Hope begged her mother to let her go to dances and movies with the rest of her friends. At that point Mrs. Hughes became flooded with feelings and memories of Jake's sexual abuse and was overwhelmed by fears that Hope would be raped. I did my best to help Mrs. Hughes separate her own experience and feelings from those of her daughter, but we were making little headway. At that point I recommended that she reconsider taking the fluoxetine (Prozac), and she agreed to take the medicine. Within several weeks, Mrs. Hughes's appearance and ways of relating to me and others changed dramatically. Before beginning to take the medication, she appeared supersensitive to me and to her environment. She would flinch when I would change positions in my chair and would almost jump out of her chair if my telephone should ring. On taking the medication, Mrs. Hughes was not only calmer and less vigilant, but she was also far less combative with me and others. She began to have pleasant and thoughtful interactions with my office staff, who in turn were starting to like her. For example, she learned in the newspaper that one of my secretaries had lost a parent, and she brought her a sympathy card and a beautiful plant. I perceived that she was more able to explore sensitive events of her past and to have insight about the meaning of these events. Most importantly, Mrs. Hughes recognized that she felt better—or, as she put it, "I feel better than I have ever felt. The Prozac makes me feel better than normal!" Her response was not unique. Certain people such as Mrs. Hughes have what is termed **double depression.** This is a condition in which a person has chronic, low-grade depression (termed **dysthymia**) as a baseline and dips into major depression during times of crisis or great stress. For example, the person might routinely have problems of poor self-esteem, great guilt, difficulties having fun, and sadness; during a crisis these symptoms would intensify to feelings of self-loathing, hopelessness, and suicidal thoughts and plans that would meet the DSM criteria for major depression. The medication not only treats the major depression, but also raises the patient's mood beyond its baseline. Commenting on her experience of being lifted from her chronic low-grade depression by an antidepressant, another patient (paraphrasing an old blues song by Furry Lewis) said to me, "I had been down so long, it looked like up to me." Mrs. Hughes's experience is a fine example of how psychotherapy and medications can be mutually beneficial in helping patients with personality disorders and other psychiatric illnesses. In other words, the psychotherapy helps the patient to accept the use of medications, which in turn enhance the patient's motivation and confidence to work in psychotherapy.

Current Status of Mrs. Hughes

More than 11 years have passed since Mrs. Hughes first entered treatment. She remains on medication and in treatment with me, although the frequency of her sessions is now reduced to about four visits a year. Over those years, however, there have been periods of time when I saw her much more frequently, as much as three sessions a week. Eight years ago, when her mother died, Mrs. Hughes had to be hospitalized briefly because she experienced auditory hallucinations telling her to kill herself. At that time she was given an antipsychotic medication for 2 weeks. At that time I also changed her antidepressant. At present she is taking the SSRI escitalopram oxalate (Lexapro).

Mrs. Hughes's changes in personality, mood, and behavior are nothing short of remarkable, compared with their status at the time she began treatment. She remains married to James Hughes and maintains regular and active involvements with his parents (whom she now adores), his siblings, and their spouses and children. In fact, Denise is now the most active person in the Hughes family in arranging get-togethers and facilitating communication. About this function she says, "As someone who was not fortunate enough to grow up in a loving family, I appreciate how important families can be. I now understand that relationships don't 'just happen,' and it is my job and pleasure to work to make sure we keep close." Both Mrs. Hughes and I are aware of the irony of her now being so positive and proactive in family activities. About this change she states, "For so long, I fought bitterly against what I had wanted the most—to be a part of a real family." In addition, she returned to school, gained her high school equivalency certificate, attended junior college, and later transferred to the University of Houston, where she maintains an excellent grade-point average. Her goal is to attend social work school and to work as a therapist with abused children. There remains little objective trace of her hostile and confrontational behavior. Rather, she is thoughtful, reflective, and appreciative. James Hughes returned to work as a teacher 9 years ago, and he has completed his master's degree in education. He has legally adopted Hope, who is now 23, is a college graduate, and is working as an intern in the Museum of Fine Arts in Chicago, where her grandparents still live.

Given the severity of Mrs. Hughes's presenting problems, I am fully aware that most people would find this treatment result unbelievable, almost like a fairy tale. Nonetheless, all clinicians with experience and expertise in treating patients with borderline personality disorder can point to therapeutic outcomes that are no less remarkable. I also realize that—for reasons related to financial resources, availability and accessibility of expert professionals, and motivation of the patient and family—such propitious therapeutic outcomes are far too few. Although outcome data support improvement of patients with borderline personality disorder who receive sustained treatment from qualified professionals, Mrs. Hughes's inordinately high level of change is perhaps the exception rather than the rule.

Key principles in the treatment of people with borderline personality disorder as exemplified by the care of Mrs. Denise Hughes are summarized in Table 10–7.

Afterword

Before her treatment, Mrs. Hughes was not capable of engaging in mature, supportive relationships. In fact, she was abusive, overcontrolling, and exploitive in her relationships with her husband, his family, and his friends. Had she refused to engage seriously in treatment or been unable to change her hostile and destructive behavior, she certainly would have qualified as having a fatal flaw of personality. Nonetheless, as do many other people with borderline personality disorder, she harbored a deep and desperate need to make intimate connections with other people. As a result of her hard work in psychotherapy and family treatment and by taking mood-stabilizing medications, she was able to make fundamental changes in her thinking, behavior, and emotions.

For a variety of reasons I will risk comparing and, more importantly, contrasting the successful treatment process of a patient with borderline personality disorder—*but certainly not the patient and degree of seriousness of the problem*—to the ground-up restoration of a fine classic automobile that had been found rusting and falling apart on a leaking

TABLE 10–7. Key principles of borderline personality disorder exemplified by the case of Denise Hughes, part II: treatment

Historical fact	Key principle	Interpretation
Mrs. Hughes was rude to the office staff of Dr. Y.	People with borderline personality disorder often alienate the very people who are in a position to help them.	By not responding to Mrs. Hughes's provocations or participating in power struggles, Dr. Y. and his staff were able to engage her in treatment.
In her initial session, Mrs. Hughes was angered when Dr. Y. denied her request that he prescribe her pain medications and call her by her first name.	Establishing clear and appropriate boundaries in the treatment of people with borderline personality disorder is an initial element of their psychotherapy and medical treatment.	Through the establishment of clear and reasonable therapeutic boundaries, Mrs. Hughes was able to express her angry feelings and did not develop the unrealistic expectation that Dr. Y. would fulfill her every need.
Mrs. Hughes believed that Dr. Y. refused to examine her breast lump because he thought her body was disgusting and because it was too much trouble for him.	As a result of being psychologically, physically, and/or sexually abused as children, people with borderline personality disorder have low self-esteem, often associated with distorted body images and impaired reality testing about being rejected and abandoned by others.	Dr. Y. encouraged Mrs. Hughes to consider alternative explanations about why he would not examine her breast. This enabled her to develop reflective functioning, or the capacity to objectively examine her own motivations and behavior and those of other people.
When Dr. Y. was out of town, Mrs. Hughes cut "I hate me" into her arm during the usually scheduled time of her therapy appointment.	Patients with borderline personality disorder develop intense transference relationships with their therapists.	Mrs. Hughes did not connect, in her own mind, the missed appointment and her rage over feeling abandoned by Dr. Y.

TABLE 10–7. Key principles of borderline personality disorder exemplified by the case of Denise Hughes, part II: treatment

Historical fact	Key principle	Interpretation
To reduce Mrs. Hughes's anxiety over her daughter's age-appropriate separation from her, Dr. Y. suggested that she keep in touch with her daughter by using a cell phone.	Effective treatment of patients with borderline personality disorder requires that the therapist be supportive and active, as well as interpretive.	Because Mrs. Hughes did not have a good parental role model, she was confused about what was in the best interests of her daughter. Dr. Y. provided suggestions and advice about how best to nurture, protect, and guide Hope.
Mrs. Hughes and her husband, James, were referred for family counseling.	As a person with borderline personality disorder changes in treatment, the dynamics (e.g., sharing of power, making decisions) of the person's marital and other important relationships also change.	Family counseling encouraged communication between Mrs. and Mr. Hughes, which helped prevent each party from misunderstanding and being threatened by their spouse's changes in behavior and personality.
The antidepressant medication fluoxetine (Prozac) was highly beneficial to Mrs. Hughes.	The symptoms of depression, irritability, anger, violence, and impulsivity of people with borderline personality disorder can be highly responsive to antidepressants, anticonvulsants, and other classes of medication.	Psychotherapy, family counseling, and medications all contributed to Mrs. Hughes's progress in treatment. Utilizing any of these interventions alone would not have been sufficient to bring about meaningful change.

TABLE 10–7.   Key principles of borderline personality disorder exemplified by the case of Denise Hughes, part II: treatment

Historical fact	Key principle	Interpretation
Mrs. Hughes remained in intensive treatment for many years.	There is no such thing as a "quick fix" for people with borderline personality disorder.	Once engaged in psychotherapy, Mrs. Hughes prioritized and worked diligently in her treatment and applied what she learned in the rest of her life.
Currently, Mrs. Hughes does not exhibit hostile or confrontational behavior, has close and positive family and personal relationships, and is no longer depressed or self-destructive.	With treatment, many people with borderline personality disorder make dramatic progress over time (Stone 1990).	The case of Mrs. Hughes exemplifies why people with borderline personality disorder, their families, and their clinicians should never give up hope.

barge. The similarities are as follows: such a restoration requires 1) experienced and motivated technicians; 2) the allocation of extensive periods of time, meticulous planning, and attention to detail; 3) the disassembly and repair of almost every part (in the case of treatment, assessment and, where required, realignment of key aspects of the person's thinking, affect, and behavior); and 4) the loving and careful reassembling of each piece (in the case of treatment, attention to providing and integrating new ways of perceiving, responding, and reacting). A further similarity is that the end result is "unbelievable," because the automobile appears to have emerged from rust and dysfunction to be almost better than new. In the case of the person with borderline personality disorder, he or she feels better than ever before, as are the relationships with people significant to him or her. The contrasts are even more important. First and foremost, a human being with an illness is far more valuable and complex than any machine. Second, people who are ill both affect and are affected by many other people—they do not exist, nor can they be treated, in isolation in some repair shop. Third, the most important work of recovery from borderline personality disorder is accomplished not by the clinician, but by the person herself or himself. (A car does not help repair itself.) This work requires trust, commitment, bravery, and motivation from those whose life experience has led them to distrust people and be wary of hope. Far from the too-prevalent, prejudicial devaluation of people with borderline personality disorder, there are no people whom I admire more than those with this condition who participate bravely and hopefully in this process of change.

References and Suggested Readings

American Psychiatric Association: Diagnostic and Statistical Manual of Mental Disorders, 4th Edition, Text Revision. Washington, DC, American Psychiatric Association, 2000, pp 706–711

American Psychiatric Association Practice Guidelines: Practice guideline for the treatment of patients with borderline personality disorder. Am J Psychiatry 158 (10 suppl):1–52, 2001

Burgess JW: Relationship of depression and cognitive impairment to self-injury in borderline personality disorder, major depression, and schizophrenia. Psychiatry Res 38:77–87, 1991

Clarkin JF, Sanderson C: The personality disorders, in Psychopathology in Adulthood. Edited by Hersen M, Bellack AS. Boston, MA, Allyn and Bacon, 1993, pp 252–274

Coccaro EF, Kavoussi RJ: Fluoxetine and impulsive aggressive behavior in personality-disordered subjects. Arch Gen Psychiatry 54:1081–1088, 1997

Fonagy P: Attachment and borderline personality disorder. J Am Psychoanal Assoc 48:1129–1146, 2000

Gardner D, Lucas PB, Cowdry RW: Soft sign neurological abnormalities in borderline personality disorder and normal control subjects. J Nerv Ment Dis 175:177–180, 1987

Gunderson JG, Links PS: Borderline personality disorder, in Treatments of Psychiatric Disorders, 3d Edition. Edited by Gabbard, GO. Washington, DC, American Psychiatric Publishing, 2001, pp 2273–2291

Kavoussi RJ, Coccaro EF: Divalproex sodium for impulsive aggressive behavior in patients with personality disorder. J Clin Psychiatry 59:676–680, 1998

Knowles JA: Genetics, in The American Psychiatric Publishing Textbook of Clinical Psychiatry, 4th Edition. Edited by Hales RE, Yudofsky SC. Washington, DC, American Psychiatric Publishing, 2003, pp 3–65

Koenigsberg HW, Kernberg OF, Stone MH, et al: Borderline Patients: Extending the Limits of Treatability. New York, Basic Books, 2000

Mann JJ, Huang YY, Underwood MD, et al: A serotonin transporter gene promoter polymorphism (5-HTTLPR) and prefrontal cortical binding in major depression and suicide. Arch Gen Psychiatry 57:729–738, 2000

Mann JJ, Brent DA, Arango V: The neurobiology and genetics of suicide and attempted suicide: a focus on the serotonergic system. Neuropsychopharmacology 24:467–477, 2001

Miles DR, Carey G: Genetic and environmental architecture of human aggression. J Pers Soc Psychol 72:207–217, 1997

Oldham JM: Integrated treatment planning for borderline personality disorder, in Integrated Treatment of Psychiatric Disorders. Edited by Kay J. Washington DC, American Psychiatric Publishing, 2001, pp 51–112

Ovsiew F, Yudofsky SC: Aggression: a neuropsychiatric perspective, in Rage, Power, and Aggression. Edited by Glick RA, Roose SP. New Haven, CT, Yale University Press, 1993, pp 213–230

Paris J: Borderline Personality Disorder: A Multidimensional Approach. Washington, DC, American Psychiatric Press, 1994

Soloff PH: Pharmacological therapies in borderline personality disorder, in Borderline Personality Disorder: Etiology and Treatment. Edited by Paris J. Washington, DC, American Psychiatric Press, 1993, pp 319–348

Soloff PH: Algorithms for pharmacological treatment of personality dimensions: symptom-specific treatments for cognitive-perceptual, affective, and impulsive-behavioral dysregulation. Bull Menninger Clin 62:195–214, 1998

Stone MH: The Fate of Borderline Patients: Successful Outcome and Psychiatric Practice. New York, Guilford, 1990

Stone MH: Clinical guidelines for psychotherapy for patients with borderline personality disorder. Psychiatr Clin North Am 23:193–210, 2000

Swartz M, Blazer D, George L, et al: Estimating the prevalence of borderline personality disorder in the community. J Personal Disord 4:257–272, 1990

Tecott LH, Barondes SH: Genes and aggressiveness: behavioral genetics. Curr Biol 6:238–240, 1996

Torgersen S: Genetic and nosological aspects of schizotypal and borderline personality disorders: a twin study. Arch Gen Psychiatry 41:546–554, 1984

Traskman-Bendz L, Alling C, Oreland L, et al: Prediction of suicidal behavior from biologic tests. J Clin Psychopharmacol 12 (2 suppl):21S–26S, 1992

van Reekum R, Conway CA, Gansler D, et al: Neurobehavioral study of borderline personality disorder. J Psychiatry Neurosci 18:121–129, 1993

Yudofsky S, Williams D, Gorman J: Propranolol in the treatment of rage and violent behavior in patients with organic brain syndromes. Am J Psychiatry 138:218–220, 1981

Yudofsky SC, Silver JM, Hales RE: Treatment of agitation and aggression, in The American Psychiatric Press Textbook of Psychopharmacology, 2nd Edition. Edited by Schatzberg, AF, Nemeroff CB. Washington, DC, American Psychiatric Press, 1998, pp 881–900

Zanarini MC, Gunderson JG, Marino MF, et al: DSM-III disorders in the families of borderline outpatients. J Personal Disord 2:292–302, 1988

11

SCHIZOTYPAL PERSONALITY DISORDER

> My eyes adored you
> Like a million miles away from me you couldn't
>   see how I adored you
> So close, so close and yet so far
>
> —Bob Crewe and Kenny Nolan,
> "My Eyes Adored You"
> (recorded by Frankie Valli
> and the Four Seasons)

Essence

Have you ever had an impassioned relationship with someone whom you have never met? In the course of this relationship, did you ask yourself the following questions?

What right does he think he has to spy on me and to learn all about my habits and personal life? Why is he so preoccupied with me, and how did I become the center of his life? How could he believe that he knows me better than any other living person, when he really doesn't understand a thing about me? Why was I so upset when he finally spoke to me? Was it his unusual appearance, strange movements, and eccentric personality, or was it the intensity of his involvement with me that frightened me so much? So secretive and quiet—does he even have a personality? Is he serious when he says that I am sending him special signals and that I can read his mind? Why does he think that I even care what's on his mind? Should I be scared of his tantrums when I tell him to stop bothering me? Does he really believe that I have been leading him on all this time? Am I in danger from him? Even though he hasn't committed any crime, should I call the police? Will they take this seriously? Will he have to kill me before anyone takes this seriously?

The Case of Robert Woods, Part One

The Prodigy

By almost every standard, Robert Woods had an advantaged, loving childhood. His father was chairman of the chemistry department at an Ivy League university, the same institution in which his mother was a full professor of art history. A middle child, Robert grew up with his older sister and younger brother in a large, historic Victorian home that was located on the university campus. All of the Woods children attended an excellent private school that was within walking distance of their home. Although they were busy with their careers, both parents were devoted to and spent ample time with their children. Unlike his two siblings, however, Robert was a loner throughout his childhood. He never had a best friend, and he preferred to stay by himself in his room to build model cities, read science fiction books, and solve mathematical puzzles. He was also a moody child who would throw tantrums when he did not get his way. For example, when he was 4 years old, Robert would almost daily resist going to pre-kindergarten classes. Before school, he would fight his mother's attempt to dress him and would refuse to eat his breakfast. He refused to walk with his sister or his father to the school. On arrival at his classroom he would start to cry and would scream when his mother departed. When he eventually calmed down, he preferred to play by himself in class rather than join in the group activities with his peers. His parents had him evaluated by a child psychiatrist, who in turn ordered psychological and aptitude testing. Not surprisingly, the psychological tests concluded that young Robert had separation anxiety disorder, but the aptitude tests took everyone aback. Robert was found to have an IQ in the genius range. Follow-up tests administered the next year, when Robert was 5 years old, indicated that he was able to perform in the high school range in mathematics. He was indeed a prodigy. Robert's parents were somewhat relieved, because they reasoned that there was a connection between his superior intelligence and his difficulties socializing with his peers.

Getting in Trouble

Over time, Robert became more comfortable attending school, and he seemed to enjoy the special attention that he received from science and mathematics teachers and his tutors for advanced study in these subjects. Nonetheless, throughout elementary school and middle school he remained aloof from most children of his own age, and he never had a best friend. By the ninth grade, Robert was taking most of his science and math classes at the university where his parents worked, and by age 16 he was accepted to several prestigious technology-intensive institutes. Even though his high school counselors advised that Robert was too socially immature to attend college, his parents hoped that he would have more in common with the college students, who were also gifted and had interests similar to those of their son's. These hopes were not fulfilled; Robert remained a complete loner. His rarely even spoke with his roommate and did not attend any college social activities. Rather, he spent most of his time by himself studying at a small cubicle in the engineering library. It was there, during his junior year, that he first saw Lois Abramowitz, a freshman engineering student. Lois would spend many hours in the same area of the library to escape the noise and distractions of the dormitory and her two roommates. Robert noticed Lois, but he never spoke to her, even when she nodded a brief hello to him on occasion. Robert's reticence was just fine with Lois, who was very attractive and had a surfeit of college suitors; she was merely seeking a quiet place in the library in which to concentrate on her studies.

In the spring of Lois's freshman year, she was visited by an underclassman from her hometown high school. He was not a beau, but he was considering applying to this college in the early admission category. Because she had an economics midterm during his visit, she had to study while he was there. He joined her on one occasion at the library while she was studying. Two days later Lois received the following unsigned, typewritten note:

WHO WAS THAT MORON WITH YOU THE OTHER DAY? HE HAS NO RIGHT TO BE AT OUR COLLEGE, AND NO RIGHT TO BE WITH YOU. I NEVER WANT TO SEE YOU WITH HIM AGAIN. YOU BETTER LISTEN TO ME.

At first Lois believed that the note was a prank from one of her girlfriends, who thought that the young man visiting from her hometown was cute. However, none of her friends would admit to having sent her the missive, and she soon stopped thinking about the unusual communication. About a month later, Lois began to date Gary Parker, a junior in the college, who was also a serious student. Gary did not accompany Lois to the engineering library. Rather, Gary preferred to study in his room in the small off-campus house that he shared with three other college juniors. He was able to access his computer at home, and he felt obligated to be with his pet terrier, which was left alone during the daytime when the young men were in classes.

The second unsigned note that Lois received was much more disturbing to her:

STAY AWAY FROM GARY PARKER, OR ELSE. I NEVER WANT TO SEE YOU WITH HIM AGAIN.

Lois showed the note to Gary, who was not at all concerned. He thought it was either a prank from one of their many friends or "just a note from some kook." Gary believed that the best thing to do was to ignore the letter, but Lois was unable to follow his well-intended advice. She wracked her brain in an effort to uncover who would care enough to send the two mean-spirited notes. She tried to remember all of the young men who had asked her out during her first 7 months of college, particularly the very few whom she had actually dated. None of them seemed likely suspects. Rather, Lois strongly suspected several of the girls whom Gary had dated before they became involved. One in particular whom she truly disliked was Delia, also a college junior. Even though Delia's relationship with Gary had supposedly ended a year ago, she attended several classes with Gary and called him regularly. Delia had also behaved very cattily on the few occasions when she and Lois met. Even though this conclusion did not fit with the content of the first note, Lois became more and more convinced that Delia was responsible. Lois's suspicions about Delia did not change on receipt of the third cryptic letter:

YOU EVIL SLUT. YOU BETRAYED ME. THIS WILL BE THE LAST TIME THAT I WARN YOU. NEVER SEE GARY PARKER AGAIN. PAY ATTENTION NOW OR YOU WILL BOTH PAY LATER.

Lois was beside herself when she read this note, which had been left in her student mailbox. She felt that both she and Gary were being seriously threatened, but she did not know what to do. She was so certain at this point that Delia was the culprit that she finally convinced Gary to speak with her about it. When Gary told Delia about the notes, she was outraged at the suggestion that she might be involved such a thing. She told Gary, "You are the most vain, self-centered person in the world to think that I care about you that much to do such a horrible thing," and she said that she would never to speak to either him or Lois again. After Delia's tirade, Gary was more convinced than ever that Lois should just ignore the notes. He told her, "If you get any more, throw them away without reading them." He strongly discouraged Lois from speaking to her college counselor about the notes: "Delia already thinks we're both nuts. Please don't make things worse by getting the college involved in this stupid prank. No one is going to get hurt from these silly notes. Let's just ignore them."

Because of Gary's strong feelings, Lois did not go to her college counselor. However, she spoke with her parents for the first time about the notes. They were alarmed and were very clear with their daughter about what they thought that she should do. They told Lois that she should speak that day with her college advisor, or else they would call the dean of the college. Lois became hysterical, because she now felt torn between what her boyfriend wanted her to do and the instructions of her parents. Suddenly she became more concerned about losing Gary than she was about the notes. She told her parents that she would think about it for a day or two and would let them know what she decided to do. She also told her parents, "If you go behind my back and treat me like a child, I will never tell you anything important about my life. I will never trust you again if you betray me."

That night neither of Lois's parents could sleep. They felt better the next day after they had spoken with Lois and learned that she was all right. Lois promised to stay near her roommates or Gary until she decided what to do. It did not take very long. This time Gary received an unsigned, typewritten note in the mailbox of his off-campus apartment:

STAY AWAY FROM LOIS. YOUR DOG IS DEAD. THE NEXT TIME IT WILL BE YOU.

The day before, Gary had found his dog, Bunjie, dead in the back yard. There were no signs of injury. He had no idea what had happened and called the veterinarian. The vet said that there would be no way to find out the cause of death without performing an autopsy, which would cost several hundred dollars. Gary reasoned, "Bunjie won't be any more alive after the autopsy, so I might just as well bury him." After he received the note, he changed his mind and called Lois. They immediately called Lois's college advisor, who arranged an emergency meeting with the college dean and the director of college security. They met for several hours and came to the following decisions:

- Both Lois's and Gary's parents would be promptly notified.
- An autopsy would be performed on the dog by university scientists.
- The local municipal police would be brought in to work with college security.

- A decision would be made by the college dean, after input from the police and the students' parents, about whether it would be safe and acceptable for Lois and Gary to remain in school.

It was soon discovered that Bunjie had been poisoned with cyanide, a highly lethal chemical that has many industrial uses and can be obtained through mail order from suppliers throughout the nation. Because no licenses or records are required for its purchase, its source is difficult to trace. Lois's parents insisted that she return home immediately to the Midwest until the perpetrator was apprehended, but Gary remained in college to complete his premed requirements. Around-the-clock surveillance was provided for Gary both on and off campus.

Getting Caught

Six days later, plainclothes campus police saw a student place a note under the windshield wiper of Gary's car. The car was parked in a student lot while Gary was attending an organic chemistry lab. Exercising caution not to be discovered, the police followed the student back to his dormitory room. The note said,

LOIS IS GONE; SO GARY'S A GONER.

The police soon determined that all the notes had been written on Robert Woods's typewriter, and Robert was arrested. When Robert's parents were notified of their son's plight, they were incredulous and outraged. At first they were convinced that the college had made a terrible mistake. To their knowledge, he had never before been in any serious trouble, and he certainly had never harmed anyone or any thing. They rushed to the campus, which was about 300 miles from their home. The received their second shock at the jail where Robert was being detained. He refused to see them or speak with them. The officer in charge explained that because Robert was 21 he had the right to deny their visitation. The police captain also revealed that Robert, who had been advised of his rights, was not speaking and had refused legal counsel. The two professors went into prompt action. They hired a prominent local attorney and, through the intervention of the president of the university where they were on faculty, arranged a meeting with the president of the university where Robert was a student. It was a university-dominated town, and the president held great sway with the local police and district attorney's office. Although Robert objected vehemently, Judge Lawrence Higgins remanded Robert for assessment and treatment to a state hospital that had a close affiliation with the medical school of the university.

The Case of Robert Woods, Part Two: Psychiatric Assessment and Treatment

Noncompliance

Robert was placed in a locked inpatient service of the state psychiatric hospital. Most of the patients on this service had severe and persistent psychotic disorders, mainly schizophrenia. Because he refused to talk to any of the doctors or other members of the professional staff, he was placed on suicide observation, which meant that he was kept in pajamas and under the watch of the nursing staff at all times—even when he went to the bathroom. Although his parents came to visit him, he was furious with them for engineering his involuntary placement in the psychiatric hospital and would not speak with them. He did, however, converse with the few inpatients who were about his age. He would write terse notes to his parents saying such things as, "You got me in here; now get me out of here." Through their connections with the president of the university, Robert's parents arranged for Dr. Flowers, the vice chairman of the department of psychiatry, to be his doctor in charge. At the time, I was a psychiatry resident assigned to that service. Only 2 years out of medical school, I had absolutely no experience with a patient like Robert Woods. Dr. Flowers indicated that because of the reasons for the patient's referral to the hospital and his refusal to communicate with us, we had to assume that he was psychotic. *Psychosis* refers to impaired reality testing that most often involves *hallucinations* (hearing, seeing, or feeling things that are not present) or *delusions* (false beliefs that seem real to the person and are not changed by logic or contradicting evidence). Often people with psychosis have *thought disorders,* which results in their inability to communicate logically with others, especially about issues with which they are preoccupied.

My job as a psychiatry resident was to meet every day with Robert and provide psychotherapy. Fulfillment of this responsibility was thwarted by the fact that he would not say a single word to me. Day after day and week after week I would sit with Robert for 45 minutes and ask him how he felt that day, how he was sleeping, if he had any issues or problems that he wished to discuss with me, etc. He did not answer me or seem to connect with me in any way. Dr. Flowers counseled me, "Just wait him out. He will come around sooner or later." Robert's par-

ents were far less patient, and they were putting intense pressure on Dr.
Flowers to discharge their son.

> **Mr. Woods:** Obviously, this hospitalization is not helping our son. If any-
> thing, we believe it is making him worse to be around such emo-
> tionally ill people. We don't believe that he belongs here. He has
> truly done nothing wrong, except perhaps to use poor judgment in
> writing that girl those silly letters. He never would have hurt her,
> as he has never hurt anyone in his life. The sooner he gets out of
> here and back into his college routine, the better off he will be.
> **Dr. Flowers:** Because Robert is not speaking with us, we have no way
> of assessing whether or not he is of danger to other people or to
> himself. Since human lives are at stake, we must err on the side of
> safety.
> **Mr. Woods:** The operant word is "err." With all due respect, Dr. Flowers,
> we don't believe our son has a psychiatric problem, and we don't
> believe that you know how to help him.

Attorneys Become Involved

Through their attorneys, Robert's parents obtained another hearing
with Judge Higgins. At that hearing, Robert spoke for the first time.

> **Robert Woods:** I made a mistake writing those notes to Lois. I think
> I was in love for the first time and got carried away. I used bad
> judgment, but I certainly am not crazy. I promise that nothing like
> this will ever happen again.
> **Dr. Flowers:** Your honor, I strongly advise you not to release Robert un-
> til he cooperates in treatment by disclosing what is on his mind to
> the hospital professional staff. Without such communication, we
> have no way of knowing what is on his mind and what he will do.
> It is not normal to say nothing for 5 weeks in a hospital, and I fear
> that we are seeing only the tip of a very dangerous iceberg.
> **Mr. Woods:** With all due respect, your honor, I believe that Dr. Flowers
> is way over his head in trying to deal with our son. He is blaming
> our son because he does not have the skills to connect with the
> boy. He is wildly speculating about some far-fetched threat that
> has no basis in Robert's past behavior, which is completely nonvi-
> olent. We beg you to release him to our custody.
> **Judge Higgins:** Robert, you have indicated in this court that you are
> fully capable of speaking coherently. However, you have not co-
> operated in the hospital by communicating with the profession-
> als. I have no choice but to return you to the hospital until such
> time as you have discussed with your psychiatrists your thoughts
> about the two college students whom you threatened and have
> convinced the psychiatrists and the court that you are of no dan-
> ger to these students or anyone else. You are remanded to return
> to the hospital for 2 more months, after which we will have an-

other hearing. At that time, if I learn that you still refuse to speak
with your doctors, you will be remanded for another 2 months,
and so on until you discuss this matter fully and seriously with
them.

Mrs. Woods: May we request another psychiatrist? We do not have
confidence that Dr. Flowers has the skills to reach our son.

Judge Higgins: All treatment decisions will remain under the responsibility of the hospital authority. I suggest, Professors, that you
find a way to work with Dr. Flowers.

Further Hospital Treatment

The following day, during my scheduled session with Robert, he spoke
to me for the first time.

Robert Woods: So, what do you want to know, Dr. Y.?

Because Robert had not spoken to a word to me during several
months of his hospitalization, I was absolutely unprepared for his question. I stuttered and relied on the stereotypical psychiatric response:

Dr. Y.: Why don't you start by telling me what is on your mind?

Robert: That's so original and so very, very helpful to me. I only have
one thing on my mind and that is getting out of this loony bin. If
you want to help me, you will help me get out of this place

Dr. Y.: O.K., let's start by telling me why you sent those threatening
notes to Lois Abramowitz.

Robert: First of all, they weren't that threatening. I just wanted to get
her attention. Secondly, she led me on.

Dr. Y.: How did she do that?

Robert: By showing up every day in my section of the library. No one
forced her to come there. She also gave me many signals that she
cared for me.

Dr. Y.: What type of signals?

Robert: She would wear certain articles of clothing that she knew
would appeal to me. She would cross her legs when I was thinking certain things about her. She held her pen in special ways to
communicate that she understood the messages that I was sending her.

Dr. Y.: Did you ever actually speak with her?

Robert (with irritation): We don't have to speak with each other. We
know what's on each other's mind. You know something, this really isn't helping me. As I said, if you want to be of help, get me
out of this place

With that Robert walked out of the small consultation room. That
day, I reported to Dr. Flowers exactly what had transpired, and he

expressed grave concern about Robert's mental status. Dr. Flowers believed that Robert was demonstrating *ideas of reference,* which are distortions of reality in which a person feels that he or she has special powers and is receiving special communications from unwitting people or from other sources. Dr. Flowers also believed that Robert remained preoccupied with Lois Abramowitz. He explained to me that Robert's impaired thinking and reality testing combined with his history of sending threatening letters to Lois and killing her boyfriend's dog portended that Lois remained in danger. He added,

> **Dr. Flowers:** We must look at the details to understand the big picture. Although he is not hallucinating and does not admit to delusions at this time, his thinking is nonetheless impaired. It just does not make sense to believe that you have an intense relationship with—and can communicate through vague signs to—a young lady with whom you have never spoken. We need to know more about the extent of his current preoccupation with Lois, and I want you to speak to the police about any other information or evidence that they gathered about this case. The true danger is that his thought disorder is subtle, and to most people he will seem a lot more sane than he truly is. I worry that if the court lets him go, he will harm Lois. It wasn't Bunjie whom Robert was really after.

At Dr. Flowers's suggestion, I wrote to Judge Higgins and asked that he remand the college security and local police to provide any information that they discovered that would aid in the better understanding of Robert Woods's preoccupation with Lois Abramowitz. Ten days later, the hospital received several of Robert's notebooks that had been found in his dormitory room. The notebooks comprised a neatly printed diary recording Robert's reactions to Lois each day of the approximately 7 months since he saw her for the first time in the engineering library. The notebook was a mixture of precise description and far-fetched fantasy. We learned that Robert followed and spied on Lois when she left the library. He kept a detailed record of everywhere that she went and almost everyone who was in her company. He carried out imaginary two-way conversations with Lois, which divulged his belief that he completely understood what was on her mind. In his notebook, Lois was quoted as if she were actually conversing with him. It was clear that her imagined responses constituted projections of what he wished her thoughts and reactions to be. It was also obvious that Robert believed each and every thought and feeling that he attributed to Lois.

The Psychodynamics of a Stalker

Dr. Flowers explained the workings of Robert's mind. His harmless fantasies grew dangerous when reality conflicted with his distortions. When he saw that Lois had become involved with Gary, Robert concluded that Lois had been lying to him and was being unfaithful. He flew into a rage—a murderous rage. The intensity of Robert's emotions was magnified by the fact that he had no real-life peer or romantic relationships. His mental life and self-esteem were wholly dependent on his imaginary involvement with Lois. Feeling betrayed and deserted by Lois, he sought to repay her for the intense pain that he was feeling; and he believed that she *deserved* to be punished for "leading him on." Of course, Lois had no idea about what was going on in Robert's mind, and Robert had no understanding that all of these intense scenarios were mental distortions. *These dynamics are typical of stalkers of famous people; but they may also apply to other types of stalkers who have never had actual relationships with their victims.*

For Robert and stalkers of this genus the bottom line is, "I have devoted so much of my true self and energies to you and our relationship. You have betrayed me and ruined my life. I have nothing left. I am in intense pain because of you. You deserve my punishment, and I will also see to it that no one else can have you."

Dr. Flowers disclosed to Robert that we had gained access to his notebooks. Dr. Flowers also expressed his deep concern that if Robert were released he would pose a threat to Lois.

> **Dr. Flowers:** Robert, in your notebook you made threats to Lois and her friends. Until you tell me exactly what is going on in your mind—precisely what you are thinking about—I will recommend to the judge that you remain in the hospital. Permanently, if necessary. I have no alternative but to conclude that you still pose a danger to Lois and to her friends.
>
> **Robert Woods:** I will talk with Dr. Y., but not to you. I don't trust you one bit. I think you dislike me and are jealous of me because of my superior intelligence. You obviously have had your mind made up about me from the very beginning. I can assure you that my parents fully agree with me.

Faking It

At that point Robert seemed to change. Although he refused to talk to Dr. Flowers, Robert appeared to be cooperating with me and the other members of the hospital treatment team. He began to attend and participate in all group meetings and talked with me about his feelings and plans in our individual sessions. He finally admitted that he had been overinvolved with Lois, but he maintained that this was a mistake and that he had gotten over her. Over time, Robert had most of the staff—including me—convinced that he had learned from his mistakes and that he deserved a chance to redeem himself as an outpatient. Dr. Flowers, however, was uniformly unconvinced.

> **Dr. Flowers:** Despite what you believe, Robert hasn't changed one bit. He is playing a game with all of us. His mind is capable of a certain type of reasoning. He is a genius at math and logic. He has figured out that if he plays along by offering vacuous expressions of understanding and remorse, at some point we will have to discharge him. I am certain that he still has disordered thinking that he has now learned to disguise. He has simple schizophrenia, a type of psychotic illness in which sufficient insight remains for him to recognize and hide what others would believe is abnormal. In the case of people with most types of schizophrenia, they are so unaware of their psychoses that they make no attempt to hide their pathology. Even though he disguises his true thoughts and beliefs, I can assure you that Robert believes that his thinking is completely normal and has always been so. My greatest concern is that he is keeping his own counsel about his continued preoccupation with Lois. Since he has not developed a capacity for honest interactions or fulfilling relationships with anyone—which is the core problem in simple schizophrenia—he remains dependent on his fantasies. In my opinion, Lois remains in great danger from Robert.

Robert also began to communicate with his parents in an effort to garner their help in getting him released from the state psychiatric hospital.

> **Robert Woods:** I made a mistake, and I learned my lesson. All I want to do is to get back to school and continue with my studies. I have decided to go to graduate school in mathematics at the University of California at Berkeley. They have a great department, and I can make a new start there.

The Wisdom of the Court

Mr. and Mrs. Woods were more convinced than ever that their son Robert was well and that Dr. Flowers was overreacting. They carefully prepared for the next hearing with Judge Higgins. They engaged their own psychiatrists, who were in full-time forensic practice. The forensic psychiatrists testified that Robert Woods was no longer—if he had ever been—of danger to others or to himself; that inpatient care was no longer required for Robert; and that they would arrange for his outpatient care.

Robert Woods: I have sincere regrets for what I have done. I now understand that I overreacted because of my affection for Lois. I am completely over that now and just want to return to college and my career in mathematics.

Dr. Flowers: Robert has a severe mental illness, a form of schizophrenia. In my opinion he has not engaged any meaningful treatment during his hospitalization.

Judge Higgins: Then what do you suggest at this point?

Dr. Flowers: I suggest that he be committed to another state hospital, one that specializes in long-term care. I believe that he should stay in a locked unit until such time as an experienced psychiatrist believes that he has fully discussed his preoccupations regarding Lois Abramowitz and has developed interpersonal skills that allow him to replace her central presence in his mental life. In my opinion that might take many years. In my opinion, Robert will remain dangerous to others until these changes occur.

Judge Higgins: We all must acknowledge that psychiatry is an imperfect science—especially when it comes to the prediction of future behaviors. Although Robert has sent threatening letters to two people, he has no history of ever injuring another person. That is no reason to keep him locked up for life. The court cannot lock people up for crimes that they might commit! I am ordering him to be discharged in the custody of his parents and for him to engage in outpatient treatment to be established by the psychiatrists of his parents' choosing. And Robert, if you ever again are proven to have threatened Lois, any of her friends, or anyone else, I will recommit you to a psychiatric hospital for the care that Dr. Flowers has recommended. Do you understand?

Robert: I understand completely, Your Honor. I will not let you down; or my parents or myself.

Dr. Flowers: I wish to go on record as stating that the court is taking a terrible risk. I ask that Miss Lois Abramowitz and her parents be notified that Robert Woods has been released.

Judge Higgins: Dr. Flowers, your reservations and contentions about this judgment are duly placed in the court record. I will see to it that Miss Abramowitz and her parents are promptly notified about the defendant's release from the state hospital. I will say, Dr. Flowers, that I am not one of those judges who "covers his derriere" by putting people away for years based on the conjectures of "experts" about what might happen. Robert, you are now free to

leave the courtroom in the custody of your parents. Court ad-
journed.

Hospitalization "Interminable"

With the help of his parents, who had petitioned the president of the university, Robert was permitted to return to college the following semester.
Through their attorneys, Lois's family had independently contacted Dr.
Flowers, who strongly recommended that she transfer to a college in the
Midwest near her hometown. Reluctantly she did as Dr. Flowers and her
parents advised. Robert's grades in math and science were, as usual, in
the superior range. He was seen weekly in supportive treatment by a
therapist who was a full-time employee of the college counseling office.
In the fall of his senior year, at the time of the Thanksgiving holiday, he
planned a trip to California to interview at University of California, Berkeley, for admission to their graduate school in mathematics. He told his
parents he would stay over the holidays with a friend who was in graduate school at Berkeley. Instead, Robert flew to the Midwest, to the town
and address where Lois lived. Undetected, he spied on Lois for 2 days before shooting her in the head and killing her with a high-powered hunting rifle that he had purchased in the town. Robert had timed her murder
to occur just before the departure of a bus that was going to Florida. En
route, as the bus stopped at Atlanta, police were waiting and took him,
without a struggle, into custody. To this day, Robert remains in a special
psychiatric hospital for the criminally insane.

DSM-IV-TR Diagnosis of Robert Woods

The portion of the life of Robert Woods described in this chapter took
place more than 30 years ago, very early in my training in psychiatry. At
that time, the second edition of the *Diagnostic and Statistical Manual of
Mental Disorders* (DSM-II) was in use (American Psychiatric Association
1968). Schizophrenia was divided into several subtypes, including simple, hebephrenic, paranoid, childhood, catatonic, and schizoaffective.
At that time, Dr. Flowers utilized the diagnosis of simple schizophrenia
to describe the psychiatric illness of people who were socially withdrawn and who, although they had impaired reality testing and illogi-
cal thinking, did not evidence active hallucinations or pervasive
delusions. These individuals were characteristically self-absorbed; and
because of grossly impaired interpersonal relationships, over time they
would exhibit a marked decline in scholastic and occupational performance. This diagnosis was ultimately changed to emphasize the deteri-

orating nature of the condition, and it is listed in DSM-IV-TR as *simple deteriorative disorder* (a proposed diagnosis included for research purposes only). The diagnostic criteria are summarized in Table 11–1 (American Psychiatric Association 2000).

TABLE 11–1.   Proposed criteria for simple deteriorative disorder (slightly modified from DSM-IV-TR)

---

1. Marked decline in occupational or academic functioning

2. Gradual appearance and deepening of negative symptoms such as affective flattening, alogia, and avolition (i.e., reduced emotional expressiveness, reduced speaking, and reduced motivation)

3. Reduced interpersonal rapport

4. Social withdrawal

Source.   Adapted from American Psychiatric Association: *Diagnostic and Statistical Manual of Mental Disorders,* 4th Edition, Text Revision. Washington, DC, American Psychiatric Association, 2000, p. 771. Used with permission.

Although over time many elements of this proposed diagnosis would apply to Robert Woods, the underlying problem of his disturbed thinking and impaired reality testing is not addressed by these criteria. The DSM-IV-TR diagnosis that most closely describes the psychiatric disorder of Robert Woods is *schizotypal personality disorder.* The diagnostic criteria for this disorder are listed in Table 11–2 (American Psychiatric Association 2000).

It is important to note that *__most__ people who have the diagnosis of schizotypal personality disorder are not dangerous to others.* Rather, they try to avoid contact with other people as much as possible. Nonetheless, within this diagnostic category are a subgroup of people who develop confused involvements with others that can become disturbing and even violent. There are many personality types—especially antisocial—among people who become dangerous stalkers and predators of other people. Unfortunately, people with schizotypal personality disorder are also common among stalkers and those who become dangerously involved with innocent others.

The discussion of the diagnostic features of schizotypal personality disorder in DSM-IV-TR is especially helpful in clarifying the criteria for this condition, so these are included, in a slightly edited form, in "Diagnostic Features of Schizotypal Personality Disorder" below. Although certain of these features do not apply to Robert Woods, they may be

---

TABLE 11–2.   Diagnostic criteria for schizotypal personality disorder

---

A. A pervasive pattern of social and interpersonal deficits marked by acute discomfort with, and reduced capacity for, close relationships as well as by cognitive or perceptual distortions and eccentricities of behavior, beginning by early adulthood and present in a variety of contexts, as indicated by five (or more) of the following:

  (1) ideas of reference (excluding delusions of reference)

  (2) odd beliefs or magical thinking that influences behavior and is inconsistent with subcultural norms (e.g., superstitiousness, belief in clairvoyance, telepathy, or "sixth sense"; in children and adolescents, bizarre fantasies or preoccupations)

  (3) unusual perceptual experiences, including bodily illusions

  (4) odd thinking and speech (e.g., vague, circumstantial, metaphorical, overelaborate, or stereotyped)

  (5) suspiciousness or paranoid ideation

  (6) inappropriate or constricted affect

  (7) behavior or appearance that is odd, eccentric, or peculiar

  (8) lack of close friends or confidants other than first-degree relatives

  (9) excessive social anxiety that does not diminish with familiarity and tends to be associated with paranoid fears rather than negative judgments about self

B. Does not occur exclusively during the course of schizophrenia, a mood disorder with psychotic features, another psychotic disorder, or a pervasive developmental disorder.

Note: If criteria are met prior to the onset of schizophrenia, add "premorbid," e.g., "schizotypal personality disorder (premorbid)."

Source.   Reprinted from American Psychiatric Association: *Diagnostic and Statistical Manual of Mental Disorders,* 4th Edition, Text Revision. Washington, DC, American Psychiatric Association, 2000, p. 701. Used with permission.

---

helpful to you in assessing whether or not you have an involvement with a person with this psychiatric condition.

Diagnostic Features of Schizotypal Personality Disorder
(Slightly Modified From DSM-IV-TR, pp. 697–698)

The essential feature of schizotypal personality disorder is a pervasive pattern of social and interpersonal deficits marked by acute discomfort with, and reduced capacity for, close relationships. Cognitive or perceptual distortions and eccentricities of behavior are also characteristics of this condition. These features begin by early adulthood and are present in a variety of contexts. Individuals with schizotypal personality disorder often have ideas of reference, which are incorrect interpretations of casual incidents and external events as having a particular and unusual meaning specifically for the person. People with schizotypal personality disorder may also be superstitious or preoccupied with paranormal phenomena that are outside the norms of their subculture. They may feel that they have special powers to sense events before they happen or to read others' thoughts. They may believe that they have magical control over others, which can be implemented directly (e.g., believing that their spouse's taking the dog out for a walk is the direct result of their thinking that it should be done) or indirectly through compliance with magical rituals (e.g., walking past a specific object three times to avoid a certain harmful outcome). Perceptual alterations may occur, such as sensing the presence of another person who is not actually there or believing that a voice is murmuring their own name.

The language used by people with this disorder may include unusual or idiosyncratic phrasing and construction. It is often loose, digressive, or vague—even though some coherence is usually maintained. Responses may be either overly concrete or overly abstract, and words or concepts are sometimes utilized in unusual ways. People with this condition are often suspicious and may have paranoid thoughts, such as believing their colleagues at work are intent on undermining their reputation with the supervisor. They are frequently unable to regulate their emotions in dealing with others, either in group settings or one on one. Therefore they often appear to others as being stiff, constricted, or even somehow weird.

People with schizotypal personality disorder are often regarded by others as being odd or eccentric because of unusual mannerisms or attire or an unkempt manner of grooming. They are frequently inattentive to the usual social conventions (e.g., the person may avoid eye contact, wear clothes that are inkstained and ill-fitting, and be unable to join in the give-and-take banter of peers and colleagues). Relating to others is difficult and uncomfortable for them. They are anxious in social situations, particularly those involving unfamiliar people. Although they may express unhappiness about their lack of relationships, their behavior suggests a diminished desire for intimate contacts. As a result, they usually have no or few close friends or confidants other than their parents or siblings. They will interact with other people when they have to, but they prefer to keep to themselves because they feel that they are different and just do not fit in. Their social anxiety does not easily abate, even when they spend more time in a particular setting.

Presented in Table 11–3 is a summary of key principles about people with this condition as exemplified by the case of Robert Woods.

TABLE 11–3. Key principles of schizotypal personality disorder as exemplified by the case of Robert Woods

Historical fact	Key principle	Interpretation
From his early childhood, Robert exhibited problems controlling his emotions and relating with peers.	Adults with schizotypal personality disorder were often socially withdrawn as children.	Robert's parents did their best to help their son and to cope with his disturbing and disruptive behaviors—at a significant cost.
Robert was a prodigy in math and science.	People with superior intelligence can also have schizotypal personality disorder.	Robert's parents and psychiatrists tried to rationalize his emotional and interpersonal problems as being the innocuous concomitant of his intellectual gifts.
In college, Robert became obsessed with Lois Abramowitz.	The rare relationships formed by people with schizotypal personality disorder are grossly impaired.	Although Robert had strong sexual feelings for Lois, he did not have the interpersonal skills to establish a real relationship with her.
Even though he never spoke with Lois, Robert was convinced that he had a close relationship with her.	A core dysfunction of people with schizotypal personality disorder is impaired reality testing, a form of psychosis.	Robert fully believed that his paranormal communications with Lois were real.
Robert became enraged when he saw Lois with another young man.	When reality clashes with delusion for people with schizotypal personality disorder, the results can range from upsetting to catastrophic.	Robert's sexual frustration and social ineptitude fueled his delusional involvement with Lois. When confronted with a real-life competitor for Lois, he became impotently enraged.

TABLE 11–3. Key principles of schizotypal personality disorder as exemplified by the case of Robert Woods *(continued)*

Historical fact	Key principle	Interpretation
Robert sent anonymous, threatening notes to Lois and to Gary Parker.	People with schizotypal personality disorder tend to avoid frontal confrontations on equal playing fields.	Robert had none of the interpersonal skills needed to compete for Lois fairly, so he chose stealth, threats, and violence by long distance.
At first, Lois and Gary minimized the implications of the anonymous, threatening notes.	*Any* threatening communication from an unknown party should be taken seriously and acted on judiciously.	The combination of fear, denial, and youthful inexperience led both Lois and Gary to make incorrect and naïve assumptions.
Robert killed Gary's dog by poisoning it with cyanide.	A history of being violent toward animals or humans is a strong predictor of future violent acts by that person. A *surreptitious* pattern of assault will also likely be repeated.	Dr. Flowers understood and emphasized the dangerous implications of Robert's killing Gary's dog. Almost everyone else involved seemed to minimize the serious implications of this act.
Although Robert's parents are fine people and highly intelligent, they never understood or accepted the severity of their son's mental illness, nor would they cooperate with his treatment team.	Parental love can be blinding. Also, when it comes to understanding and treating people with serious psychiatric illnesses, a little knowledge can be a dangerous thing.	Their love for their son and guilt over their impounded anger from dealing with him over the years distorted Robert's parents' objectivity in accepting the severity of his psychiatric illness. They displaced their anger and blamed the insightful messenger, Dr. Flowers.

TABLE 11–3. Key principles of schizotypal personality disorder as exemplified by the case of Robert Woods *(continued)*

Historical fact	Key principle	Interpretation
Robert's parents used their connections with the president of the university to influence their son's treatment.	When VIP status influences treatment, the result is usually ineffective treatment.	By pulling strings to influence the course of their son's treatment, Robert's parents were complicit in the ultimate tragedy for Lois and their son.
Robert was not honest with his parents, his attorneys, his psychiatrists, or the judge.	Don't expect honesty from someone who is capable of murder. People with fatal flaws of personality and character are dishonest in all settings.	Although his reality testing was impaired, Robert had sufficient insight to try to hide his severe psychopathology from his family, his doctors, and the attorneys.
Judge Higgins did not heed Dr. Flowers's warnings about the nature of Robert's illness and his danger to Lois.	America's adversarial judicial system is poorly conceived and equipped to help people with mental illnesses or to protect people who are endangered by those with fatal flaws of personality of character.	Judge Higgins was well intentioned, but he did not heed the warning of a true expert in understanding people with severe mental illness. The arrogance of the court was complicit in the murder of Lois.

The Brain and Schizotypal Personality Disorder

Most experts in schizotypal personality disorder believe that this condition is a component of the spectrum of schizophrenic illnesses. Genetic, epidemiological, and brain imaging research support the notion that schizophrenia is fundamentally a brain illness. Data from family studies indicate that there is an increased risk of schizotypal personality disorder in relatives of people with severe and persistent cases of schizophrenia (Kendler et al. 1993; Torgersen et al. 1993). In addition, other investigators have documented that patients with schizotypal personality disorder have increased cerebral ventricular size as demonstrated on computed tomographic scans—a phenomenon also known to occur in patients with full-blown schizophrenia (Buchsbaum et al. 1997). Finally, many components of neuropsychological tests measuring specific aspects of brain function that yield abnormal results in people with schizophrenia also show abnormal results in people with schizotypal personality disorder (Cadenhead et al. 2000; Trestman et al. 1995). The main point is that because many of the data corroborating that schizophrenia is a brain disorder also apply to patients with schizotypal personality disorder, it is also very likely that the latter condition also has important brain-based determinants. A neurobiological basis for schizotypal personality disorder would have many implications in various areas, including treatment (e.g., the use of medications that work in the brain), heredity (e.g., genetic counseling for prospective parents), and legal matters (are people with this diagnosis who commit violent crimes capable of understanding what they are doing and controlling their behavior?).

Treatment of People With Schizotypal Personality Disorder

As exemplified by the case of Robert Woods, people with schizotypal personality disorder rarely seek out psychiatric or psychological treatment for themselves. Three principal factors result in their reluctance to seek or accept help from mental health professionals. First, basic to the disorder are social anxiety, social isolation, and problems with establishing close and trusting relationships—which must occur for psychotherapeutic treatments to be successful. Second, people with schizotypal personality disorder have impaired reality testing that includes paranoid thinking patterns, odd beliefs, and ideas of reference (defined above under "Further Hospital Treatment"). These thinking disturbances lead them to distort and distrust the motives of clinicians and to be guarded in what they would reveal in treatment. Third, people with this condition invariably have poor insight. What this means is that they do not recognize that they have psychological problems and related difficulties in understanding their own role in creating significant problems for themselves and others. They are much more likely to believe that well-intentioned and even unrelated actions of others negatively affect them. It is also a great challenge for them to understand how past experiences might affect their currently confused thinking and behavior. Another way of saying this is that people with schizotypal personality disorder are notoriously non–psychologically minded. For the most part, many people with this diagnosis truly do not believe in or accept the entire process of treatment. The ultimate result is that, as in the case of Robert Woods, mental health professionals have a difficult time helping people with schizotypal personality disorder. When people with schizotypal personality disorder are remanded by courts or coerced by their families to seek treatment, they will typically resist through nonengagement and nonparticipation. Even the most experienced and gifted of practitioners may often fail to engage a patient under these circumstances.

Despite the aforementioned challenges, psychiatrists and other mental health professionals make valiant attempts to help people with schizotypal personality disorder. Although he notes that most studies of long-term treatment of young men with the diagnosis of schizotypal personality disorder indicate that their core symptoms persist, psychiatrist Michael Stone (2001) has documented five successful results in patients whom he has treated personally. I wholeheartedly endorse Dr. Stone's conceptual therapeutic approach.

Dr. Stone advocates choosing from among a broad range of treatment options and individualizing the type of treatment to the specific symptoms and psychological capacity of each patient.

Psychotherapies

Dr. Stone believes that the most important goal of *insight-oriented psychotherapy* is to help people with schizotypal personality disorder achieve stable, close personal relationships. For treating these patients on an outpatient basis, he suggests that the clinician meet with the patients less frequently than might be the case for patients with different diagnoses—once a week is an ambitious goal. The structured rules of psychotherapy—limiting outside personal contact with the therapist, communicating thoughts and feelings about the therapist, and analyzing the reasons that problems occur between patient and therapist—can help the patients understand how they confuse communications in their other relationships.

Supportive psychotherapy is especially valuable to patients with this diagnosis. The therapist is active with the patient in helping solve problems with family, work, and relationships; with encouragement; and with helping the patient correct his or her distortions of reality. As a rule this type of treatment proceeds at a slow pace, and many patients require such care over the course of their lifetime. *Cognitive-behavioral therapy* focuses on flawed basic assumptions of the patient that lead to their dysfunctions and discomfort. For example, one group of investigators believe that there are three characteristic misassumptions of a person with schizotypal personality disorder (Beck and Freeman 1990):

1. "I feel like an alien in a frightening environment."
2. "Things don't happen by chance."
3. "Relationships are threatening."

These assumptions will be challenged and reframed in the therapeutic interchange, as well as in relationships in the patient's outside life. The therapist also works with the patient to call attention to and modify personal habits, ways of speaking, and ways of acting that might seem unusual or weird to other people. There is an emphasis on educating the patient about what behaviors and responses are socially appropriate.

Family and group therapies can be most helpful to patients with schizotypal personality disorder. In these treatments, they are encouraged to participate in social discourse, and they are corrected in a supportive way when they distort the communications of others. They become practiced at listening carefully to what other people are saying, and they are cautioned not to add overly personalized meanings to the messages of others. The goal is that over time they will become less shy and more forthcoming about their own feelings and ideas in the full range of social settings.

Medications

If patients with schizotypal personality disorder will agree to take them, psychiatric medications can be of great benefit. However, there is a "Catch-22" problem with their taking psychiatric medications. Patients with this diagnosis are distrustful both of psychiatrists and of "chemicals" that the "shrinks" want to put in their body to change how they think, feel, and behave. In fact, the patient may also have paranoia and would fear that the doctor is trying to kill him or her through poisoning. Therefore, a trusting relationship is required for the patient to be compliant in taking any psychiatric medication, and a trusting relationship with someone who has impaired reality testing might depend on the administration of an antipsychotic medication. The bottom line is that the psychiatrist must move slowly and first try to develop a trusting relationship before encouraging the patient to take medications. I have found that newer-generation antipsychotic medications such as risperidone (Risperdal), olanzapine (Zyprexa), and quetiapine (Seroquel), in *low dosages,* are especially helpful for people with this condition. The medications can be invaluable in organizing psychotic thinking, enabling the psychotherapeutic treatments to move along faster and be more effective. Should patients with schizotypal personality disorder have concomitant depression, antidepressant medications are highly effective, as are antianxiety agents for their severe anxiety.

What to Do When Threatened or Stalked by a Person With Schizotypal Personality Disorder

In the case of Robert Woods, the victim, Lois, never knew her assailant. This is not an uncommon circumstance. Most vulnerable to this form of predation are people who are in the public eye, such as actors, newscasters, musicians/singers, athletes, models, politicians/public officials, writers/journalists, and socialites. In addition, people who stand out, for almost any reason, can become targets. Examples would include a charismatic business leader, an inspiring lecturer, or a beautiful and intelligent young woman such as Lois.

It is also common for people who have had some form of relationship with a person with schizotypal personality disorder to become the objects of their obsessions and, later, enmity. Potentially, such relationships can run the full gamut from casual acquaintances to intense involvements of all varieties. Because people with schizotypal personality disorder are often evaluated at some point in their lives by mental health professionals, these clinicians can become targets. I know of many examples of this, because a large number of my colleagues have called on me for counsel after being threatened by current or former patients. What leads to their becoming targets of their patients is the intense feelings that are engendered on the part of the patient/client toward the professional. These feelings may either be negative, as exemplified by Robert's feelings toward Dr. Flowers, or they may be positive. It is the *intensity* of the patient's feelings that is the most important variable. People with schizotypal personality disorder are not able to modulate such feelings though direct communication or normative relationships with the objects of their intense feelings. It hardly matters whether the initial feelings are intensely negative or strongly positive; they are all destined to become angry feelings. The intense positive feelings of a person with schizotypal personality disorder are soon transmuted to rage toward that person for failing to reciprocate accordingly. The combination of self-absorption and impaired reality testing leads the person with schizotypal personality disorder to believe that he or she has been deceived and disrespected. At that point, either of two disparate dynamics can prevail: the person can internalize the rage, in which case he or she will become despondent or depressed and will usually retreat further into a solitary existence, or the rage can be externalized, leading to threats and violence.

Specific Steps To Take When You Are Threatened or Stalked

This chapter has been specifically crafted so that you will be able to recognize the characteristic features and behavioral patterns of a person who has schizotypal personality disorder. The following are guiding principles about what to do when you feel you are threatened by a person who may have this diagnosis. These principles, which I have developed over many years of advising both endangered colleagues and patients, also apply if you are threatened by dangerous people with other types of personality disorder, such as paranoid or antisocial. These guiding principles are summarized in Table 11–4.

TABLE 11–4. Guiding principles for people who are being threatened or stalked by a person with a personality disorder

---

1. Take any threat seriously.
2. Until you are certain of the source of the threat, do not rule out any possibility.
3. Obtain help from *experienced* professionals.
4. Once you have engaged competent professionals, follow their advice.
5. Do *not* try to reason with or confront the person who has threatened you. Use professionals and intermediaries to deal with this person.
6. Even after a favorable resolution, keep your guard up.
7. You must follow *each* principle (1–6) to be safe.

Given the potentially serious consequences to people who are threatened or stalked, each of these seven principles merits separate discussion.

Principle 1: Take Any Threat Seriously

As a general rule, the more frightening a possibility of our being harmed, the greater becomes our level of denial. For example, even highly trained and experienced psychiatrists frequently fail to ask their patients who have high risk of future violence whether or not they have access to guns or other weapons. (One of the first questions I ask a colleague who seeks my help on being threatened by a patient is, "Does this person own or have access to guns or other types of dangerous weapons?" Most of these colleagues reply that they have never asked their patient about weapons.) The reason for this critical omission in their workup of these patients is that the professionals unconsciously sensed the danger to themselves but denied this risk out of great fear. Unfortunately, such denial can be—and often is—disastrous. Take any threat seriously by pursuing all responsible avenues to assess the risk and avoid harm.

Principle 2: Until You Are Certain of the Source of the Threat, Do Not Rule out Any Possibility

One form of denial is to seize on the least threatening possibility to re-assure ourselves that we are not in great danger. Such an approach also gives us the illusion of control over the terrifying unknown. Recall from the case history presented in this chapter that Lois did not even know Robert, so of course she did not suspect him of sending her the threatening notes. Rather, Lois incorrectly concluded that one of her female classmates was jealous of Lois's relationship with her boyfriend and was the perpetrator. Jumping too quickly to firm conclusions without the necessary confirmatory evidence will not only cause hard feelings among those who are wrongly accused, but will also waste valuable time and resources. Any delay in identifying and apprehending the true culprit can be fatal.

Principle 3: Obtain Help From Experienced Professionals

Anyone who is being threatened requires help from experienced professionals. You should not try to deal with threats on your own. Because the threat involves you personally and in such a fundamental and dangerous way, there is no way that you can maintain your objectivity. Even if you are an expert in psychology or police work and believe that you can best handle this threat by yourself, you are wrong! Because you cannot be objective, you will not be aware of your blind spots. What you miss can be fatal. Rather, you must secure the appropriate help from professionals who know what they are doing when it comes to dealing with threats from people who are dangerous for whatever reason. These experts might include the local police, your district attorney, tough-minded and available private attorneys or mental health professionals, licensed and responsible private investigators, and even well-referenced private security professionals. Even though you don't deserve and don't want to face this problem, it is nonetheless real. Finding capable experts to help you usually requires considerable time, effort, and often funds. Such professionals are well worth your time, effort, and money. Your life may depend on your engaging the appropriate professionals.

Principle 4: Once You Have Engaged Competent Professionals, Follow Their Advice

You might be reluctant to follow the advice of the professionals whom you engage. This is understandable. These professionals may ask that you disrupt your life in order to be safe. They might advise you to change your residence or job. They might encourage you to press charges against or seek a restraining order on a person of whom you are afraid. Certainly you will have the realistic concern that such firm actions might provoke the potential assailant. All experienced professionals will carefully assess the risk of taking direct actions toward the potential assailant with the alternative tack of your maintaining a low profile. Each case is different, and there are no all-encompassing formulas. Be aware, however, that most people in your circumstances would much rather take a passive approach and hope that the problem will go away on its own. This may or may not be the correct decision. Recall from the case history that Gary wanted to ignore the threatening notes entirely, and his dog was killed. Robert was not angry with Gary's dog; he just as easily could have killed Gary. Even more disturbing in the case history was that neither Robert's parents nor the judge listened to Dr. Flowers's strong admonition that Robert should remain in a mental institution until such time as a *knowledgeable* psychiatrist advised that he had become safe. After all, who would want to think that a young college student was a potential murderer, or who would want to lock him up in a state mental hospital for an indefinite period of time? Prospectively, it seemed that only Dr. Flowers wanted to take this definitive action. With the benefit of hindsight, *everyone* wished they had listened to the true expert. In cases of threats and stalking, the *easiest* way is often not the *safest* way. My bottom-line recommendation, which I know will not be easy for you to follow, is: ***Make the effort to find the best professionals, and then follow their advice.***

Principle 5: Do Not Try to Reason With or Confront the Person Who Has Threatened You; Use Professionals and Intermediaries to Deal With This Person

If you are threatened, particularly by a person who has a severe personality disorder, do not try to confront or reason with this person directly. Please understand that this person is *inherently unreasonable,* probably as the result of a brain-based mental illness. This illness will affect the potential assailant's reality testing, level of rage, and ability to control violent impulses. No matter how logical and reasonable the case you offer may be, it will be distorted and turned against you. In most instances when a person who is threatened takes matters into his or her own hands, the situation is made far worse. The reason is that the perpetrator seeks this intense and intimate engagement with you through the threats, and he or she will intensify the threats and level of danger to keep you engaged.

A professional intermediary changes this dangerous dynamic for several reasons: 1) the intermediary deflects the perpetrator's attention from you to himself or herself; 2) the professional will understand how best to assess and manage the risk; 3) the perpetrator will understand that you are now protected and less vulnerable; 4) the perpetrator will, for the first time, recognize that *the risk is now shared!* The person who threatens you will now realize that he or she has a great deal to lose by further threats or violent acts toward you. On many occasions I have seen this change in dynamics—from the person threatened to an empowered professional—reduce the risk significantly. When this shift occurs, you will begin to feel better almost immediately.

Principle 6: Even After a Favorable Resolution, Keep Your Guard Up

Once you have been seriously threatened by a person with severe flaws of personality and character, your life has been changed forever. Even if a satisfactory resolution occurs—such as the person's being put in jail for a life term—the danger may not have ended. That person, for example, can escape from prison or be paroled and come back to harm you. Although you will want to put the whole episode out of your mind and bury it in your past, you cannot afford to do so. There are so many examples of perpetrators maintaining and acting on violent obsessions and delusions after many years of being separated from their victims. *You* must assume the responsibility of trying to know what is going on with the person who has threatened you. Certainly, in most cases it will be necessary for you to work through your professional intermediaries. Their responsibility will be to take the direct actions required keep you current on the disposition of the potential assailant. They will accomplish this in a dispassionate way that is part of their professional duties. They should perform their duties while keeping you as removed as possible from awareness of the person who has threatened you in the past. *Your job* is to make sure that your representatives *stay on the job.*

Principle 7: You Must Follow Each Principle (1–6) to Be Safe

First the good news: If you follow *all* of my principles, your crisis will almost always abate. Your professionals will advise you of the correct actions to take, and if you follow their recommendations, these actions will usually be successful in stopping the threats and mitigating the danger.

Now the bad news: If you follow only *some* of my principles and do not adhere to others, you will remain in danger. In the case of Robert Woods, a tragic outcome occurred because all but one of my principles was violated, as indicated below:

1. Lois and Gary did *not* take Robert's initial threats seriously.
2. Lois and Gary *jumped to conclusions* about who was issuing these threats.
3. Lois and her parents *did not enlist the help* of experienced experts to protect themselves. They were far too passive in the entire process. On the other hand, Robert's parents enlisted the help of adversarial forensic psychiatrists, who in this case were "guns for hire." In other words, as so often happens in courtroom situations, the so-called experts who were available for hire testified according to the views of the people who paid them.
4. Because Lois and her parents, Mr. and Mrs. Abramowitz, did not participate in the court hearings of Robert Woods, they were not in a position to adhere to the advice of an expert. This is too bad, because it turned out that they had an excellent advocate, Dr. Flowers, a knowledgeable and reputable professional. Had the Abramowitz family remained active and supported Dr. Flowers's clearly defined recommendations, it is possible that they could have helped sway Judge Higgins to protect Lois rather than to "convenience" Robert Woods and his parents.
5. Lois and her family did not know Robert Woods, nor did they directly confront him. Thus they unwittingly adhered to Principle 5. This makes my point that you have to follow *all* of the principles to be safe, not just some of them. Nonetheless, please trust me, adhering to Principle 5 is extremely important: Your direct confrontation

of people with fatal flaws of personality and character who threaten you will almost always backfire and intensify your risk of being harmed.

6. Although Lois moved to a new school near her home, neither she nor her parents kept abreast of what was happening with Robert Woods once he was put away in a psychiatric hospital. Even though Dr. Flowers insisted that they be notified that the court had released him from the protection and care of the hospital, the Abramowitz family did not take special precautions to assure Lois's protection and safety. More than a year after the Abramowitz family thought that their problem had been resolved, Lois was killed by Robert.

Afterword

On April 4, 1996, my secretary opened the door of my office during a treatment session with a patient. She told me that an FBI agent calling me from San Francisco said that it was urgent that I be interrupted. The FBI agent revealed to me that the bureau believed that it had just captured a person whom it believed to be the Unabomber. "Unabomber" was the name given to a person who, over a period of 17 years, dispersed through the mail a series of at least 16 bombs that had killed 3 people and wounded or maimed 23 others. The agent went on to say that in the suspect's Montana cabin a short "hit list" of potential targets was found and that my name was listed near its top. The person who was suspected and later convicted of being the Unabomber is Ted Kaczynski, who is now serving a life sentence in a federal prison. Mr. Kaczynski had primarily targeted (and killed) scientists, and the FBI found in Mr. Kaczynski's cabin a volume of the journal *Scientific American* in which my work on the neurobiology of aggressive disorders was extensively referenced. As recommended by the FBI, for 6 months thereafter all packages addressed to me that were delivered to my office at Baylor College of Medicine, to my home, or to the Washington address of the *Journal of Neuropsychiatry and Clinical Neurosciences*, of which I am the editor, had to be x-rayed before being opened. Initially, the FBI also expressed some concern about "copycat" bombings from a rogue member of the many fringe groups that shared Mr. Kaczynski's antipathy for people in high-profile positions in science, medicine, and technology. The extensive local and national media coverage of me and the other people on Mr. Kaczynski's hit list proved to be upsetting to my three school-age daughters, and it frightened my office staff and several of my patients. All in all, even though I and my office staff were fortunate not to be physically harmed by Mr. Kaczynski, this was a disturbing and distracting intrusion by someone whom I have never even met. Because I was never Mr. Kaczynski's psychiatrist and therefore have not evaluated him clinically, it would certainly not be ethical for me to speculate on any psychiatric diagnosis that he may or may not have. Nonetheless, in the bibliography for this chapter, I have referenced a popular biography of Mr. Kaczynski (Waits and Shors 1998). I believe that his childhood history, his personality patterns, and his adult lifestyle reveal many similarities with other people who stalk and prey on the innocent from the shadows and safety of their anonymity.

References and Suggested Readings

American Psychiatric Association: Diagnostic and Statistical Manual of Mental Disorders, 2nd Edition. Washington, DC, American Psychiatric Association, 1968

American Psychiatric Association: Diagnostic and Statistical Manual of Mental Disorders, 4th Edition, Text Revision. Washington, DC, American Psychiatric Association, 2000, pp 697–701

Battaglia M, Torgersen S: Schizotypal disorder: at the crossroads of genetics and nosology. Acta Psychiatr Scand 94:303–310, 1996

Beck A, Freeman A: Cognitive Therapy of Personality Disorders. New York, Guilford, 1990

Bender DS, Dolan RT, Skodol AE, et al: Treatment utilization by patients with personality disorders. Am J Psychiatry 158:295–302, 2001

Buchsbaum MS, Yang S, Hazlett E, et al: Ventricular volume and asymmetry in schizotypal personality disorder and schizophrenia assessed with magnetic resonance imaging. Schizophr Res 27:45–53, 1997

Cadenhead KS, Perry W, Shafer K, et al: Cognitive functions in schizotypal personality disorder. Schizophr Res 37:123–132, 1999

Cadenhead KS, Light GA, Geyer MA, et al: Sensory gating deficits assessed by the P50 event-related potential in subjects with schizotypal personality disorder. Am J Psychiatry 157:55–59, 2000

Checkley H: The Mask of Sanity, 4th Edition. St. Louis, MO, CV Mosby, 1964

Gabbard G: Cluster A personality disorders: paranoid, schizoid, and schizotypal, in Psychodynamic Psychiatry in Clinical Practice, 3rd Edition. Washington, DC, American Psychiatric Press, 2000, pp 385–410

Kalus O, Bernstein DP, Siever LJ: Schizoid personality disorder: a review of its current status. J Personal Disord 7:43–52, 1993

Kendler KS, McGuire M, Gruenberg AM, et al: The Roscommon family study, III: schizophrenia-related personality disorders in relatives. Arch Gen Psychiatry 50:781–788, 1993

Phillips KA, Yen S, Gunderson JG: Personality disorders, in The American Psychiatric Publishing Textbook of Clinical Psychiatry, 4th Edition. Edited by Hales RE, Yudofsky SC. Washington, DC, American Psychiatric Publishing, 2003, pp 803–832

Stone MH: Schizoid and schizotypal personality disorders, in Treatments of Psychiatric Disorders, 3rd Edition. Edited by Gabbard GO. Washington, DC, American Psychiatric Publishing, 2001, pp 2237–2250

Torgersen S, Onstad S, Skre I, et al: "True" schizotypal personality disorder: a study of co-twins and relatives of schizophrenic probands. Am J Psychiatry 150:1661–1667, 1993

Trestman RL, Keefe RS, Mitropoulou V, et al: Cognitive function and biological correlates of cognitive performance in schizotypal personality disorder. Psychiatry Res 59:127–136, 1995

Voglmaier MM, Seidman LJ, Salisbury D, et al: Neuropsychological dysfunction in schizotypal personality disorder: a profile analysis. Biol Psychiatry 41:530–540, 1997

Voglmaier MM, Seidman LJ, Niznikiewicz MA, et al: Verbal and nonverbal neuropsychological test performance in subjects with schizotypal personality disorder. Am J Psychiatry 157:787–793, 2000

Waits C, Shors D: Unabomber: The Secret Life of Ted Kaczynski. Helena, MT, Farcountry Press, 1998

Zuckerman M: The psychobiological model for impulsive unsocialized sensation seeking: a comparative approach. Neuropsychobiology 34:125–129, 1996

ADDICTIVE PERSONALITY DISORDER

O thou invisible spirit of wine, if thou hast no name to be known by, let us call thee devil!

O God, that men should put an enemy in their mouths to steal away their brains! that we should, with joy, pleasance revel and applause, transform ourselves into beasts!

It hath pleased the devil drunkenness to give place to the devil wrath; one unperfectness shows me another, to make me frankly despise myself.

—William Shakespeare,
Othello, Act II, Scene 3

Essence

Have you ever had a relationship with someone whom you believe is really two different people? The "real" person is kind, thoughtful, considerate, even-tempered, reliable, capable, and unselfish. The "other" person is just the opposite: entirely self-centered, dishonest, and irritating, and almost always failing to come through on commitments. You respond lovingly to the "real" person and become elated and hopeful when this persona appears. You have missed him so much. For many years you also feel compassion for the "other" person, and try to believe in and help him. Over time, however, you become disillusioned and worn out from the emotional roller coaster that rumbles from optimism to deep disillusionment. Even the hurt that you feel when the "other" person breaks promises, ignores you, or embarrasses you begins to deaden, to be replaced with an intensifying anger. At first you feel guilty over your anger, and you continue to make excuses for him. "It's an illness. He can't help himself. He'll get better. He's trying harder and will really make it this time." You finally understand that you are only kidding yourself, and you feel like a fool. You have waited so long. The "real" person now appears less and less often, and you begin to wonder if that person ever really existed in the first place. Did you make him up entirely? You find that you are giving up. It is so hard to care for someone who does not seem to care about you, about himself, or about anything else that matters. You finally get it. You have not had a relationship with this person for a very long time. You ask yourself two troubling questions: Can you have a true relationship with someone who is dependent on alcohol or drugs? And which one is the "real" person: the individual addicted to alcohol or drugs, or the other one?

The Case of Dr. Maria Torres, Part One: Background History

If there ever was someone who understood what it might mean to lose everything, it was Dr. Maria Torres. She grew up in abject poverty in Texas's Rio Grande Valley. Her father, an undocumented migrant worker from Mexico afflicted by chronic alcoholism, was only occasionally employed. Her mother supported Maria and her three younger sisters by working as a maid in ramshackle motels that in many ways resembled the stubborn cacti that somehow cling to the dry, crumbling earth along the Texas–Mexico border. Often when the economy was bad in the valley, Mrs. Torres would be laid off, and the family would be unable to pay the rent for their meager apartment. During those times, they would live for many months at a time in abandoned, rusting buses that reddened the dust and briars of vacant fields on the outskirts of their small town. That was how Maria discovered books. Because she had no place to go after school, Maria would spend her evenings at the local library until it closed at 9:00 P.M. It was only a small library, but it had a bathroom, books, and Mr. Simon Zimmerman. Under the guidance of this gentle and scholarly librarian, Maria became an active and disciplined reader.

Only a small percentage of the students in Maria's town completed high school, and going on to college was a rarity. Very few of those who were interested could afford college. Nonetheless, Mr. Zimmerman encouraged Maria to take the College Board Entrance Examination (the SAT). Because she had been so shy and withdrawn in high school, her teachers were surprised when they learned that Maria's SAT scores were nearly perfect. Soon thereafter, she became the first student in her school's 30-year history to qualify as a National Merit Finalist. Solely on the basis of her love for the novels of F. Scott Fitzgerald, she decided to apply to Princeton. Maria recalls only too well that she had to request special dispensation on her application to Princeton, because she could not afford the $50 application fee. "To that point in my life, I had never seen 50 dollars in one place," Maria recollected.

Maria was accepted to Princeton with a full scholarship. She excelled in all of her classes, but she felt self-conscious about her impoverished background when she was around her classmates. While attending a fraternity party during her third week at college, she discovered that she could relate much more comfortably with her peers after drinking several cans of beer. Maria vividly recalled that experience: "For the first time in my life, I wasn't paralyzed by anxiety when I was with people of my own age."

To earn extra money for clothes and sundries, Maria worked weekday evenings and many weekends at the Princeton Faculty Club. It was there that she began to drink hard liquor. At first she would drink only what remained in the glasses that were brought back to the kitchen. Thereafter, whenever the opportunity arose, she would steal partially empty bottles of liquor from the bar area. This gave Maria the opportunity to drink every evening—whether or not she was going to be in the company of her friends. Despite the fact that Maria drank every night throughout college and would become inebriated several times a week, she maintained high grades in her premedical courses. At the medical school that she attended in the Houston region, she dated men—mostly medical students—based on whether or not they were regular drinkers. She stated, "I still didn't have enough disposable income to afford the half-bottle of Jack Daniels that I would like to drink every night, so I would go out with the medical students who were drinkers and ask them to buy 'us' bottles of bourbon." As she had been in college, however, Maria was also serious about her studies, and her scholastic performance remained in the superior range. During her senior year of medical school, Maria met Dr. Jonathan Ungar, who at that time was a resident in orthopedic surgery. The kindly and hard-working young physician reminded her somewhat of Mr. Zimmerman. Maria soon fell in love with Dr. Ungar, the first man she ever dated seriously who hardly ever drank alcohol. About her relationship with Dr. Ungar, Maria stated, "I am great at hiding myself. My classmates in high school never knew that I lived in a bus. My girlfriends at Princeton, some of whom took me on vacations in their families' private planes, never knew that I owned only two pairs of shoes and one overcoat—that I bought at Goodwill—during my entire four years at college. For the first few years that we knew each other, Jonathan had no idea how much I drank." Maria added, "In medical school, I would get drunk when he was on call at the hospital; and I would also drink heavily after he fell asleep on his nights off. Jonathan is such an honest and trusting man that even after we were married, he never suspected that I had a drinking problem. I simply covered up all the evidence and lied to him as necessary."

Maria and Jonathan were married during the second year of her residency in anesthesiology. When she became pregnant 1 year later, she tried to stop drinking to prevent the occurrence of developmental disorders in her child. She accomplished that by switching from alcohol to the antianxiety drug alprazolam (Xanax), which, although highly addictive, is thought not to be damaging to the developing fetus. To acquire the Xanax, Dr. Torres began to steal medications from the pharmacy trays on the units and in the operating rooms of the hospital where she worked. As her tolerance for and dependency on Xanax increased over time, she persuaded several physicians whom she knew to prescribe her large quantities of the drug for "migraine headaches" and for "back pain." After the birth of their son, who had no developmental abnormalities, she continued to take high daily doses of Xanax while returning to drinking Jack Daniels at night. Early one Saturday morning, when Jonathan returned from performing emergency surgery on a person who had been injured in a car accident, he found their infant son soiled and crying in his crib and Maria in a comatose state in their bed. Later, Dr. Ungar was dumbfounded and incredulous when the emergency room physician communicated to him that his wife was intoxicated with dangerous levels of both alcohol and alprazolam. When she awakened, Dr. Torres explained to her husband that that what had occurred was an accident. She explained, "I was only trying to get some rest from a hard week at work and with our baby." Maria easily dissuaded her husband from following the recommendation of the emergency physician that they consult a psychiatrist about a potentially serious problem.

Several weeks later, Dr. Torres was observed by an operating room nurse to be dozing off while she was administering anesthesia to a patient for a cardiovascular surgery procedure. The nurse reported the incident to Dr. Kelley, the chairman of the hospital's anesthesiology service. Dr. Kelley was outraged over Dr. Torres's endangerment of her patient. He did not buy Dr. Torres's excuse that she was overworked from her job and her caring for a young child. Furthermore, Dr. Kelly said, "Although I don't have proof, I believe that you are taking drugs. I'll give you two choices: either accept the psychiatric consultation of my choice, or resign your position with the hospital."

Without even discussing the options with her husband, Dr. Torres chose to leave her job. She told Jonathan that she wanted to spend more quality time with their son. He readily agreed. Soon Maria was drinking and taking Xanax heavily during the day, and she did not stop when she again became pregnant. Her daughter was born prematurely and was soon recognized to have fetal alcohol syndrome along with serious physical and intellectual impairments. Among the infant's problems were a heart defect that would require surgery and mild mental retardation. As a physician, Maria recognized her responsibility for causing the lifelong disability of her daughter, and she drank literally day and night to blot out this bitter realization. She began to take the pain medication hydromorphine hydrochloride (Dilaudid) and began to forge her husband's triplicate-form prescriptions that are required in Texas for any medications that are highly addictive. Before long, Dr. Ungar was summoned before the Texas State Board of Medical Examiners for prescribing alprazolam in such high quantities to a family member. When Jonathan confronted Maria with this disclosure, she denied taking alprazolam or forging his prescriptions. The gentle doctor was as upset over his wife's blatant lying in the face of such evidence as he was over her substance abuse. Against Maria's strongest objections, he sought my consultation. Presented in Table 12–1 is a summary of key principles in the treatment of people with addictive personality disorders as exemplified by the case of Dr. Maria Torres.

Defining Addiction and Substance Dependence

Substance Dependence

The World Health Organization and the U.S. Alcohol, Drug Abuse, and Mental Health Administration have agreed on a definition of substance dependence that includes the elements summarized in Table 12–2 (World Health Organization 1992).

Several other definitions are important in the understanding of substance abuse. *Tolerance* refers to the progressive diminution of the

TABLE 12–1.   Key principles of addictions exemplified by the case of Dr. Maria Torres, part 1: presenting history

Historical fact	Key principle	Interpretation
Dr. Torres's father had chronic alcoholism.	There are strong familial and genetic predispositions to alcoholism and chemical dependencies.	Dr. Torres's genetics was probably the key determinant of her addictions.
Dr. Torres was highly intelligent and hardworking and had achieved considerable academic and professional success.	Many people with addictive disorders are intelligent, hardworking, and successful.	Equal-opportunity discriminators, addictive disorders afflict both the advantaged and the disadvantaged; those who succeed and those who fail.
Dr. Torres began using alcohol as an attempt to deal with her social anxiety.	Psychosocial factors commonly trigger the initial addictive behaviors in people with genetic predispositions to alcohol and chemical dependencies.	Biological, psychological, social, and spiritual factors are all involved in the development of alcoholism and chemical dependencies.
Dr. Torres's addiction progressed from the episodic use of beer, to the daily drinking of bourbon, to the mixing of hard liquor with prescribed medications.	One type of addiction typically leads to others.	Patterns of addiction often involve the progression from "gateway drugs" like alcohol and marijuana to other drugs that are even more addictive and endangering to the person's health and safety.
Dr. Torres hid the extent of her addictive behavior from her friends and family.	People with addictive behaviors characteristically engage in secretive activities, lie to loved ones and others, and violate the trust of family and friends.	People with dependencies first deny—to themselves—the nature and extent of their addiction. This extends to their lying about and hiding their addictions in all important relationships.

TABLE 12–1. Key principles of addictions exemplified by the case of Dr. Maria Torres, part 1: presenting history *(continued)*

Historical fact	Key principle	Interpretation
Dr. Torres stole bottles of alcohol, abused prescription medications, and forged prescriptions as the result of her drug-seeking behavior.	Addictions often lead to felonies.	From driving while intoxicated to impulsive violence, people with alcoholism and chemical dependencies have impaired judgment and poor impulse control.
By drinking heavily during her pregnancy, Dr. Torres permanently injured the brain of her child.	People with addictive disorders commonly cause irreversible harm to others.	The self-involvement of people with addictive disorders leads them to endanger and harm others.
Dr. Torres intensified her abuse of alcohol and prescribed medications in an unsuccessful attempt to assuage her guilt over harming her child.	The destructive consequences of addiction-related behaviors frequently lead to vicious cycles of increased alcohol and/or drug abuse.	The cycle of increasing use of alcohol and drugs to deal with guilt and shame will not be interrupted until the person is completely withdrawn from the substances of abuse.
Dr. Ungar's faith in his wife and belief in his marriage was shattered by Dr. Torres's addiction-related behavior.	Alcoholism and chemical dependencies destroy trust and ruin relationships.	The indirect effects of addictions—such as dishonesty and neglect of responsibilities—damage relationships more than the direct effects of intoxication.

TABLE 12–2.   Summary of World Health Organization definition and U.S. Alcohol, Drug Abuse, and Mental Health Administration definition of substance dependence

1. The abused substance is *psychoactive,* meaning it alters the brain to affect mood, perception, thinking, and behavior.

2. There is drug-seeking behavior.

3. The use of the abused substance and obtaining the substance are given a higher priority than what had previously been the important aspects of everyday life.

4. There is dependence on the substance, which means the person has a strong desire to take the substance and requires increasing amounts to gain the desired effect, and there are uncomfortable physical and emotional responses when the drug is withdrawn. One important aspect of dependence is that the person continues to take the drug in an effort to avoid the withdrawal effects.

5. The person persists in using the drug despite harmful consequences.

6. The person is unsuccessful in trying to reduce the dosage or discontinue using the substance.

---

desired effects of the drug with each successive use—hence the drive to take the drug more frequently and in higher doses. *Sensitization* is the opposite effect of tolerance, wherein repeated use of the drug results in an intensification of the desired effect. This phenomenon often occurs after a person has been free from the drug for a prolonged period of time. The intense responses on reintroducing certain drugs after periods of abstinence can account for the high relapse rates associated with these addictive substances.

Presented in Table 12–3 are the DSM-IV-TR diagnostic criteria for substance dependence (American Psychiatric Association 2000).

Substance Intoxication and Withdrawal

For the most commonly abused substances, the signs and symptoms associated with intoxication and withdrawal are defined in DSM-IV-TR. The diagnostic criteria for alcohol intoxication are summarized in Table 12–4 (American Psychiatric Association 2000).

When an individual has been dependent on a substance for a prolonged period of time, he or she will experience psychological symptoms and physical signs when that substance is abruptly withdrawn. Withdrawal effects vary depending on the nature and extent of the

TABLE 12–3.   DSM-IV-TR diagnostic criteria for substance dependence

A maladaptive pattern of substance use, leading to clinically significant
impairment or distress, as manifested by three (or more) of the following,
occurring at any time in the same 12-month period:
(1) tolerance, as defined by either of the following:
    (a) a need for markedly increased amounts of the substance to achieve
        intoxication or desired effect
    (b) markedly diminished effect with continued use of the same amount of
        the substance
(2) withdrawal, as manifested by either of the following:
    (a) the characteristic withdrawal syndrome for the substance (refer to
        Criteria A and B of the criteria sets for withdrawal from the specific
        substances)
    (b) the same (or a closely related) substance is taken to relieve or avoid
        withdrawal symptoms
(3) the substance is often taken in larger amounts or over a longer period than
    was intended
(4) there is a persistent desire or unsuccessful efforts to cut down or control
    substance use
(5) a great deal of time is spent in activities necessary to obtain the substance
    (e.g., visiting multiple doctors or driving long distances), use the substance
    (e.g., chain-smoking), or recover from its effects
(6) important social, occupational, or recreational activities are given up or
    reduced because of substance use
(7) the substance use is continued despite knowledge of having a persistent or
    recurrent physical or psychological problem that is likely to have been
    caused or exacerbated by the substance (e.g., current cocaine use despite
    recognition of cocaine-induced depression, or continued drinking despite
    recognition that an ulcer was made worse by alcohol consumption)
Specify if:
With Physiological Dependence: evidence of tolerance or withdrawal
    (i.e., either Item 1 or 2 is present)
Without Physiological Dependence: no evidence of tolerance or withdrawal
    (i.e., neither Item 1 nor 2 is present)
Course specifiers:
Early Full Remission
Early Partial Remission
Sustained Full Remission
Sustained Partial Remission
On Agonist Therapy
In a Controlled Environment

Source.   Reprinted from American Psychiatric Association: *Diagnostic and Statistical Manual of Mental Disorders*, 4th Edition, Text Revision. Washington, DC,
American Psychiatric Association, 2000, p. 197. Used with permission.

TABLE 12–4. Diagnostic criteria for alcohol intoxication (slightly modified from DSM-IV-TR)

A. Recent ingestion of alcohol

B. Clinically significant maladaptive behavioral or psychological changes (e.g., inappropriate sexual or aggressive behavior, mood lability, impaired judgment, impaired social or occupational functioning) that developed during, or shortly after, alcohol ingestion

C. One (or more) of the following signs, developing during, or shortly after, alcohol use:

  1. slurred speech

  2. poor coordination

  3. unsteady gait

  4. nystagmus

  5. impairment in attention or memory

  6. stupor or coma

D. The symptoms are not due to a general medical condition and are not better accounted for by another mental disorder

---

Source. Adapted from American Psychiatric Association: *Diagnostic and Statistical Manual of Mental Disorders,* 4th Edition, Text Revision. Washington, DC, American Psychiatric Association, 2000, p. 215. Used with permission.

abuse of the substance and the health status of the abuser. The diagnostic criteria for alcohol withdrawal are summarized in Table 12–5 (American Psychiatric Association 2000).

Addictive Disorders as Flaws of Personality and Character

The Destructive Behaviors of Some People With Addictive Disorders Occur Only When They Are Under the Influence of Alcohol or Drugs

The American Psychiatric Association does not include a category of addictive personality disorders in its official publication, DSM-IV-TR. However, people who persistently abuse substances share the pattern of symptoms and signs that would ordinarily qualify a person for a diagnosis of a personality disorder. The hallmark of personality disorders—persistent patterns of feeling, thinking, and behavior that result in problems with relationships, in controlling impulses, and in functioning in social, school, and occupational settings—are prevalent

TABLE 12–5. Diagnostic criteria for alcohol withdrawal (slightly modified from DSM-IV-TR)

A. Cessation of (or reduction in) alcohol use that has been heavy and prolonged

B. Two (or more) of the following, developing within several hours to a few days after Criterion A:

1. autonomic hyperactivity (e.g., sweating or pulse rate greater than 100)

2. increased hand tremor

3. insomnia

4. nausea or vomiting

5. transient visual, tactile, or auditory hallucinations or illusions

6. psychomotor agitation

7. anxiety

8. grand mal seizures

C. The symptoms in Criterion B cause clinically significant distress or impairment in social, occupational, or other important areas of functioning

D. The symptoms are not due to a general medical condition and are not better accounted for by another mental disorder

Source. Adapted from American Psychiatric Association: *Diagnostic and Statistical Manual of Mental Disorders,* 4th Edition, Text Revision. Washington, DC, American Psychiatric Association, 2000, p 216. Used with permission.

among people with dependencies on alcohol or other addictive substances. Among my many difficult conceptual and editorial decisions required in the writing of this book was whether or not to include people with alcoholism and addictive disorders within the category of fatal flaws of personality and character, particularly when it is not a sanctioned DSM diagnostic category. I invite you into my thinking process as I made this determination. First and foremost, I have known many people who have been afflicted for years and years with alcoholism and other types of substance dependence who have recovered. Almost to a person, these people, when free from the mind-numbing and mind-distorting effects of alcohol and drugs, do not have fatal flaws of personality or character. Many, in fact, are among the most accomplished, productive, ethical, and generous people whom it has been my privilege to know. However, when they were under the influence of alcohol or other substances, their stories were much different. Each of them would certainly have qualified on the Fatal Flaw Scale (see Appendix A in Chapter 2, "Does This Person Have a Fatal Flaw?") as having fatal flaws of personality and character. It is my firm belief that their brain-based cravings for alcohol and drugs, combined with the biochemical alterations in their brains caused by alcohol, led to the destructive changes in their personality, values, and character. For example, people who would never be dishonest when sober were pathological liars under the influence of alcohol or other drugs. The husband of one of my patients who, while drinking regularly, had deceived both of us many times with her fabrications and distortions, once asked me, "When my wife is drinking, do you know how you can tell when she is lying?" I responded that I was not able to determine whether she was lying or being truthful. He then said, "Over the 15 years of my marriage I have learned that you can tell that my wife is lying if her lips are moving." Similarly, I have known men to be verbally and physically abusive to their wives and children only while intoxicated. Many people with multiple arrests and convictions have never broken a law outside the context of intoxication or their drug-seeking behaviors. There are many women who are among the most caring and responsible mothers but will nevertheless risk the lives of their children by driving while intoxicated or under the influence of other drugs. I have known men whose infidelity to their wives took place exclusively during circumstances in which they were intoxicated. Finally, in my psychiatry practice I have evaluated many people who do not have fatal flaws of personality and character but who, exclusively under the influence of alcohol or drugs, have committed the most serious criminal acts, including impulsive violence and murder. To the purists in psychiatric diagnosis, these examples would make the case that the personality changes that occur in people under the influence of substances are secondary to brain alterations brought on by chemicals and should therefore not be considered primary personality disorders.

Addiction as a Personality Disorder

Although the American Psychiatric Association does not classify substance dependence as a personality disorder per se, certain highly regarded investigators have shown that there is an association between addictions and certain personality traits and types. The research of psychiatrist Dr. C. Robert Cloninger (1998) has demonstrated that aggressive personality traits of children and adolescents predict the early-life abuse of substances. Novelty seeking, risk taking, impulsiveness, and antisocial personalities in adolescents are also associated with high incidences of substance dependence and alcoholism among young adults. Other investigators and experienced clinicians have indicated that people who are perfectionists and who have obsessive-compulsive personalities are also prone to alcoholism and substance abuse. These investigators point out that such people require the depressant effects of alcohol and depressant substances such as marijuana to relax their churning minds. If these individuals stop abusing alcohol or other psychoactive substances, their personality disorders and other problems may become more prominent. Therefore, treatment must involve more than the discontinuation of the abused substance; otherwise social, occupational, or relationship problems will emerge. Unless the underlying personality disorders associated with people with addictions are addressed, recidivism to the original substance of abuse ("falling off the wagon") is high. Finally, many studies have documented that people with antisocial personality disorders are at high risk to abuse alcohol, prescription medications that are addictive, and the full range of illegal drugs.

In summary, I believe that it is practical and useful to include addictions as a category of personality disorders for *Fatal Flaws*. The thinking, behavioral, emotional, and interpersonal problems experienced by people with addictive disorders closely resemble those brought about by the personality disorders officially recognized in DSM-IV-TR. Most important, clinicians and other people who are attempting to understand, help, and deal with people with chemical dependencies can be benefited by the information and principles imparted in this book.

The Enormous Toll on Individuals and Society Taken by Addictive Disorders

Alcohol and substance abuse are among the foremost public health problems in America. About 20% of the population of the United States will, at some point in their lives, have a substance use disorder. Conservatively, this means that at least nine million people in the United States meet DSM-IV-TR criteria for alcohol dependence, and approximately six million others abuse alcohol periodically. Tragically, even though it is illegal, more than ten million Americans under 21 years of age drink alcohol on a regular basis, and of these, about seven million engage in binge drinking that results in serious intoxication. About 20% of people in general hospitals and about one-third of patients being treated on inpatient psychiatric services have primary diagnoses of substance dependence. Regarding alcoholism alone, approximately one in five intensive care unit (ICU) admissions are the direct result of alcohol abuse, and two in five Americans will be harmed by an alcohol abuse–

related accident at some point during their lives. *It is estimated that alcohol abuse alone accounts for more than half of the fatal automobile accidents in the United States and for more than 50% of deaths by violence. More than 5% of people who are alcohol dependent will complete suicide, and overall about half of suicides occur in the context of alcohol or substance abuse* (Miller and Adams 2005). Let us think for a moment about the grief and pain of parents who lose an adolescent child in a fatal traffic accident, about the terror of a child who loses a parent who was killed by an armed robber seeking money for a drug habit, about the fright and confusion of a child who is sexually abused by her intoxicated uncle, about the miserable deaths of the untold millions of Americans who have developed acquired immune deficiency syndrome (AIDS) or infected livers from the contaminated needles they used to inject heroin or cocaine, and about the illnesses and the costs to society of those who have alcohol-related illnesses such as cirrhosis of the liver, dementia, bleeding ulcers and stomach cancer, anemia, strokes, and fractured bones from falls—to name just a few. The fiscal cost of addictive disorders is about $170 billion just for treatment and lost wages. The costs for related matters such as damages to other people and to property, the protection of property, the maintenance of personal safety, and law enforcement (police, courts, jails, federal drug-prevention programs) would be even higher.

Determining Whether Addictive Disorders Qualify as Fatal Flaws of Personality and Character

If one were to complete the Fatal Flaw Scale (Appendix A in Chapter 2, "Does This Person Have a Fatal Flaw?") for almost any person who is dependent on alcohol or other substances, the scores on this test would almost always qualify him or her as having flaws of personality or character. As discussed at the end of this chapter ("Afterword"), when Dr. Ungar first presented to me the psychological history of his wife, Dr. Maria Torres, she would have had sufficiently high scores on the scale to have placed her in the range of "Highly Likely" to have fatal flaws of personality and character. For almost everyone with addictions, questions in the scale regarding trust, fulfillment of commitments, prioritization of the needs of other people, honesty, open communication, safety, and obedience to rules and laws would almost always be answered "No." In addition, the ubiquitous and persistent denial of addiction-related problems by people with alcoholism and chemical dependencies, their refusal to accept professional help or consider changing their behavior, their endangerment of others through the effects of substances on their judgment and impulse control, and the persistence of their dependencies despite multiple treatment regimens would qualify the flaws of many people with addictions as "fatal."

Mental health professionals commonly treat patients and clients who are family members or are in other types of important relationships with people who are dependent on alcohol or other substances of abuse. These clinicians are often called on to help their patients and clients make informed and realistic decisions about whether or not to continue their relationships with these individuals who are dependent on alcohol and other substances. Invariably, these decisions are difficult to make and heart-wrenching to carry out. As a rule, people display remarkably different personalities and exhibit far more destructive behaviors when they are on drugs and alcohol than when they are abstinent. Subgroups of people who are dependent on alcohol and substances manifest fatal flaws of personality and character exclusively during the times when they are abusing alcohol or drugs. Family members of such individuals find themselves on emotional roller coasters wherein their hopes and spirits are buoyed during the times of abstinence, only to be repeatedly dashed when their loved one returns to the substances of abuse.

A second category of people who abuse alcohol and substances also qualify as having some type of personality or character disorder during times of abstinence. Their dysfunctional traits only intensify during times of intoxication and abuse. For all practical purposes, the behaviors of most people who are chronically or episodically dependent on alcohol and other substances would qualify them as having fatal flaws in which their personality and character are prominently affected. Therefore, if you have an important relationship with a person with alcohol or substance dependencies, you must be realistic about the emotional toll that these disorders will take on you. Under these circumstances a mental health care professional with special expertise in treating people with substance use disorders should be helpful in your determination about whether or not it makes sense for you remain in the relationship. Such a professional will also be in the best position to make recommendations for treatment options for the person who abuses substances, should that individual be willing to accept professional help. In the following section ("Addiction: Personal Choice or Brain Illness?") I consider whether alcoholism and chemical dependencies qualify as medical illnesses or whether such conditions are best understood as personal choices.

TABLE 12–6.   The relevance of conceptualizing addictive disorders as brain illnesses

1. Such a conceptualization will affect how society and family members regard and treat people with addictive disorders: as people who have illnesses or people who are "weak-willed" and self-indulgent.

2. Such a conceptualization will affect how people with addictive disorders regard and treat themselves.

3. Such a conceptualization will affect whether or not the biological relatives of people with addictive disorders should take special precautions (e.g., avoidance of alcohol and addictive medications) because they and their progeny might be predisposed to alcoholism and chemical dependencies.

4. Such a conceptualization will affect how research scientists explore the causes of these conditions: focus resources on brain research or on psychological determinants of addictions? Clearly, if addictive disorders are personal choices, substantial funds should not be focused on brain research.

5. Such a conceptualization will guide the approach to the treatment of people with addictive disorders. If all addictions are personal choices, use of medications to prevent or reduce craving for drugs and alcohol does not make much sense.

Addiction: Personal Choice or Brain Illness?

Whether addiction is a behavior that leads to physical and psychological illnesses or is a primary brain illness that results in impaired thinking, mood, and behaviors has been debated and studied intensively during the past two decades. Informed scientists and scholars come to diverse conclusions about this question. Although at first the question might seem like an irrelevant academic exercise (such as "which came first, the chicken or the egg?"), its answer has far-reaching implications. Summarized in Table 12–6 are the principal arguments on the relevance of determining whether or not addictive disorders are brain illnesses.

Those who argue that addiction is a personal choice often maintain that people who attribute their addictive behaviors to an illness will not recover because they do not accept personal responsibility. A thorough review of this point of view can be found in the book *Addiction Is a Choice* by Dr. Jeffrey A. Schaler (2000). On the other hand, a growing number of behavioral scientists, clinicians, and those with addictive disorders now conclude that even though personal choice has critical importance, addictive behaviors have all the hallmarks of any other type of brain-based medical illness. I firmly hold this belief and will endeavor to present the available evidence for this conclusion. If there is evidence for hereditary predispositions to alcoholism and drug addictions, that would indicate that these conditions have strong brain-based components. I hasten to add, however, that biological bases for behaviors do not preclude important psychological determinants, such as willpower and personal responsibility. Just as with many other types of medical illness, personal responsibility plays an important role in the development, course, and outcome of alcoholism and chemical dependencies. Please consider diabetes mellitus, which all informed physicians agree is a medical illness with strong genetic factors. Patients who ignore their diet and personal hygiene and who are not compliant with their medication regimen are at significantly higher risk for associated features of diabetes such as stroke, heart attack, and gangrene of the feet and toes. However, this does not mean, in most cases, that their diabetes is caused by poor behavioral choices.

Determining Whether Addictive Disorders Are Brain Illnesses

Genetics

The most compelling evidence that alcoholism and chemical dependencies are brain illnesses comes from studies documenting that these conditions have strong hereditary and genetic components. This evidence is derived primarily from three types of investigation: family studies, adoption studies, and twin studies.

Family studies. There is broad acceptance among behavioral scientists and experienced clinicians that alcoholism and other chemical addictions run in families. In the case of alcoholism, a careful review of epidemiological studies of families demonstrated that biological children of people with alcohol dependencies have a risk of developing the condition that is seven times greater than that of close relatives of a person without alcoholism (Merikangas 1989). In another large study, the siblings of people with alcoholism were found to have almost the same dramatically higher rates of alcohol dependence compared with siblings of people without alcohol dependence (Beirut et al. 1998). Of course, the question must be raised whether or not these very high familial rates of alcohol addiction are the result of children modeling after their parents and siblings or whether the increases are based in heredity. The following paragraphs will help answer that question.

Adoption studies.   Adoption studies are designed to determine whether or not a predisposition to a psychiatric condition derives from genetic transmission or from the influences of the behavior of the relatives. Studies consistently demonstrate that male children of a biological parent or parents with alcoholism have much higher rates of alcohol dependence—even when they are raised by adoptive parents (Goodwin 1979). Of great significance, in these and several other studies, the presence of alcoholism in adoptive parents does not increase the risk of alcoholism in their adopted children, which indicates that genetics, not the family environment, is the major determinant of the development of alcoholism (Cadoret et al. 1980).

Twin studies.   Twin studies compare the incidence of medical conditions in identical twins (who have exactly the same genetic makeup) with fraternal twins (who share about 50% of their genes, as do all biological brothers and sisters). If large studies prove that identical twins have much greater incidences of certain illness than fraternal twins, it is inferred that the predisposition for that illness is transmitted genetically. In a broad range of large twin studies conducted internationally, it has been clearly demonstrated that if one identical twin of the pair has alcoholism or drug dependence, there is a multifold greater incidence of the disorder in the other twin than in the general population. Similarly, if one of a pair of adult identical twins does *not* have alcoholism or drug addiction, the risk of dependence for the other twin is equal to that in the general population. Specifically, if one identical twin has alcoholism or drug addiction, the risk of dependence for the other is greater than 50%, as opposed to about 15% if the twins are fraternal (Prescott et al. 1999).

Adoption studies and twin studies provide proof that there is a strong hereditary component to alcoholism and other addictive disorders. What this means is that genes predispose certain people to be vulnerable to dependencies on brain-altering substances. Most likely, the genes alter the brains of vulnerable people to become dependent on certain substances. This scenario closely parallels other types of medical illnesses. For example, women with genetic predispositions to breast cancer have increased vulnerabilities to the cancer with exposure to certain hormones, such as estrogens. Ingestion of table salt in quantities that are harmless to other men can be dangerous to certain men with a genetic predisposition to hypertension. The conceptual difference between substance abuse and these other medical conditions is that addictive substances in turn further alter the brain to intensify and aggravate the illness (the dependency).

TABLE 12–7. Guiding questions for brain research regarding addictive disorders

1. Why are certain substances more addictive than others?

2. What specific parts of the brain and what brain systems do addictive substances affect?

3. What specific brain transmitters are involved in addictions?

4. What changes occur in the brain cells of people who have chronic addictions?

5. How does stress change the brain to make people more vulnerable to dependencies?

6. How do genes affect the human brain to make it more vulnerable to alcohol and drug dependence?

7. Where does the brain store the memories of past drug highs?

Brain Biology

Science is entering an exciting new era for understanding the role of the brain in addictive disorders. Although a comprehensive review of this subject would require another book, I will try to summarize the major research questions and opportunities. New technologies—such as functional brain imaging of living people with alcoholism and chemical dependencies—are being employed, and novel avenues of investigation—such as utilizing the mapping of the human genome to link addictions to other human traits and illnesses—are now being explored to seek answers to the questions posed in Table 12–7.

In recent years, the fields of cellular and molecular biology, functional brain imaging, genetics, and neurobiology have uncovered evidence confirming that addictive disorders are true brain illnesses. The specifics of this evidence provide exciting new opportunities for the understanding, treatment, and prevention of alcoholism and substance abuse. Readers who are interested in an excellent overview of this topic should refer to the review chapter by Drs. Eric J. Nestler and David W. Self (2002).

Effects of Alcohol and Other Abused Substances on the Brain and Other Organs

Although there may be some remaining controversy about whether or not addictive disorders are in fact *primary* brain illnesses, all informed physicians and scientists agree that alcohol and substances of abuse can adversely affect the human brain—acutely and chronically. The dangers of the brain-altering drugs associated with acute intoxication cannot be underestimated; these dangers include impaired judgment, diminished alertness and attention, and poor impulse control. Such functional disruptions can lead to sudden, life-changing events such as unplanned and unwanted pregnancies, injurious falls, fatal car accidents, and precipitous violence and other so-called crimes of passion. With episodic intoxication, once the brain-altering substance is out of the person's system, the brain and its functions *usually* return to normal. However, certain abused substances—such as the mind-altering drugs lysergic acid diethylamide (LSD), phencyclidine (PCP), and methylenedioxymethamphetamine (MDMA; Ecstasy)—can cause irreversible brain changes with only a few uses. Unfortunately, the results of these alterations in brain structure and chemistry can be—and often are—devastating and permanent problems with mood regulation, motivation, learning and memory, and even sensory perception.

Long-term use of alcohol results in many brain illnesses. When heavy drinkers abruptly discontinue the use of alcohol, delirium tremens (DTs) can occur. This can involve extreme confusion in which a person does not know the date, the time of day, or his or her location at that time. Visual and auditory hallucinations also occur. In addition, tactile hallucinations, in which people with DTs feel things crawling all their bodies, are characteristic of this condition. People with DTs tend to be paranoid and agitated and to have fever, insomnia, and great anxiety. In extreme cases people with DTs experience seizures, dehydration, and salt depletion that can be fatal. Because alcohol lowers the brain's seizure threshold, seizures are relatively common in heavy drinkers. Studies show that about 10% of all heavy drinkers will have what are called grand mal epileptic attacks that are not a component of DTs. Irreversible changes to the tissues and structure of the brain occur with heavy drinking. These changes can lead to persistent problems with memory that interfere with the person's ability to perform on a job or to meet family or social responsibilities.

Finally, heavy and prolonged alcohol use affects many other organs of the body in addition to the brain. For example, heavy drinkers can develop inflammation of the liver (hepatitis), which will be fatal over 5 years in half of those who develop the condition. Irreversible destruction of the cells of the liver (cirrhosis) occurs in 10% of heavy drinkers, and this results in more than 10,000 deaths each year. Pancreatitis, an inflammation of cells the pancreas, is one of the most painful and life-threatening of all medical illnesses. Seventy-five percent of all patients with pancreatitis have a history of alcoholism.

Narcotics Addiction

Preparing the Ground for Chemical Dependence

Maria Torres's abuse of substances began with a dangerous—but legal—substance, alcohol. It is worth noting, however, that because she was under 21 years old when she began drinking, her alcohol use was illegal. Recall that Maria was first exposed to "institutionalized" beer drinking as a college freshman at Princeton fraternity parties. Clearly, many other Princeton students also were exposed to beer at that time without disastrous results. We can also be sure that Maria Torres was not the only student in her class with genetically based, biological propensities to alcoholism and chemical dependencies who began, during that year, such a spiral of self-destruction. I believe that the tacit approval given by parents and the passive permission by college professors and staff for alcohol use by underage people is reprehensible. In addition to the monumental waste of time, the dissolution of personal and professional opportunities, and the resulting physical and mental illnesses, many of those who survive teenage alcohol abuse extend their practice of breaking the law to the abuse of illegal substances. In keeping with our biopsychosocial-spiritual model (see Chapter 6, "Narcissistic Personality Disorder, Part II: Treated Narcissism") for the causes and treatments of psychiatric conditions, we must understand the powerful psychological and social message and implications delivered when an authority figure permits a teenager to break the law by using an addictive substance. Thus the genetic predispositions to dependence (i.e., biology) and the addictive qualities of alcohol (i.e., biology) combine with the permissiveness and poor examples of authority figures (i.e., psychology) to create patterns of illegal behavior (i.e., social factors). In the next section ("Opioid Addiction") I briefly review narcotics abuse, a form of substance abuse that almost always entails criminal behavior and self-destruction.

Opioid Addiction

Narcotics is a general term for drugs—both prescribed and illegal—that are both sedating and highly addictive. In this category are sleep medications such as **barbiturates,** including pentobarbital (Nembutal), secobarbital (Seconal), amobarbital (Amytal), butalbital (Fiorinal), and phenobarbital; **prescription pain medications** such as hydrocodone (Vicodin), oxycodone (Percodan), hydromorphone (Dilaudid), sustained-release oxycodone (OxyContin), meperidine (Demerol), tramadol (Ultram), codeine, and morphine; and illegal substances like heroin. The prescription pain medications listed above (and heroin) are classified in DSM-IV-TR as *opioids,* because they are natural and synthetic deriva-tives of opium-producing poppy plants. A recent survey indicated that about 7% of American men and about 5% of American women have used this class of drug illegally. Even more disturbing is a high use among young people: 2% of high school seniors have used heroin and about 10% have abused prescription-type narcotics. Not surprisingly, opioid dependence is highly associated with criminal activity other than the substance abuse—such as drug dealing, burglary, forgery, and violent crimes. Opioid intoxication is associated with drowsiness, poor coordination, impaired attention and memory, apathy and low motiva-tion, and impaired judgment. Opioid withdrawal is characterized by significant physical and emotional problems, including nausea and vomiting, muscle aches, insomnia, depression, agitation, anxiety, and intense drug craving. When people inject opioids there is a high danger of their developing infections such as human immunodeficiency virus (HIV) and hepatitis from sharing needles. The high rate of accidental deaths from overdosing with opioids is the result of the drugs' interfer-ence with breathing regulation and other brain functions.

The Case of Dr. Maria Torres, Part Two: Treatment Phase

Dr. Ungar's Report

Dr. Ungar was both embarrassed and uncomfortable when he re-counted his dire concerns about his wife, Dr. Maria Torres. We both agreed with Dr. Torres's preliminary diagnoses—alcohol and opioid de-pendence and major depression. We also were like-minded about the seriousness of her illnesses and her immediate need for an outpatient psychiatric diagnostic assessment and treatment plan. Our problem was that Dr. Torres did not acknowledge abusing alcohol and drugs or having any psychiatric symptoms. She also told her husband, "Psychi-atrists are worthless. They *know* nothing and *do* nothing. I have never known a psychiatrist who wasn't crazy himself."

Addiction, Psychiatry, and the Profession of Medicine

Dr. Ungar and I mused about the differences between his medical spe-cialty, orthopedics, and mine, psychiatry. In orthopedics, patients readily accept and act on their need for professional help—even though their misbehavior or misjudgment may have been responsible for their medical condition. Consider a 60-year-old man who broke his leg by landing on rocks while surfing in a restricted zone of a California beach. Even though his injury was the result of poor judgment and even involved breaking a law, he would have no hesitation in seeking the help of an orthopedist to repair his fracture. On the other hand, people with painful and life-threatening mental illnesses often will not accept help from psychiatrists. There are two reasons for this disparity. First, all psychiatric illnesses involve some element of *brain dysfunction.* Such brain dysfunctions can also impair the insight and judgment required to accept the need for professional help. Second, there is a *stigma* associated with having a mental illness and requiring psychiatric help. Please note that the stigma of mental illness overflows to mental health professionals. Psychiatric and psychological treatments are commonly viewed to be ineffective, and psychiatrists and psychologists are thought to be weird or crazy themselves. The data show that psychiatric medicine is as necessary and effective as that of any other medical specialty. Dr. Ungar and I agreed that psychiatrists and psychologists are, in general, no more weird or crazy than orthopedists or any other type of medical specialists. Nonetheless, many patients requiring psychiatric help will use prejudicial misconceptions and misperceptions to bolster their denial of their illness and their refusal to accept help. One thing we knew for sure: Dr. Maria Torres would adamantly refuse to see any kind of mental health professional.

Dr. Ungar's Resistance to Accepting a Definitive Treatment Plan for Dr. Torres

The following discussion took place between me and Dr. Ungar regarding a treatment plan for Dr. Torres:

> **Dr. Ungar:** We are in complete agreement about Maria's diagnoses and her desperate need for treatment. The problem is that we are talking to ourselves. Maria wants no part of either of us at this point. What do you suggest?
>
> **Dr. Y.:** We have two options. If we believe that she is of imminent danger to herself or others, Texas law allows us to commit her to the general hospital psychiatric unit against her will. We will have to sign a petition for the police to go to your home and take her to the hospital involuntarily. Within 2 days, a judge will adjudicate our contention. In court we will contend that Dr. Torres endangers your children while intoxicated and high on drugs and that she could endanger her own life by taking an accidental overdose.
>
> **Dr. Ungar:** I am not sure I could do that. Maria has so much pride. I know that she will never forgive me for bringing the police to our home or for having her locked up on a mental unit. What

would happen if she convinces the judge that she is fine; that all of this is an overreaction on our part? What is the second option?

Dr. Y.: Dr. Torres has committed a felony that, by law, should be reported. She has forged your triplicate prescriptions to obtain narcotics for herself. You could have her arrested. No judge would side with her in the face of that type of evidence. I am sure that since this is her first offense, she could plea bargain for an extended stay in a psychiatric hospital.

Dr. Ungar: Are you telling me that I should have my own wife arrested? It would be the end of our marriage. Maria would never forgive me. I could never do that. Don't you think that is a bit of an overreaction?

Dr. Y.: Not at all. As an orthopedist, how many people have you cared for who have severely inured themselves or even paralyzed others from driving while intoxicated?

Dr. Ungar: Countless cases. But I still won't have her committed like an insane person, and certainly I won't participate in her being locked up like a criminal. She's sick, she's not a criminal. Can't you help me find some middle ground? One of my friends told me about something called "interventions." What's that?

Dr. Y.: Intervention is a therapeutic process that helps family members deal with a person who is highly resistant to accepting or changing their problems with alcohol and substance abuse. First, a therapist works with the family to understand and cope with the effects of the addictive behavior on the family system and on the individuals. Second, where indicated, external support is provided to the family members in need, such as therapists for the children and support groups. Third, the family and therapist meet with the person with the dependency and endeavor to confront the person's denial of the problem and encourage him or her to pursue treatment. If the person refuses the treatment plan, the family pursues a plan of distancing and detachment from the person with addictions.

Dr. Ungar: Let's do that!

Dr. Y.: Maria requires hospitalization. Any other course is too risky. You would not prescribe a cast for a patient with a fractured arm that requires an open surgical reduction.

Dr. Ungar: Are you saying that you won't help us?

Dr. Y.: It is not helping Maria or you to underestimate the seriousness of her pathology or to minimize the level of treatment needed.

Dr. Ungar: We aren't getting anywhere. With all due respect, I am going to seek out a second opinion. I have the name of another psychiatrist, and I will get back to you about how we decide to move forward.

Dr. Ungar was clearly angry with me over what he called my "inflexibility." Once more I communicated what I believed about the dangerousness of Maria's clinical state—to herself, to her children, and to others—and encouraged him to seek the second opinion that very day on an emergency basis. He said that he would do so.

I did not hear from Dr. Ungar over the next two days, so I called him at his office. With a somewhat irritated tone, he told me that he and Maria would be working with the psychiatrist whom he had contacted for the second opinion. He told me that this psychiatrist had made a house call to Maria, and that he agreed with him that outpatient care was "in everyone's best interest." I stated that between well-intentioned and well-informed people there can be differences of opinion, and that I would be available to him and Maria should that ever become necessary.

Emergency Call From Dr. Ungar

About 3 months later I received an emergency page from Dr. Ungar. He stated that Maria was in the ICU in a near-fatal coma. Laboratory tests confirmed potentially lethal levels of alcohol and Vicodin. We met that afternoon.

> **Dr. Ungar:** Let me catch you up with what has happened. As we agreed, I contacted Dr. Riley. Maria consented to meet with him once a week in his office for psychotherapy. After about 2 weeks, she stopped seeing him. She said that Dr. Riley was not helping her. Maria also said that she had had a "wake-up call" and that she would never drink again. As absurd as it sounds, I believed her. I guess I wanted to believe her. If she survives this overdose, I'm asking you to treat her.

Dr. Torres survived the overdose, and I was by her bedside shortly after she regained consciousness. Her first words to me were, "When can I go home?"

> **Dr. Y.:** I am admitting you to the psychiatry inpatient service as soon as it is safe for you to leave the ICU.
> **Dr. Torres:** Like hell you are. I want to see my husband right this minute.

I asked the ICU administrator to call Dr. Ungar, who soon joined us.

> **Dr. Torres:** Jonathan, I want you to sign me out of this hospital right now. This doctor is threatening to lock me up on the psych ward.
> **Dr. Ungar:** Calm down, Maria. You almost died. You are in no condition to go home. We have to do something about your drinking problem.
> **Dr. Torres:** I haven't had a drink of anything for over 3 months. I swear to you.

> **Dr. Ungar:** Maria, you were admitted with a blood alcohol level over 200, not to mention a toxic level of Vicodin.
>
> **Dr. Torres:** No way. They mixed up my labs with someone else's. You know that happens all the time in this hospital. I swear I haven't had a drink in months. Get me out of here or get me a lawyer.
>
> **Dr. Ungar:** Dr. Yudofsky, What do you suggest that I do? She won't go along with this.
>
> **Dr. Y.:** Do as Maria has requested. Get her a lawyer. I am writing up commitment papers to our inpatient unit.

For over an hour Dr. Torres tried to convince her husband not to participate in her involuntary commitment to the locked psychiatry unit of the general hospital. For this entire time—despite the wealth of laboratory, clinical, and historical evidence to the contrary—she argued that everyone else was wrong, that she had no problems with substance abuse. Almost swayed to believe her, Dr. Ungar was finally persuaded to leave the ICU and to go back to work. Once her husband was gone, Dr. Torres's first words to me were the following:

> **Dr. Torres:** I must have hit my head when I had my seizure. My head feels like it is about to explode. I need some Vicodin right now. If you will get it for me, I will keep you on as my psychiatrist.
>
> **Dr. Y.:** You experiencing the effects of withdrawal from alcohol and addictive pain killers. I will prescribe some medications to help you withdraw from these drugs safely and comfortably.
>
> **Dr. Torres:** Then order me some Vicodin, and taper that. I feel like I am about to die.
>
> **Dr. Y.:** We have many more important and interesting things to talk about than the medications that I choose to use to withdraw you from alcohol and drugs. We have had our last conversation on that subject, unless it comes up in court.
>
> **Dr. Torres:** If you are the type of doctor who doesn't believe that it is important to communicate with his patients about their treatment, I need someone else. I need a doctor who was trained in the twentieth century. Get me the list of psychiatrists on the hospital's active staff. Is Dr. Riley on the staff? Also get me my cell phone right now so I can call my attorney. I believe that I am being kidnapped and illegally held.

Dr. Torres Turns the Corner

Over the next 2 weeks, Dr. Torres was a reluctant participant in her treatment. As promised, she hired an attorney and contested her involuntary commitment to the psychiatry service. When possible, I chose to avoid all power struggles over medications and privileges such as having visitors and obtaining passes to leave the hospital. Another staff psychiatrist was assigned to deal with Dr. Torres on these issues, and

I would talk with her only about feelings and issues that were not blatant aspects of her drug-seeking behavior. Dr. Torres had her day in court. Despite hiring a highly qualified attorney, Dr. Torres, sadly, was not able to find a single person other than her husband who would be a character witness. Manifestly, her dependencies had resulted in her almost complete isolation; her only "friends" were alcohol and drugs. The judge remanded her to my care for a month. Although I had legal authority to prescribe and administer medications against her will, I chose to taper her from all medications. At first Dr. Torres was silent and withdrawn. Seemingly depressed, she did not speak with other patients or participate in the group therapeutic activities. At the beginning of her fourth week of hospitalization, it seemed as if a window shade had been lifted in the dark room of her personality. For the first time, she asked to meet with me and said the following:

> **Dr. Torres:** Do you realize that this is the first time I haven't been on alcohol or drugs in 16 years? Since I was a freshman in college. This is the first time that I have been a "real person" since I was in high school. I have two questions for you. First, have I irreparably fried my brain with the drugs and alcohol? Second, have I done irreversible damage to my children by never being there for them as a mother?
>
> **Dr. Y.:** Welcome back, Dr. Torres. I agree that you have been away from yourself and from everyone else for a very long time. Now, about your questions. I believe that your considerable intellectual gifts have somehow been spared. I will confirm my conjecture with an extensive battery of neuropsychological tests, which you must be motivated to take. The remarkable preservation of your intellect is a true blessing: you will need every cell in your brain and every point of your IQ to come back to yourself and to the world. This brings us to your second question. Although you somehow may have dodged the bullet of brain destruction, there are far-reaching consequences of what you have done to your family, friends, patients, and yourself. How you deal with this, literally will define your future. I don't want to be overly dramatic, but I believe that how you deal with these consequences will determine your fate. I am certain that if you choose, again, to anesthetize your feelings with drugs and alcohol, you will lose everything—probably even your own life. Said another way, you are one drink away from losing everything. You should never take one swallow of alcohol again or accept into your body any addictive substance. The second thing of which I am certain is that despite your obvious brilliance and capacity for hard work, you cannot stay abstinent by yourself. You will have to change your lifelong pattern of putative self-sufficiency, which, in truth, is a pattern of being a loner. It will take many people to help you stay alive. Let's now begin.

In a family meeting with Dr. Torres and Dr. Ungar that was held several weeks after this exchange, I suggested that Maria consider accepting my referral of her to the Professionals in Crisis program of the Menninger Clinic, then located in Topeka, Kansas.

> **Dr. Torres:** Why do I need that? I am making great progress with what we are doing now. I accept that I have alcoholism, I am going to our church's AA [Alcoholics Anonymous] program, and I am even reduced to working with you, who are meaner than any surgeon I have ever known. What I should be doing is going back to work to help pay for all this recovery stuff.
>
> **Dr. Y.:** The Menninger program focuses on the special problems associated with addiction in professionals like doctors, lawyers, and the clergy. They combine addiction-recovery treatments with intensive, psychoanalytically oriented psychotherapy. I believe that you need both. Let's not make the mistake again of underestimating the seriousness of your addiction and psychological problems, which cannot be separated.
>
> **Dr. Torres:** We'll think about it. But I also think you can "create a crisis by becoming a professional patient."

Laughing at Dr. Torres's clever parody of the Professionals in Crisis appellation, I responded as follows:

> **Dr. Y.:** Let's try to use your incredible wit and intelligence in the service of insight into how you can change, as opposed to finding reasons to resist changing.

Ultimately, Dr. Torres convinced Dr. Ungar that she was making progress and that she had "learned her lesson." They decided not to participate in an intensive residential treatment program for recovery from alcohol and chemical dependencies. Because Dr. Torres was no longer drinking and was not depressed, she had every legal right to decline my recommendation. On her discharge from the general hospital psychiatry service, the treatment plan outlined in Table 12–8 was agreed on.

Dr. Torres Looks at Herself

In psychotherapy, Dr. Torres began to explore the implications of her abandonment of her children and her responsibility for her daughter's developmental disabilities. Beyond her guilt and grief, she gained insight into her problems with nurturing children. Maria realized that her mother had been far too tired and demoralized to take care of her when she was a child. Rather, as the oldest, it was Maria's responsibility to take

TABLE 12–8. Outpatient treatment plan for Dr. Maria Torres

- Weekly laboratory testing for alcohol and drugs

- Episodic, unscheduled laboratory testing for alcohol and drugs on her psychiatrist's or her family's recommendation

- Regular (i.e., at least five times a week) attendance at Alcoholics Anonymous meetings

- Twice-weekly psychotherapy with her psychiatrist

- Twice-monthly family treatment with a family counselor

- Church attendance on Sunday mornings and Wednesday evenings

- Immediate readmission to the inpatient psychiatry service if she failed to adhere to any of the items listed above

care of her two younger siblings. She began to understand that she resented her maternal responsibilities and that her drinking represented, in part, a type of "maternal replenishment." These were not reassuring insights. She also figured out that her relationship with her husband was partly a replication of her previous relationship with Mr. Zimmerman, the town librarian. This reality carried several divergent implications. On one hand, both Mr. Zimmerman and Dr. Ungar are people of great integrity, humility, commitment, loyalty, and intelligence. However, because Maria had been abandoned by her father, she tended to discount unconsciously her husband's elevated opinion of and loving behavior toward her. During one psychotherapy session she stated,

> **Dr. Torres:** I never realized this before I became sober: I love Jonathan but I never have been *in* love with him. He is a rescuer, which means I must always remain a victim for the relationship to work.
>
> **Dr. Y.:** This is true but not quite the whole story. Because of the circumstances of your childhood, you don't feel worthy of being loved. Consequently, you are terrified about being abandoned by Jonathan, so you test his loyalty to you incessantly. Through everything, he has stayed by you. Since you don't think highly of yourself, you unconsciously discount him for loving you. The old Groucho Marx line about "not wanting to belong to any club that would accept him as a member" applies to you.
>
> **Dr. Torres:** Enough psychobabble. How is this supposed to help me?
>
> **Dr. Y.:** "This" won't help you. You must help yourself by working on your relationship with Jonathan. You have to risk committing to him as he has to you. At the same time you must work at real involvement with your children; and it is probably a good idea for you to get back into medicine—maybe research. If you work at all of these, you will begin to feel worthy of being loved by Jonathan.

Dr. Torres: And if I don't work on this stuff?

Dr. Y.: You have already run that experiment. Endless self-loathing and self-destructiveness through alcohol and drugs. The only thing missing, perhaps, is a relationship or two with narcissistic men who devalue you.

Dr. Torres Reconstructs Her Life: Ups and Downs

Always the outstanding student, during the next two years Dr. Torres not only worked in psychotherapy on understanding herself and her relationships, but also worked tirelessly and successfully to reconstruct her life as a mother, wife, and physician. Both areas of work are essential for recovery. Treatment entailed a balancing act: simultaneous with Dr. Torres's progress was her sadness over the significant losses that had occurred during her 16 years of substance dependence. On one occasion, Maria learned that her daughter, Lois, had not been admitted to the private school that her son, Jason, attended. The principal of the private school said that Lois's aptitude tests showed that she was not capable of handling the schoolwork. On that day, for the first time in 3 years, Dr. Torres had a drink. After missing her appointment with me 2 days later, I called her at home. She answered the phone and said that she had the flu and was too weak to call me to cancel her appointment. When she missed her next appointment without notifying me, I called Dr. Ungar and told him that per our agreement I wanted Dr. Torres to have an unscheduled laboratory evaluation for the presence of alcohol and drugs in her system. After some protest, he acquiesced. Dr. Torres was found to have high levels of both alcohol and Vicodin (which she had kept hidden away for 3 years), and she was readmitted to the psychiatry service. She admitted to wanting to kill herself. The day after her hospitalization the following dialogue occurred:

Dr. Torres: I hate myself. Through my own indolence and irresponsibility, I have destroyed my daughter's brain. I have no right to live.

Dr. Y.: First of all, Lois's brain is not destroyed. She is a wonderful, happy child. And of all people, you should know that being a genius doesn't guarantee happiness.

Dr. Torres: Dr. Y., are you feeling well? You are actually offering me reassurance!

Dr. Y.: You should not allow yourself to escape your responsibilities to Lois or yourself by using Lois's brain injury as an excuse. That, indeed, is true indolence.

Dr. Torres: You scared me for a second, Dr. Y., with your uncharacteristic reassurance. Thank God you are back to your mean and miserable self.

For the first time, Dr. Torres met DSM diagnostic criteria for major depression, clearly a reaction to her grief and shame over her responsibility in Lois's intellectual deficiency. Her suicidal intent resolved after her first day in the hospital. She was administered an antidepressant in the hospital and was discharged after 5 days under the structure and conditions of the outpatient therapeutic regimen previously indicated. At that point Dr. Torres requested that I meet with her more frequently (three times a week) to provide support until her depression remitted and to help her work through her deep-seated feelings of loss associated with her 16 years of addiction. It was not lost on her that for the first time in her life, she felt sufficient self-worth to ask for help. Far from becoming, as she had once joked, "a professional patient," Dr. Torres progressively became stronger and more independent. She risked commitment and close feelings with her husband and children, and she maintained, "I am feeling true intimacy for the first time in my life." Over the ensuing 5 years, Dr. Torres gained a position on the department of anesthesiology of an excellent medical school and has since achieved great success as an educator and research scientist in the field. At the time this chapter was written, she had not drunk alcohol or taken an addictive substance for 62 months, 3 weeks, and 5 days. Summarized in Table 12–9 are key principles in the treatment of patients with addictive disorders as exemplified by the case of Dr. Maria Torres.

Afterword

Dr. Torres did not exhibit disorders of personality and character when she was not under the influence of alcohol or substances. Until her intensive psychotherapy and regular attendance at AA meetings, alcohol and drugs had prevented her from growing as a person and from surmounting the deep-seated insecurities that stemmed from the circumstances of her childhood. At the time of our initial consultation, her husband, Dr. Ungar, was far too upset with my treatment recommendations to fill out the Fatal Flaw Scale (Appendix A in Chapter 2, "Does This Person Have a Fatal Flaw?") for Dr. Torres. Therefore, based on the information provided by Dr. Ungar, I have completed the scale. On Part A of the scale, Dr. Torres's behavior would have merited a score of 10, which indicates that she has the highest measurable level of flawed personality and character; and on Part B her score would have been 4 out of a possible 6, which indicates a high likelihood that her personality and character flaws would be "fatal," or persistent and intractable. Six

TABLE 12–9. Key principles about patients with addictive disorders as exemplified by the case of Dr. Maria Torres, part 2: treatment

Historical fact	Key principle	Interpretation
Initially, Dr. Torres refused to acknowledge her illness or accept treatment.	Don't expect a sick brain to make a healthy decision.	Alcohol and drug abuse impaired Dr. Torres's brain function in ways that reinforced her dependencies and resistance to treatment.
Initially, Dr. Ungar refused to go along with Dr. Y.'s treatment recommendations.	Always a part of the problem, it is difficult for family members of people with addictive disorders to become a part of the solution.	Although Dr. Ungar functioned in the role of rescuer for his wife, it was always on her terms.
The family intervention and outpatient treatment plan of Dr. Riley failed.	In the treatment of patients with addictive disorders, any therapeutic compromise is destined to fail.	No treatment plan could be successful until Dr. Torres was first withdrawn from alcohol and drugs.
Even in the face of the overwhelming evidence of laboratory proof of drugs and alcohol in her blood, Dr. Torres denied her addictions.	Never, never underestimate the addictive power of alcohol and opioids.	When Dr. Torres awoke from her coma, the only thing she cared about was getting more alcohol and drugs.
Despite her superior intelligence, strong work ethic, and medical training, for 16 years Dr. Torres was unable to discontinue alcohol and drugs by herself.	Don't expect a broken brain to fix itself by itself.	Dr. Torres required a locked psychiatric unit, a trained and tough medical team, and a court order to be withdrawn from alcohol and drugs.

TABLE 12–9. Key principles about patients with addictive disorders as exemplified by the case of Dr. Maria Torres, part 2: treatment (continued)

Historical fact	Key principle	Interpretation
For her court hearing, Dr. Torres was not able to find a single friend to testify on her behalf.	People who are addicted to alcohol and drugs alienate all friends who are not themselves chemically dependent.	After 16 years of uninterrupted alcohol and substance abuse, the only friends whom Dr. Torres could find were inside a bottle.
Once Dr. Torres was off of alcohol and drugs, her many assets enabled her to benefit from a broad range of therapies.	Combining other personality disorders with addictive disorders is like combining jet fuel with a match.	Dr. Torres has many strengths. She does not have character or personality flaws other than her addictive disorder.
Dr. Torres's outpatient therapeutic regimen was highly structured, with clear consequences for noncompliance.	It takes one physician to *withdraw* a person from alcohol and drugs. It takes a "therapeutic village" to *prevent* his or her return to alcohol and drugs.	Notwithstanding Dr. Torres's many strengths, a multifaceted, multidisciplinary treatment team was required to sustain her recovery.
Upon attaining abstinence from alcohol and drugs, Dr. Torres had to face, for the first time, both old and new psychological and interpersonal problems.	Although a person with addictive disorders cannot recover without total abstinence, total abstinence does not constitute recovery.	Freed from the obfuscations of alcohol and drugs, Dr. Torres encountered, for the first time, key issues and problems within herself, her marriage, her family, and her professional life.
As Dr. Torres made fundamental changes in herself, her relationship with her husband changed.	When a person with addictive disorders begins to recover, the dynamics of all important relationships also change.	Family therapy with Drs. Torres and Ungar was required to enable their relationship to change and to grow.

TABLE 12–9. Key principles about patients with addictive disorders as exemplified by the case of Dr. Maria Torres, part 2: treatment (*continued*)

Historical fact	Key principle	Interpretation
Dr. Torres's realization that she had injured her daughter through her alcohol abuse triggered a relapse.	The discontinuation of alcohol and drugs lifts the veil of denial covering over the tragic consequences of addiction-related misbehavior.	Individual, group (Alcoholics Anonymous), and family treatments were essential in helping Dr. Torres make the decision to work toward a better future rather than using her past misdeeds as an excuse to return to drinking and taking drugs.
Dr. Torres developed major depression as a consequence of insights gained in her treatment.	Even though the reasons for depression are understandable, treat the person for depression.	Antidepressants may be required at any phase of the treatment of patients with addictive disorders. In the case of Dr. Torres, medications became necessary 3 years into her recovery from alcohol and drug abuse.
Dr. Torres has now gone 5 years without using alcohol or addictive drugs. She has achieved success in almost every facet of her personal, family, and professional life.	Alcohol and drugs of abuse will poison a person's assets.	Once she was free from drugs and alcohol, Dr. Torres's many fine qualities and personal attributes reemerged.

years later, Dr. Torres would score zero on both components of the scale.

The unusual reversal in Dr. Torres's score on the Fatal Flaw Scale can be understood and explained by several factors. First, beyond her addictive disorders Dr. Torres did not exhibit any other type of personality disorder, an exception rather than the rule. *Comorbidity* refers to the presence of two or more psychiatric disorders in a single person. People with addictive disorders have approximately a 50% prevalence of comorbidity for at least one additional psychiatric condition. Many people with addictive disorders have additional personality and character problems, such as antisocial or narcissistic personality disorder. The combination of personality disorders with addictive disorders intensifies the psychopathology and exponentially diminishes the chances of recovery. Second, Dr. Torres is advantaged with many personal gifts and positive attributes. She is intelligent and a hard worker, and she chose a wonderful person for a husband. (Consider how difficult her recovery would have been had her husband also been dependent on substances or demonstrated character flaws.) Third, she had the familial and financial resources to seek out and pay for reputable treatment, which is often not the case. People with addictive disorders waste money on drugs and usually lose their source of income by being fired from their job or divorced from their spouse.

It is not uncommon for people with fewer financial resources than were available to Dr. Torres to go to prison for their illegal activities associated with their drug-seeking behavior. Going to prison for drug-related crimes (which certainly could include forging prescriptions) usually marks a point of precipitous social and occupational decline from which people almost never return. Most often, people with addictive disorders who have been incarcerated become chronically dependent on some form of social welfare, and all too commonly, after their release from prison, they soon return to drugs, to crime, and to prison. What this indicates to me is that as a society we need to find better ways to help people with addictive disorders. I believe that both individuals who have chemical dependencies and society would be far better off if the astronomical amount of money that our government (i.e., "we") spends on so-called drug enforcement would be utilized instead for brain research and treatment programs for people who have these conditions.

References and Suggested Readings

American Psychiatric Association: Diagnostic and Statistical Manual of Mental Disorders, 4th Edition, Text Revision. Washington, DC, American Psychiatric Association, 2000

Beirut LJ, Dinwiddie SH, Begleiter H, et al: Familial transmission of substance dependence: alcohol, marijuana, cocaine, and habitual smoking: a report from the Collaborative Study on the Genetics of Alcoholism. Arch Gen Psychiatry 55:982–988, 1998

Cadoret RJ, Cain CA, Grove WM: Development of alcoholism in adoptees raised apart from alcoholic biologic relatives. Arch Gen Psychiatry 37:561–563, 1980

Cloninger CR: Genetics and psychobiology of the seven factor model of personality, in Biology of Personality Disorders. Edited by Silk KR. Washington, DC, American Psychiatric Press, 1998, pp 63–87

Cloninger CR: Genetics of substance abuse, in The American Psychiatric Press Textbook of Substance Abuse Treatment, 2nd Edition. Edited by Galanter M, Kleber HD. Washington, DC, American Psychiatric Press, 1999, pp 59–73

Goodwin DW: Alcoholism and heredity: a review and hypothesis. Arch Gen Psychiatry 36:57–61, 1979

Kupfermann I, Kandel ER, Iversen S: Motivational and addictive states, in Principles of Neural Science, 4th Edition. Edited by Kandel ER, Schwartz JH, Jessell TM. New York, McGraw-Hill, 2000, pp 998–1013

Mack AH, Franklin JE, Servis ME: Substance use disorders, in The American Psychiatric Publishing Textbook of Clinical Psychiatry, 4th Edition. Edited by Hales RE, Yudofsky SC. Washington, DC, American Psychiatric Publishing, 2003, pp 309–377

Merikangas KR: Genetics of alcoholism: a review of human studies, in Genetics of Neuropsychiatric Diseases. Edited by Wetterberg I. New York, Macmillan, 1989, pp 269–280

Miller NS, Adams BS: Alcohol and drug disorders, in Textbook of Traumatic Brain Injury. Edited by Silver JM, McAllister TW, Yudofsky SC. Washington, DC, American Psychiatric Publishing, 2005, pp 509–529

Nestler EJ, Self DW: Neuropsychiatric aspects of ethanol and other chemical dependencies, in The American Psychiatric Publishing Textbook of Neuropsychiatry and Clinical Neurosciences, 4th Edition. Edited by Yudofsky SC, Hales RE. Washington, DC, American Psychiatric Publishing, 2002, pp 899–921

Prescott CA, Aggen SH, Kendler KS: Sex differences in the sources of genetic liability to alcohol abuse and dependence in a population-based sample of U.S. twins. Alcohol Clin Exp Res 23:1136–1144, 1999

Schaler JA: Addiction Is a Choice. Chicago, IL, Open Court, 2000

Shuckit MA: Alcohol-related disorders, in Kaplan & Sadock's Comprehensive Textbook of Psychiatry, 7th Edition. Edited by Sadock BJ, Sadock VA. Philadelphia, PA, Lippincott Williams & Wilkins, 2000, pp 953–971

World Health Organization: Mental and behavioral disorders, in International Statistical Classification of Diseases and Related Health Problems, 10th Revision. Geneva, World Health Organization, 1992, pp 371–387

Ziedonis D, Krejci J, Atdjian S: Integrated treatment of alcohol, tobacco, and other drug addictions, in Integrated Treatment of Psychiatric Disorders (Review of Psychiatry Series; Oldham JM, Riba MB, series eds.). Edited by Kay J. Washington, DC, American Psychiatric Publishing, 2001, pp 79–111

Part III
Conclusion

13

GETTING HELP

Overview

Goals of This Book

A principal goal of this book is to provide information and impart skills to help mental health professionals and trainees understand and care for their patients or clients who have personality disorders or character flaws. Chapters 4 ("Hysterical [Histrionic] Personality Disorder"), 6 ("Narcissistic Personality Disorder, Part II: Treated Narcissism"), 8 ("Obsessive-Compulsive Personality Disorder"), 10 ("Borderline Personality Disorder"), 11 ("Schizotypal Personality Disorder"), and 12 ("Addictive Personality Disorder") focus on patients who are treated for these respective conditions. A related, primary goal of this book is to impart knowledge and proficiency to clinicians for treating patients or clients who are currently in painful, troubling, or destructive relationships with people with personality disorders or character flaws. Chapters 5 ("Narcissistic Personality Disorder, Part I: Untreated Narcissism"), 7 ("Antisocial Personality Disorder"), and 9 ("Paranoid Personality Disorder") focus on the treatment of people—family members and professional colleagues—trying to cope with painful and dangerous relationships with people with these problems.

Flawed Relationships

As they are initially revealed in relationships, fatal flaws are subtly sensed as almost imperceptible filaments of fragility in people who appear to all the world as attractive, substantive, and safe. Such flaws may initially add the flavor of individuality and identity to the person, and although they are not without consequence, they may even appear captivating. An example would be the initial enticing and exciting flirtations of a person whose psychology inhibits the establishment and sustenance of truly intimate and committed relationships. Thus, seemingly harmless flaws may be only the perceptible extensions of deeper crevices and caverns of weakness and negativity that undermine the integrity of the relationship and commitment with that individual.

Many people initially seek professional help because of their agonizing involvements with people who have flaws of personality or character. Often people in these circumstances enter treatment believing that their problems derive entirely from the "flaws" of the other party involved. They are convinced that if they are able to gain through their therapy a clear understanding of the nature of personality disorders and character flaws, they will be able to change the other parties involved or disengage from their destructive relationships with the people with these conditions. This perspective can have a detrimental impact on their treatment. The patients or clients with such a perspective will tend to focus on the problems of the other person but not gain sufficient insight about themselves to effect meaningful change in their circumstances. Manifestly, they must first change themselves before changing the nature and status of their dysfunctional relationship. In this concluding chapter, my intention is to help place the focus of treatment where it will be most helpful to the goals of the patient or client. For the reasons stated in the introduction to the book, I will now address directly—i.e., in the first person—people in such circumstances.

Understanding Yourself

To escape, avoid, and survive destructive people, you must understand how and why you became involved with such people in the first place. The conception of your power in an impaired relationship is a clear understanding of your role in that relationship. Don't fool yourself or waste too much of your time and your energies by trying to change the other person if he or she refuses to acknowledge or does not wish to change the flawed behavior. It will be hard enough to change yourself. The good news is that changing yourself and your situation, while difficult, is entirely possible. Although it is not always fun, the process of self-discovery and true change is inherently intellectually stimulating and emotionally fulfilling. Throughout this book, I have done my best to lead you through a process of change that is respectful, rational, and realistic.

Why Trust Is So Important in a Relationship

The fulfillment of all important commitments requires predictable and trustworthy relationships. Your vital commitments with other people depend on their coming through on your mutual agreements. Such commitments will also depend on your ability and motivation to maintain and fulfill your part of the agreement, as do commitments that you make with yourself. Assuming that you are maturely committed— whether considering a proposal of marriage or hiring a divorce attorney; whether evaluating a job offer, hiring an employee, or accepting a retirement plan; whether assessing a day care center for your 4-year-old or selecting a nursing home for your parent—the ultimate success of your decisions and the quality of your future will reside in your ability to assess accurately the character of the *other* person or people involved and to act accordingly.

Questions to Ask When Your Relationships Fail

Over the three decades of my practice of psychiatry, I have listened to my patients detail the devastating consequences that inevitably occur when trust is violated, leading important relationships to go bad. I have had patients who have been betrayed, abandoned, or abused by their spouses; who have been mistreated by their bosses or cheated in business deals by their friends; or who have been deceived and injured by people whom they should have been able to trust, such as their physicians, attorneys, ministers, financial advisors, teachers, housekeepers, and even their parents, siblings, or children. Patients who have had these experiences should be asking themselves the questions summarized in Table 13–1.

This book, coupled with excellent treatment, should help you answer many of these questions. If the answers to the first three questions are affirmative, the answer to the remaining four questions is, also: "Yes, but you must be willing to open your mind to new ways of understanding others and yourself." A goal of this book is to help you accomplish this.

Although a main focus of this book is how to recognize, avoid where possible, and deal with other people who have severe personality and character flaws, inevitably, these discoveries will also engender the need for self-exploration. Questions that you should ask about your role in the impaired relationship are summarized in Table 13–2.

TABLE 13–1. Questions to raise when you think you might be in a relationship with a person who has a flaw of personality or character

1. Is there something very wrong with the character or personality of this person?

2. Is this person's problem correctable?

3. Is the nature of the person's problem so dangerous and destructive that I should end our relationship?

4. Could I have foreseen this problem and my bitter disappointment about the relationship?

5. Can I figure out a sane and safe way to end or escape this relationship?

6. Is there something that I could have done differently to have prevented getting into this situation?

7. Can I prevent the recurrence of a similarly destructive relationship in the future?

TABLE 13–2. Questions to ask yourself after you have determined that you are in a relationship with a person with a flaw in personality or character

1. Why did I become involved with this person to begin with?

2. Why do/did I respond so intensely to this person?

3. Why, despite such pain and personal cost, did I not try to break away sooner?

4. After being deceived and hurt so deeply, how will I ever be able to trust anyone else?

5. Could I benefit from the help of a mental health professional to answer these questions?

The Process of Change and Escape

First Look Inward

First, and foremost, the key to prevention or remediation of personal tragedies resides in making decisions based on your understanding of your own psychology. Second, you must learn how to evaluate the personalities and characters of other people—the strengths that enable relationships to succeed and the flaws that augur and guarantee failure. It is naïve and foolish for you to believe that the world is populated entirely by people who are kind, well-intentioned, honest, and fair. (It is also dangerously dysfunctional to live as if the world were so beatific.) Understanding your own psychology and that of significant others is not a simple task. Because of how the mind works (which involves the complex commingling of biology, conscious and unconscious thoughts and feelings, and the subjective resistance to insight), it is usually less difficult to understand others than it is to understand oneself. To prevent or disentangle yourself from a relationship with a person with a personality flaw, you will need to understand both yourself and the nature of the disordered personality of the other person involved. In *Fatal Flaws* I have endeavored to provide a clear and rational method for going about the exhilarating and liberating process of self-discovery, which, for those of us who so embark, can enable the most important journey of our lives—the journey toward being a centered, independent, and self-actualized person. I have also tried to delineate how to go about determining whether or not it makes sense for you to engage a guide (e.g., an ethical, well-trained, and competent mental health professional) for such a journey. Presented in the remainder of this section are some suggestions on how to go about finding such a person.

Beware of Bias

Unfortunately, as I emphasize in this book, many people with severe personality flaws neither seek nor accept professional help. Rather, they may demean mental health professionals and do everything in their power to discourage those whom they exploit from seeking such help. Points of view other than their own are often threatening to them. Be careful not to permit people with severe personality flaws to be the arbiters of your decision or route to change. This road inevitably must lead to *their* loss of power over you, something that they will not encourage or readily permit. In medicine we call this a **bias**, which means that their objectivity is influenced by their personal gains.

For a similar reason, it may or may not be wise for you to recommend this book, or relevant parts of this book, to persons with disorders of personality or character. I fully understand that (for many reasons) you might be inclined to share sections of this book that precisely delineate the forms and consequences of their flaws. However, they might find little incentive to gain insight about their personal failings or the many ways in which they have hurt you. They may not accept that such revelations are in their interest. Rather, people with such flaws will continue to want and to expect many things from you. Therefore, they will wish to discount and discourage any insights or avenues that will lead to rational expression of your will and to the liberating actions that will ensue. They will only be concerned with how your change will affect them. In the highly unlikely event that they develop a sincere desire for self-improvement and change, they will find, on their own, this book or other routes toward recovery. If you are committed to a path of understanding and change, be very, very careful about whom to entrust with the validation of your escape route to safety, self-sufficiency, and self-actualization. Similarly, it is imperative that mental health professionals be free of bias or personal gain involving the critical choices and changes you make during your treatment with them.

Learn to Identify Fatal Flaws of Personality, Character, and Behavior

A goal of this book has been to provide the needed information and to impart the requisite skills to enable you to identify the most subtle and the most superficial revelations of fatal flaws. These skills should help you avoid establishing relationships that will inevitably lead to destructive entanglements. Because no one is perfect, we must learn how to distinguish between harmless imperfections and the tips of icebergs of more serious and severe psychopathology. A second goal has been to help you delve more deeply into the psychology and biology that underlie fatal flaws so that you will appreciate the full measure of their destructive potential. With this awareness you will not only recognize the deleterious consequences of fatal flaws, you will also comprehend how they came about and how resistant they can be to change. It is difficult (if not impossible) to begin to take the arduous steps for change and independence without this understanding.

Commit to the Process of Change

If you have voluntarily entered a relationship with a person or people with fatal flaws of personality, character and behavior, meaningful change requires the insights and understandings that are summarized in Table 13–3.

If your life circumstances—as opposed to personal choice—have led to an ongoing involvement with a person with fatal flaws (such as your having to work under the authority of a newly recruited chief executive officer who has severe narcissism), insight into and understanding of the psychology of this person and how your psychology is affected by him or her may help preserve both your job and your peace of mind.

TABLE 13–3. Requirements for change

1. Recognition that there is a significant problem in your relationship

2. Realization that the source of the problem involves a flaw of personality or character in the other person involved

3. Acceptance that nothing will change in the relationship unless *you* change

4. Motivation to obtain and entertain new insights and points of view about yourself and the other person in the relationship

5. Willingness to make the necessary changes, based on what you have learned about the flawed psychology of the other individual involved and the problems that you bring to the relationship

---

Should You Seek Professional Help?

My Bias

I must admit to my own strong bias in favor of using a qualified and competent (these are not necessarily one and the same) mental health professional for help in understanding and changing relationships with persons who have significant flaws of personality and character. I am also aware of people who, without professional counsel, have made lasting and positive changes in themselves and who have successfully extricated themselves from entangled, destructive relationships. Nonetheless, I believe in the value and economy of gifted and experienced coaches and of specialists. Although each of us is born with special talents and insights, none of us is born with the requisite skills and knowledge that can be gained from education and experience. No matter how gifted an athlete you are, you cannot train yourself to be a swimmer or tennis player who is even competitive at the college level, much less at Olympic or professional levels. To achieve these levels, you require, at minimum, an experienced coach who will help transfer to you the enormous base of knowledge of the sport that has been gained over many decades, and who will be able to observe you objectively to help you overcome your inevitable weaknesses. I believe that the same need for professional help most often applies to changing yourself and overcoming significant and destructive interpersonal relationships. However, what does it take to become a competent mental health professional?

Professional Competence

Unfortunately, in the field of mental health, many people erroneously regard themselves as experts based on their own limited life experience, or even as the result of a single positive experience in personal counseling. This is dangerous. Understanding and helping others with behavioral and emotional problems is a deceptively difficult and demanding profession. Extensive classroom education, supervised clinical experience, and continuing learning are required—even for those who were born with the intellectual, emotional, and intuitive gifts essential to provide useful professional help to others. The hubris of self-proclaimed expertise and professional qualifications is particularly clear in the realm of sports competition, where performance is more easily measured than in other realms such as mental health counseling. You may recall that the legendary basketball player Michael Jordan left basketball for a time to try to become a professional baseball player. Ted Williams, one of the greatest hitters in the history of baseball, saw Michael Jordan swing at some pitches during his practice sessions. A reporter asked Ted Williams what he thought of Michael Jordan as a baseball player. In response Mr. Williams stated that although Mr. Jordan was obviously a great athlete, "he will never hit a fastball thrown by a major league pitcher, much less a curve." Ted Williams was absolutely correct, because Michael Jordan never made it to the major leagues as a baseball player. Ted Williams understood what it takes to play baseball at a professional level: not only raw talent, but years of being coached, practicing, and learning from mistakes. One more example from sports. Ed "Too Tall" Jones was the intimidating Hall of Fame linebacker for the Dallas Cowboys. At one point in his professional football career, he decided to take up professional boxing. Despite his extraordinary size, power, and coordination, his promoters found it hard to dig up heavyweight boxers who were sufficiently unskilled to keep from knocking out the football player in the early rounds of the fight. Unfortunately, the damage that results from inexperienced and poorly trained mental health professionals falls mostly on their clients.

What Some Therapists Don't Know Can Hurt You Very Much: The Case of Elliott Mayer

Elliott Mayer is a married, 45-year-old corporate attorney who was referred to my care by his family for evaluation and treatment of his depression that did not respond to antidepressants. Mr. Mayer was employed in a large company that had downsized drastically as the result of gross mismanagement at a senior level. Although Mr. Mayer had not himself been a party to any wrongdoing, he was greatly concerned about losing his job at a time in Houston when there were poor prospects for corporate attorneys. He had been in twice-a-week psychotherapy for almost a year under the care of a spiritual counselor to whom he had been referred by his minister at church. He had received his antidepressants from a general practitioner to whom the spiritual counselor had referred him specifically for that purpose. The general practitioner had spent less than 15 minutes with Mr. Mayer before prescribing the antidepressant sertraline (Zoloft). His wife had insisted that Mr. Mayer see me, because he was not improving and had fallen far behind in his job responsibilities. (Interestingly, Mr. Mayer had resisted seeing a psychiatrist because of his concern that it might someday damage his employment opportunities.)

Several aspects of the formal neuropsychiatric mental status examination that I administered to Mr. Mayer led me to be concerned about a biological change in his processing of information. His ability to think clearly was compromised, but not in the ways that are the result of depression. Also, he did not fully meet the formal DSM criteria for major depression. From my history of his medical and psychiatric symptoms (which required two visits of an hour each), I also learned that he had ulcer symptoms, which had been treated for 2 years with cimetidine (Tagamet), a commonly used medication to reduce gastric acidity. This medication works by blocking histamine-2 receptors in the stomach that are involved with the release of digestive acids. There are also histamine-2 receptors in specific regions of the brain involved in sequencing and processing abstract information, such as numbers. In very rare cases, the antagonism of these histamine-2 receptors by a drug like cimetidine can lead to mental confusion and impaired information processing. Working closely with Mr. Mayer's wife and a trusted colleague from his company (for another 2 hours), we were able to determine that Mr. Mayer's psychological problem began after the institution of the cimetidine. In addition, his inability to handle his work preceded most of his worries and mental preoccupations for which he was being treated by the spiritual psychotherapist. Three weeks after the discontinuation of both the cimetidine and the antidepressant, Mr. Mayer again was able to handle his job responsibilities. Simultaneously, his anxieties and the symptoms that might have resembled depression completely abated. Unfortunately, this is an example of the commonplace malpractice that occurs when a poorly educated and inexperienced therapist misdiagnoses, and therefore mistreats, a person with a serious psychiatric condition. I believe that had Mr. Mayer continued in his psychotherapy without the correct diagnosis and treatment being made, he would have lost his job and not had the cognitive capacity to pursue a similar position. I hesitate to speculate how often this happens and how much damage to patients and their families is the consequence.

Even though I have admitted to my bias in favor of coaches and specialists, there are also problems when mental health professionals become too specialized. These are reviewed in the next section below.

The Dangers of Limited Conceptual Approaches Among Mental Health Practitioners

With so many different disciplines of mental health professionals offering consultation and treatment, people seeking such help are often confused and uncertain about how to go about choosing the professional whose training and treatment philosophy is best suited to solve their problems. Please understand that this is a different issue from your finding a compassionate person with whom you can form a trusting relationship. Both of these aspects are important for the success of your treatment.

I am often concerned when a clinician, usually a so-called specialist, adheres rigidly to a particular theory or approach to the understanding and treatment of a particular clinical problem, such as eating disorders. I can assure you that any specialist who believes so strongly in the conceptual reality of the object of his or her specialization is significantly limiting his or her understanding of the subject. For example, to treat successfully the full range of people with serious eating disorders, the clinician must have expertise in the psychopharmacology of mood and anxiety disorders, because depression and obsessive-compulsive disorder so often occur with these conditions. Often the interpersonal and psychosocial aspects of care cannot be optimized until depression, obsessions, and compulsions are first mitigated with the appropriate medications. This clinician must also be accomplished in psychotherapy and family therapy, because these components of care are invariably essential to successful treatment. Expert knowledge in diet and nutrition, endocrinology, and gastrointestinal functioning is also required.

In my specialty, certain psychiatrists believe so strongly that the role of traumatic life experience affects the psychology of their patients that they neglect the prominent role of genetics and other biological factors. Such subspecialists devote all of their energies and those of their patients to exploring painful childhood events and problems in key relationships. However, these psychiatrists often miss the biological aspects of illnesses and symptoms—such as depression—that must be treated with medications for their patients to get well. As a consultant, every year I diagnose serious neurological illnesses—including brain tumors—in patients who have spent many months and even years in psychotherapy for symptoms directly caused by a neurological disorder.

Cases similar to that of Elliott Mayer are almost everyday occurrences in my practice and those of other psychiatrists. Conversely, I also regularly evaluate patients who are being treated exclusively with psychiatric medications for psychological problems. Limited by their own concepts of illness and conceptualization of their own professional role (e.g., psychopharmacologist), these specialists do not discover important psychosocial and experiential stresses, such as their patient's being physically and emotionally abused by her spouse. They are also unaware of fundamental factors in the development and continuation of their patients' conditions because of their narrow concepts of illness and their professional roles. Given their strong belief in medications as "magic bullets" in the treatment of psychiatric disorders, these practitioners often do not establish the therapeutic relationship necessary for their patients to reveal to them their dependence on alcohol or prescription painkillers. Thus the limited and limiting concept of themselves as clinicians and of the illness they purportedly treat prevents them from asking their patients the relevant questions that would provide the requisite information that would lead to personal change and clinical improvement. When I encounter any limiting professional designations such as "spiritual counselor," "holistic therapist," "aroma therapist," and the like, my antennae of suspicion are raised. Although I may be wrong, I am concerned that these individuals do not have the training or knowledge to know what they don't know. They so often miss important medical disorders and psychological issues related to their clients' problems and do not have the panoply of therapeutic tools necessary to effect meaningful recovery. They are dangerously limited by their myopic concepts of illness and recovery, and they endeavor to wedge and chop every patient or client into the short and narrow procrustean beds of their unidimensional professional identities.

Inpatient Care

When people with personality disorders become so severely ill or disturbed that they are of danger to themselves or others, psychiatric hospitalization is indicated. Denise Hughes (in Chapter 10), who had borderline personality disorder, was admitted to acute inpatient services of general hospitals when she inflicted severe wounds on herself on feeling abandoned by loved ones. During her hospital stay, she was medicated and placed on continuous suicidal observation until she calmed down and was no longer intent on harming herself. Robert Woods (Chapter 11) was committed to state psychiatric hospitals, both for the treatment of his schizotypal personality disorder and to protect

Lois Abramowitz and others from his homicidal intent. Dr. Maria Torres (Chapter 12) was hospitalized on the acute psychiatric service of a general hospital on two occasions: the first time to withdraw her safely from alcohol and prescription narcotics, and the second time to protect her from suicide. People with severe and persistent personality disorders who do not respond to outpatient treatment may also be referred to psychiatric hospitals that specialize in intensive inpatient treatment. Often such patients have not only a personality disorder, but also some other psychiatric condition such as bipolar illness, major depression, or alcohol dependence. The best of these hospitals use a multidisciplinary approach in which psychiatrists, psychologists, social workers, and nurses work as a team with patients and their families in both individual and group settings. Psychoeducation is emphasized, wherein patients and their families learn about their psychiatric conditions and treatments. Stays in such facilities can range from weeks to months, and costs can be quite high. Notwithstanding the time and expense, I have seen many people with personality disorders and other psychiatric conditions derive great benefit from intensive inpatient treatment in well-regarded psychiatric hospitals, and this option should be considered when outpatient care is not achieving the desired results.

Self-Help, Support, and Advocacy Groups

Self-help, support, and advocacy groups can be an important source of information and care for people with almost any type of mental disorder and for their families. As indicated in Chapter 12, Alcoholics Anonymous was an integral component of Dr. Maria Torres's treatment plan, and AA has been critical in her recovering from the abuse of and dependency on alcohol and prescription medications. Many people with personality disorders also develop alcohol dependencies, and Alcoholics Anonymous, with approximately two million active members in almost 100,000 groups in more than 100 countries, should be considered to address this aspect of their problem. Al-Anon, Alateen, and Adult Children of Alcoholics are companion support, information, and self-help groups for the family members of people with alcoholism. Narcotics Anonymous is a self-help program for people with drug dependencies.

Many people with personality disorders, as well as people in important relationships with those with these conditions, may also have depression. There are several excellent national organizations that provide support and information for people with depression and their families. These organizations are listed below. Because of the pervasive stigmatization of people with personality disorders, there are very few support and advocacy groups for people with personality disorders and their families. I expect this to change in the near future, in part because of our increasing understanding of the genetic and other biological aspects of these conditions. The National Education Alliance for Borderline Personality Disorder is a wonderful new organization that is developing local chapters around the United States to provide scientific information about the assessment and treatment of people with borderline personality disorder, while providing support to people with this condition and their families. The following are key resources that you may wish to consider contacting:

1. **National Education Alliance for Borderline Personality Disorder (NEA-BPD)**
   P.O. Box 974
   Rye, NY 10580
   (914) 835-9011
   NEABPD@aol.com
   http://www.borderlinepersonalitydisorder.com
2. **National Mental Health Association (NMHA)**
   2001 N. Beauregard Street, 12th Floor
   Alexandria, VA 22311
   (703) 684-7722
   (800) 969-NMHA
   http://www.nmha.org
3. **National Alliance for the Mentally Ill (NAMI)**
   Colonial Place Three
   2107 Wilson Blvd., Suite 300
   Arlington, VA 22201
   http://www.nami.org
4. **Depression and Bipolar Support Alliance (DBSA)**
   730 N. Franklin Street, Suite 501
   Chicago, IL 60610
   (312) 642-0049
   (800) 826-3632
   http://www.dbsalliance.org

Concluding Advice

Emotional and behavioral problems are inherently complex and multifactorial conceptualizations. The sophisticated and experienced clinician is always far more concerned and impressed by what he or she does not know than by the limited understandings encompassed by the theories that guide his or her causal explorations and therapeutic actions. The serious harm that stems from what we do not consider in trying to diagnose and treat the disorders of our patients lingers longer in our memories than any diagnostic or therapeutic success. Nearly every day in the large treatment programs of the medical school where I work, our faculty diagnose a severe neurological condition—such as a brain tumor, brain infection, or seizure disorder—that causes the depression or psychosis of a patient who was treated endlessly and unsuccessfully for these conditions with psychotherapy. And nearly every day our psychiatry faculty recommend psychotherapy for the complex psychological problems in patients whose disabling psychological dysfunctions have not responded to years of treatment with a broad range of medications.

The bottom line is this: if your symptoms are not improving or you are not making positive changes in your life during your current treatment, it is time to consider a second opinion from a clinician with broadly based training and conceptualizations of causality and treatment. This advice is especially warranted if you are currently being treated by a mental health professional who is limited by a single theory of the causality and treatment of your problem. Professionals with limited concepts of the causes and treatments of mental illness literally do not know what they are missing. And neither do you! And in this case, what you don't know can hurt you. On a more positive note, I firmly believe that what you do know about disorders of personality and character can be of great help in salving the dysfunctions, pain, and suffering associated with these conditions. I hope that this book has provided understanding, knowledge, and skills that will help you accomplish just that.

INDEX

*Page numbers printed in **boldface** type refer to tables or figures.*